Pitfalls in Cervical Spine Surgery

Luca Denaro
Domenico D'Avella
Vincenzo Denaro (Eds.)

Pitfalls in Cervical Spine Surgery

Avoidance and Management of Complications

Springer

Dr. Luca Denaro
Prof. Dr. Domenico D'Avella
Department of Neuroscience
University of Padua
Via Giustiniani 5
35128 Padua
Italy
lucadenaro@hotmail.com
domenico.davella@unipd.it

Prof. Dr. Vincenzo Denaro
Department of Orthopaedic
and Trauma Surgery
Campus Bio-Medico University
Via Alvaro del Portillo 200
00128 Rome
Italy
denaro@unicampus.it

ISBN: 978-3-540-85018-2 e-ISBN: 978-3-540-85019-9

DOI: 10.1007/978-3-540-85019-9

Springer Heidelberg Dordrecht London New York

Library of Congress Control Number: 2009935689

Illustrations: Alessia Perseghin-Illustrazioni Scientifiche, Via Milano 172/3 - 39100 Bolzano, Italy

Cover design: Frido Steinen-Broo, eStudio Calamar, Figueres/Berlin

Printed on acid-free paper

Springer is part of Springer Science+Business Media (www.springer.com)

Foreword

Over the last 20 years there has been a marked increase in spinal surgery and in particular procedures on the cervical spine; the increase is expected to continue for the next several decades. The results of surgery for cervical radiculopathy and myelopathy have been good on the one hand, and on the other, the public no longer are content to live with spinal deformity; both will result in an increase of surgery. The general availability of CT and MRI scans have outlined the pathology for both the surgeon (who can plan exactly) and the public (who wish for more); the latter are extremely well informed of the expected benefits and the possible complications of surgical intervention, from the internet.

So this book by Professor Denaro and his colleagues is timely in that it faces up squarely to the avoidance of complications and their rapid and appropriate treatment.

The book begins with the important philosophical approach that the cervical spine is imbedded within a complex soma, whose general health or lack of it, will influence greatly the expected outcome of any surgical intervention. This cannot be over-emphasised as, too often in the past, the temptation has been to "operate on the X-rays and not the patient". With rising costs, healthcare providers, both hospitals and national health services, require information on the "value" for a specific procedure; complications requiring prolonged hospital care or inability to work will negatively influence allocations of resources.

In the second section, they emphasise the importance of a detailed anatomical knowledge on which to base the surgical approach. The risks to the vertebral artery, recurrent laryngeal nerve and the sympathetic chain are obvious examples of structures that are vulnerable when there is scanty anatomical knowledge. Newer approaches, particularly those to the upper two vertebrae and the cervicodorsal junction, require knowledge not usually part of conventional neurosurgical or orthopaedic curriculum. In these areas, collaboration with other disciplines (head and neck, and maxillofacial and thoracic surgery) cannot be over-emphasised.

The subsequent sections cover the potential "pitfalls" associated with trauma, tumours, inflammatory bone diseases and rarer vascular abnormalities and spinal cord problems such as syrinogomyelia. The knowledge base is expanding at an intimidating pace and the authors' reference lists are wide and very up to date.

As the society reflects its demands for (sometimes instant) "cures" for conditions related to neck pathology, it requires information on the risks and benefits of a proposed surgical intervention. They now come as individual patients to surgeons with much better information than ever before. It is essential that spine surgeons prepare themselves to carry out the procedures with minimal complications and also be able to put in context for the individual patient the advantages and potential drawbacks of their personal treatment plan.

This book sets about addressing such issues. I warmly commend it.

London, UK Prof. Alan Crockard, Dsc, FRCS, FRCS (Ed.) FDSRCS (Eng.)

Foreword

Cervical spine surgery has been largely used in the last decade following the refinement and continuous development of new instrumentation. Young surgeons are more widely familiar with these techniques and attend training practical courses. As a consequence, there is a high risk of enlarged surgical indication for cervical disease. A wise evaluation of suitable candidates and a correct choice of the best surgical technique on an individual basis are the main strategies to avoid complications in the surgical management of these patients. This book deserves highest consideration because it presents a wide range of possible complications allowing the reader to be aware of them and helping in the decision-making process.

The volume content is based on the large surgical experience and the skilful technique of the authors.

This is an outstanding contribution added to the related literature because only the thorough knowledge of the pitfalls helps to prevent them. The complication avoidance is crucial and can be considered an essential adjunct to the surgical armamentarium.

The authors have to be congratulated for the excellent focus on important aspects of this surgery. They deserve our appreciation because they emphasise several tips and tricks useful in achieving greater chances of clinical success.

References are reported providing further support to the knowledge.

Definitely, this volume will be of paramount interest for spine surgeons, both neurosurgeons and orthopaedists.

Messina, Italy Prof. Francesco Tomasello, MD

Preface

This book aims to guide the reader through the myriad of complications that may occur in patients undergoing cervical spine surgery: in this way, the surgeon can learn how to try to avoid them, when possible, and to tackle them when they have occurred.

It is important to understand the pitfalls from the patient's perspective. Patients seem better disposed to understand that some complications can be intrinsic in this surgery if their original symptoms were more debilitating, and can find a causal link between the symptoms and the complication. On the other hand, it is difficult for patients to accept complications when symptoms leading to surgery were not serious, even though imaging and electrophysiology studies confirmed the correct indication to surgery.

A very important moment in the preparation of the patient to surgery is the process of informed consent.

From my yearly experience in the field of cervical spine surgery, I learned that pitfalls in cervical spine surgery may be divided into unpredictable and predictable. Obviously, only the latter can be considered as avoidable.

A classical example of an unpredictable pitfall is the deep venous thrombosis following technically well-performed surgery on the correct patient, with the correct diagnosis, indication, and with adequate prophylaxis.

The pitfalls defined as avoidable may arise from several factors: wrong diagnosis, wrong indication and wrong surgery (both in excess – i.e. when performing wide stabilisation – or in defect – i.e. performing incomplete decompression).

There are also difficult situations, when the surgeon is forced to operate because the pathology, for example, a tumour, imposes to perform adequate resection of the tumoural mass with the sacrifice vascular or myelo-radicular structures. These pitfalls are predictable, but unavoidable.

Another common pitfall is a false-positive investigation, interpreted as pathological before considering the presenting signs and symptoms. In tertiary referral practice, many patients are seen for the first time after a host of tests have already been performed. Diagnoses formulated only on the basis of tests, which do not take into account the history and clinical examination of the patient, may induce to operate on the images, and not on the patient. At times, we are guilty of not taking a thorough history and not performing a thorough physical examination, and of relying too much on investigations. This can be particularly true for patients who are anxious and afraid, in whom the inexperienced surgeon may be led to operate.

Also, the anatomy of the spine is complex, but the language used to describe pathology may be even more complex. The absence of universal standardisation of spinal nomenclature with respect to the definition of a disk herniation and its different categories, especially regarding type and location, is still a major problem. Classically, in the presence of a report describing a bulging disk as an herniation, the patient will find sooner or later a surgeon who will operate on him/her.

In this era of high technology in clinical medicine, new devices (i.e. cervical arthroplasty) and minimally invasive techniques are proposed for the management of disorders of the cervical spine. However, classical techniques should not be abandoned until strong evidence in favour of new techniques is available.

Surgery is not the only solution to patient's problems: often conservative management is the best solution!

Padua, Italy
Rome, Italy

Dr. Luca Denaro
Prof. Dr. Domenico D'Avella
Prof. Dr. Vincenzo Denaro

Contents

Contributors

Felice Eugenio Agrò Department of Anesthesia, University School of Medicine Campus Bio-Medico, Via E. Longoni 83, 00155 Rome, Italy
f.eugenio@unicampus.it

Ombretta Annibali Department of Hematology, University Campus Bio-Medico, Via Àlvaro del Portillo 21, 00128 Rome, Italy
o.annibali@unicampus.it

Serena Antonelli Department of Anesthesia, University School of Medicine Campus Bio-Medico, Via E. Longoni 83, 00155 Rome, Italy
s.antonelli@unicampus.it

Massimiliano Carassiti Department of Anesthesia, University School of Medicine Campus Bio-Medico, Via E. Longoni 83, 00155 Rome, Italy
m.carassiti@unicampus.it

Elisabetta Cerchiara Department of Hematology, University Campus Bio-Medico, Via Àlvaro del Portillo 21, 00128 Rome, Italy
e.cerchiara@unicampus.it

Domenico D'Avella Department of Neuroscience, University of Padua, Via Giustiniani 5, 35128 Padua, Italy
domenico.davella@unipd.it

Marianna De Muro Department of Hematology, University Campus Bio-Medico, Via Àlvaro del Portillo 21, 00128 Rome, Italy
m.de muro@unicampus.it

Luca Denaro Department of Neuroscience, University of Padua, Via Giustiniani 5, 35128 Padua, Italy
lucadenaro@hotmail.com

Vincenzo Denaro Department of Orthopaedic and Trauma Surgery, Campus Bio-Medico University, Via Alvaro del Portillo 200, 00128 Rome, Italy
denaro@unicampus.it

Alberto Di Martino Department of Trauma and Orthopaedic Surgery, University Campus Biomedico of Rome, Via Alvaro del Portillo 200, 00128 Trigoria, Rome, Italy
a.dimartino@unicampus.it

Umberto Vespasiani Gentilucci Clinical Medicine,
University Campus Bio-Medico, Via Alvaro del Portillo 200, 00128 Rome, Italy
u.vespasiani@unicampus

Giuseppe Avvisati Department of Hematology, University Campus Bio-Medico,
Via Àlvaro del Portillo 21, 00128 Rome, Italy
g.avvisati@unicampus.it

Rosa Greco Department of Hematology, University Campus Bio-Medico,
Via Àlvaro del Portillo 21, 00128 Rome, Italy
r.greco@unicampus.it

Umile Giuseppe Longo Department of Orthopaedic and Trauma Surgery,
Campus Bio-Medico University, Via Alvaro del Portillo 200, 00128 Rome, Italy
g.longo@unicampus.it

Nicola Maffulli Centre for Sports and Exercise Medicine,
Barts and The London School of Medicine and Dentistry, Mile End Hospital,
275 Bancroft Road, London E1 4DG, England
n.maffulli@qmul.ac.uk

Francesco Marchesi Department of Hematology, University Campus Bio-Medico,
Via Àlvaro del Portillo 21, 00128 Rome, Italy
f.marchesi@unicampus.it

Carolina Nobile Department of Hematology, University Campus Bio-Medico,
Via Àlvaro del Portillo 21, 00128 Rome, Italy
c.nobile@unicampus.it

Odoardo Olimpieri Department of Hematology, University Campus Bio-Medico,
Via Àlvaro del Portillo 21, 00128 Rome, Italy
o.olimpieri@unicampus.it

Demetrio Panzera Department of Anesthesia, University School of Medicine
Campus Bio-Medico, Via E. Longoni 83, 00155 Rome, Italy
d.panzera@unicampus.it

Rocco Papalia Department of Orthopaedic and Trauma Surgery,
Campus Bio-Medico University, Via Alvaro del Portillo 200, 00128 Rome, Italy
r.papalia@unicampus.it

Antonio Picardi Clinical Medicine, University Campus Bio-Medico,
Via Alvaro del Portillo 200, 00128 Rome, Italy
a.picardi@unicampus.it

Azzurra Romeo Department of Hematology, University Campus Bio-Medico,
Via Àlvaro del Portillo 21, 00128 Rome, Italy
a.romeo@unicampus.it

Daniele Santini Medical Oncology, University Campus Bio-Medico,
Via Alvaro del Portillo 200, 00128 Rome, Italy

Chiara Spoto Medical Oncology, University Campus Bio-Medico,
Via Alvaro del Portillo 200, 00128 Rome, Italy

Maria Cristina Tirindelli Department of Hematology, University Campus Bio-Medico, Via Àlvaro del Portillo 21, 00128 Rome, Italy
m.tirindelli@unicampus.it

Giuseppe Tonini Department of Medical Oncology, University Campus Bio-Medico, Via Alvaro del Portillo 200, 00128 Rome, Italy

Bruno Vincenzi Medical Oncology, University Campus Bio-Medico, Via Alvaro del Portillo 200, 00128 Rome, Italy
b.vincenzi@unicampus.it

Section I

General Complications

Complication Related to Medical Conditions

1

Umberto Vespasiani Gentilucci and Antonio Picardi

Contents

1.1 Introduction

In this chapter, we discuss the medical conditions that can complicate the perioperative period and postoperative outcome of cervical spine surgery. In particular, we discuss about comorbidities determining an increased risk of perioperative complications and cardiac events, and about medical conditions associated with postoperative spinal infections, failure of spinal fusion, and poor neurologic recovery after surgery. When the published studies specific for cervical spine surgery were scanty, such as in comorbidities associated with spinal infections and poor neurologic recovery, we have referred to studies on thoracic and lumbar spine surgery.

1.2 Comorbidities Increasing the Risk of Major Perioperative Complications

The studies on the long-term outcomes of cervical spine surgery focus mainly on outpatient factors, such as return to work, subjective ratings of pain improvement, neurologic outcome, and overall functional status. However, cervical spine surgery can be associated with major perioperative complications, and the medical conditions predisposing to these complications should be recognized.

Wang et al. reported on the incidence of complications and mortality associated with surgery for degenerative disease of the cervical spine by using data from the Nationwide Inpatient Sample, a nationally representative sample of hospital discharges in the United States [1]. They found a 4% incidence of perioperative complications, and a 0.14% incidence of in-hospital mortality, ranging from 0.03% for patients aged 20–34 years

U. V. Gentilucci (✉)
Clinical Medicine, University Campus Bio-Medico, Via Alvaro del Portillo 200, 00128 Rome, Italy
e-mail: u.vespasiani@unicampus

L. Denaro et al. (eds.), *Pitfalls in Cervical Spine Surgery*,
DOI: 10.1007/978-3-540-85019-9_1, © Springer-Verlag Berlin Heidelberg 2010

to 1.33% for those aged 75 years and older. A similar overall incidence of perioperative complications, ranging from 5 to 6.7%, and mortality, ranging from 0 to 0.8%, had been reported in previous studies [2–4].

The most important patient-related factors are age and preexisting comorbidities. The age factor has been well-established and has the effect on the number of comorbid conditions. Some studies suggest a linear correlation between the number of comorbid conditions and complication rates, whereas others found an increased risk only when two or more comorbidities were present. The most frequently cited comorbid conditions include cardiovascular diseases, pulmonary diseases, hypertension, and diabetes. Moreover, preexisting myelopathy in the operated patients carries a higher risk of complications.

Harris et al. attempted to identify clinical factors associated with unexpected critical care management and prolonged hospitalization after elective cervical spine surgery by reviewing their center's experience with 109 cases performed between 1995 and 1999 [5]. They found that the following diseases were significantly linked to the need for perioperative critical care management and prolonged hospitalization: pulmonary diseases, hypertension, cardiovascular diseases, and diabetes mellitus. Romano et al. found that congestive heart failure, alcohol/drug abuse, chronic lung disease, previous spine surgery, psychological disorders, and chronic musculoskeletal disorders were independently associated with perioperative complications [4]. In this study, the authors stressed that important comorbidities should be identified and treated, if possible, before surgery. Finally, Emery et al. identified a small group of patients who required intubation after anterior cervical surgery [6]. Five of these seven patients made a normal long-term recovery, but two died. Myelopathy and smoking were identified as preoperative risk factors by these authors. Indeed, the presence of pulmonary disease or myelopathy is often associated with the need for intermittent respiratory care [7].

1.3 Comorbidities Specifically Increasing the Risk of Perioperative Cardiac Events

A successful strategy for diagnosis and management significantly reduces the risk of cardiac events in patients undergoing noncardiac surgery. Indeed, among approximately 25 million patients undergoing noncardiac surgery every year in the United States, 50,000 patients have postoperative myocardial infarctions and 20,000 die of this event [8]. The most frequent systemic complications for patients undergoing cervical spine surgery aged >65 years are cardiac, which are second only to respiratory ones in younger subjects [1].

Risk stratification of these patients often relies on noninvasive tests for myocardial ischemia, but analyses suggest that test results are most useful in patients whose clinical data suggest moderate risks for complications, and that they have limited impact on high- or low-risk groups [9, 10]. Among the tools for clinical risk stratification are the Cardiac Risk Index and other decision aids [11, 12] (Table 1.1). More recently, new guidelines have been developed by the American College of Physicians [13, 14], both to classify each patient as being at low, moderate, or high risk for perioperative cardiac events, and to guide management strategies. Here, we will analyze only the criteria by which the risk profile can be determined, while the original guidelines should be checked for the evaluation of management strategies.

The original Cardiac Risk Index was the first validated multivariate model developed to predict cardiac complications in a general surgical population [11], and it was subsequently modified by Detsky et al. with the adjunct of angina as a new variable and simplification of the score [12]. Table 1.2 shows the variables that should be assessed and the three classes of risk corresponding to the cumulative score.

Class II and Class III patients have a high risk (>15%) of perioperative cardiac events, i.e., myocardial infarction, death, and congestive heart failure, and should be further assessed as indicated by the American College of Physicians [14]. Low modified Cardiac Risk Index scores (Class I) still do not reliably identify patients who have low-risk for perioperative cardiac events. Class I patients should be further evaluated according to the five variables in the clinical model by Eagle et al. [15, 16]: age > 70 years, Q-wave on ECG, any angina, history of ventricular ectopy, and history of diabetes. Patients with 0 or 1 factor should be considered at low risk (<3%), while the risk of those with two or more factors is intermediate (3–15%).

Table 1.1 Modified cardiac risk index [12]

Variable		Points
Age	>70 years	5
History of MI or Q-wave on ECG	Within 6 months	10
	> 6 months previously	5
History of angina	CCS class III	10
	CCS class IV	20
Left ventricular dysfunction or CHF	Pulmonary edema within 1 week	10
	Any previous pulmonary edema	5
Arrhythmia	Any rhythm other than sinus	5
	>5 PVCs	5
Other heart disease	Critical aortic stenosis	20
Other medical problems	Any of the following: pO_2 < 60 mmHg, pCO_2 > 50 mmHg, K^+ concentration < 3 mmol/L, BUN level > 50 mmol/L, creatinine concentration > 260 μmol/L, bedridden	5
Type of surgery	Emergency	10
	CLASS I	0–15
	CLASS II	20–30
	CLASS III	>30

MI myocardial infarction; *CHF* congestive heart failure; *PVC* premature heart contraction; *CCS* Canadian Cardiovascular Society; *BUN* blood urea nitrogen

Table 1.2 Comorbidities/Conditions associated with a proven increase in the risk of perioperative and postoperative complications of cervical spine surgery

Comorbidity/condition	Major perioperative complications and cardiac events	Postoperative infections	Failure of spinal fusion	Poor neurologic recovery
Age	X		X	
Hypertension and cardiovascular diseases	X			
Smoking and pulmonary diseases	X	X	X	
Diabetes	X	X	X	X
Osteoporosis			X	
Malnutrition	X	X	X	
Early postoperative use of NSAIDs			X	

NSAIDs nonsteroidal antiinflammatory drugs

1.4 Comorbidities Increasing the Risk of Postoperative Infections and Their Management

Improvements in surgical techniques and instrumentation have allowed for enhanced patient outcomes for many difficult spinal conditions. However, as many spinal procedures require long operating times, extensive approaches, and implantation of significant amount of instrumentation, they continue to carry a significant risk of postoperative infections, ranging from 0.7 to 11.9% [17–21]. Postoperative infections can have devastating sequelae, including failure of fixation, osteomyelitis, pseudoarthrosis, and significant medical problems.

Recognition of preoperative risk factors may allow for optimization, and if possible, modification of the patient's preoperative condition, and adjustment of antibiotic prophylactic therapy. Comorbidities that have been consistently associated with the risk of infection after spinal surgery are malnutrition, diabetes, pulmonary diseases, smoking, immunocompromised hosts, and obesity [22–26]. Independent from comorbidities, other factors that have shown to contribute to the risk of infection are extended prehospitalization, high blood loss (>1,000 ml), and prolonged operative time [27].

Protein and protein-calorie malnutrition are associated with poor wound healing, increased postoperative infections, and immune suppression. Klein et al. found that 25% of the patients in their study undergoing elective lumbar surgery were malnourished, and that 11 of 13 wound complications occurred in these patients [28]. Assessment of the nutritional status of a patient should include measurement of albumin and transferrin levels, total lymphocyte count, skin-antigen testing, anthropometric measurements, and nitrogen balance studies.

Several studies have shown that diabetic patients are more prone to surgical wound infections, independent of the type of surgery, and similar results have been obtained in patients specifically undergoing spine surgery [26–29]. In the study by Simpson et al., 24% of the diabetic patients undergoing lumbar spine surgery had a superficial wound complication characterized by delayed healing and persistent drainage [26]. Moreover, in a retrospective analysis of 1,629 spinal procedures, Fang et al. found that 5 of the 48 (10.5%) patients who developed a postoperative infection (defined by the need of surgical incision and drainage, and positive deep cultures) were diabetics, while no diabetic patient was present in the control group [29]. In contrast, the role of obesity in contributing to the risk of postoperative infection varies from study to study [22, 24, 26], and only larger samples will contribute to clarify this issue.

Antibiotic prophylaxis has been supported by several studies from the neurosurgical literature, and is particularly indicated in patients at high risk of postoperative infection. Savitz et al. reported that the antistaphylococcal agent, lincomycin, reduced the infection rate from 5.1 to 2.3% [30], and clindamycin from 10.9 to 1.2% [31]. Malis et al. reported no case of postoperative infection when 80 mg of gentamycin was given intramuscularly, when 1 g of vancomycin was given intravenously at the induction of anesthesia, and when streptomycin was added to the irrigating saline [32]. However, in later works, cefazolin given before skin incision was found to be effective against all staphylococcal infections [33], and prophylaxis with a first-generation cephalosporin is both logical and supported in the literature. However, the duration of antibiotic prophylaxis postoperatively is less clear, and the decision should rely on patient's risk factors, the extent of surgery, and the presence of instrumentation.

Postoperatively, patients frequently complain of discomfort associated with incision and muscle dissection. However, when pain increases or occurs after a period of comfort, postoperative wound infection should be considered. Signs and symptoms of infection usually present after a mean of 15 days from surgery: pain and wound inflammation/drainage are typical, while fever is less frequent [21]. Even if not specific, significant elevations of C-reactive protein and erythrocyte sedimentation rate are quite sensitive [27].

Plain radiography, CT scanning, and MRI can support the diagnostic process. Early implant loosening, rapid loss of adjacent-level disk space height, and abnormal soft-tissue swelling are indirect indicators of spinal infection, which can be detected by plain radiography. Both CT and MRI can reveal the presence of fluid collections, even if the distinction between postoperative sterile seromas and abscesses can be difficult. Early-onset postoperative discitis is well recognized by gadolinium-enhanced MRI, but the possibility that the operation itself produces an increase in postcontrast MRI signal intensity should always be kept in mind.

Staphylococcus aureus is the most common organism found in postoperative spinal wound infections, followed by *Staphylococcus epidermidis* [34]. Gram-negative organisms are the only causative agents in nearly 10% of the cases, while another 10% of infections are mixed (Gram-negative and Gram-positive bacteria).

When the infection occurs, careful debridement is nearly always required. Debridement should consist of aggressive removal of all necrotic tissue and foreign materials such as sutures. Once the superficial layer has been debrided and irrigated copiously, the fascial layer should be inspected. This may be left unopened only if the surgeon is absolutely sure that the infection is only superficial, and if opened, debridement of necrotic muscle and necrotic bone graft should be performed. Repeated debridements may be necessary depending on the extent of the infection, the appearance of the wound, and the causative organism. At the time of debridement, additional cultures should be obtained, and the patient should then be administered with appropriate broad-spectrum antibiotics until culture and sensitivity results are obtained. Bone graft and instrumentation should be left in place if the fusion is not solid. If the instrumentation is removed too soon, the patient may develop pseudoarthrosis, persistent infection, and unstable spine. Large pieces of allograft, if free in the wound, can be removed and replaced with autogenous bone graft [35].

1.5 Comorbidities Complicating Spinal Fusion

Osseous spinal fusion remains a cornerstone of surgical treatment of severe spinal disorders, and its success results in the elimination of movement across an intervertebral motion segment after bony union. The rate of nonunion has been reported to range from 5 to 35%, with a myriad of factors thought to affect this rate [36, 37]. The important influences include local factors (mechanical environment, fusion site preparation, blood supply, bone graft source, and quantity), patient-related factors (mainly comorbidities and drugs), and biologic enhancement (electrical stimulation, growth factors). Here, we will discuss patient-related factors that can affect spinal fusion, and, as little data are available specifically for spinal arthrodesis, much of the information reviewed pertains to the effects on bone healing in general.

First, the individual biological factors governing spinal fusion are related to bone homeostasis and thereby, to age. Little is known about the individual capacity to achieve spinal fusion, although it is accepted that young patients heal well. In skeletally-mature individuals, advancing age may have a significant impact on skeletal repair [38]. A recent investigation in rats reported age-related changes in fracture healing [39], consisting of delayed periosteal reaction, cell differentiation, and angiogenic invasion of cartilage, decreased bone formation, protracted period of endochondral ossification, and impaired bone remodeling. The decline in healing capacity continued throughout the life span of the animal. In the elderly humans, Robinson et al. and Parker et al. reported an increased risk of nonunion of clavicular and femoral fractures, respectively [40, 41]. One probable cause for reduced healing potential with increasing age is the reduction in the number of mesenchymal stem cells in the bone tissue with increasing age [42], and some evidence also exist that even the growth factor levels within the bone matrix decline with age [43]. Osteoporosis is the most prevalent metabolic bone disease, affecting nearly 25 million Americans. It leads to a decreased bone volume, especially in areas with trabecular bone tissue, compromising on the bone's mechanical properties and increasing the risk of fractures. Osteoporotic vertebrae are weak and difficult to adequately stabilize with internal fixation for sufficient time for union to occur. Moreover, while osteoporotic bone was classically thought to have the same healing potential as nonosteoporotic one, recent evidences demonstrated reduced fracture healing in osteporotic rats [44].

Several clinical studies have shown a significantly higher incidence of delayed union, nonunion, and a doubling of the time to healing of the fracture in diabetic patients when compared with nondiabetic patients [45, 46]. Adequate glycemic control has been regarded as the key for the treatment of fractures in diabetics [47]. Different hypothesis have been postulated on how diabetes negatively affects fracture healing: inhibition of growth factor production, macro- and microangiopathy, and neuropathy. Diabetes-associated microangiopathy can certainly have a major negative effect on spinal fusion, as the entire fusion process depends on the ingress of osteoprogenitor and inflammatory cells from the recipient bed and from the few surviving bone cells transplanted when autogenous bone is used. Moreover, the vascularity of the fusion bed is a source of nutrients to the healing fusion and a vehicle for endocrine stimuli, which are essential for the successful incorporation of graft material and the inhibition of infection.

Nutritional status affects bone healing in orthopedic patients, and nutritional and metabolic requirements increase during bone healing. The importance of dietary protein, calcium, phosphorous, vitamin D, and vitamin C in the healing process has been clearly shown in experimental studies [48, 49]. Particular attention to nutritional status and optimization of deficiencies should be considered as a key step in favoring fracture repair and spinal fusion, especially in the elderly.

The rate of nonunion after spinal fusion in cigarette smokers has been shown to be higher than in nonsmokers [50, 51]. In a spinal fusion model in rabbits, nicotine stimulation resulted in nonunion in all cases, as opposed to only 44% in the control group [52]. Reduced blood supply, calcitonin resistance, increased bone resorption at fracture ends, inhibition of osteoblastic function, high levels of reactive oxygen intermediates, low concentrations of antioxidant vitamins, and the effects of nicotine on arteriole endothelial receptors are amongst the mechanism by which smoking has been considered to affect bone healing [53]. Not only nicotine is responsible for these deleterious effects, a tobacco extract not containing nicotine is also found to significantly reduce the mechanical strength of healing femoral fractures in rats, while nicotine alone did not affect the mechanical properties [54].

Various drugs taken during the perioperative period can inhibit or delay bone formation. Chemotherapeutic agents, such as methotrexate and adriamycin, inhibit bone formation and healing if administered early in the period after surgery [55, 56]. In experimental and clinical situations, corticosteroids have shown deleterious effects on bone healing as a result of increasing bone resorption and decreasing formation [57, 58]. It appears that long-term corticosteroid therapy is detrimental for bone healing, while short-term administration displays less clear effects. Also, nonsteroidal antiinflammatory (NSAID) drugs have been consistently associated with poor bone repair [59, 60]. Both animal and human studies attempted to address the failure rate of spinal fusion with NSAID therapy. Lebwohl et al. showed that ibuprofen was able to inhibit the healing of spinal fusion in rabbits [61], and Dimar et al., in a rat model of posterior spine fusion, demonstrated a fusion rate of 10% if indomethacin was given for 12 weeks postoperatively vs. 45% in control animals [62]. In humans, Glassman et al. reviewed the cases of 288 patients who had undergone posterior spinal fusion procedures from L4 to S1 over a 3-year period. Two demographically equivalent groups were compared – one group received ketorolac postoperatively and the other group did not. The authors showed a statistically significant adverse effect of ketorolac on fusion, and reported that nonunion was approximately 5 times more likely to occur if ketorolac was administered postoperatively [63]. Deguchi et al. in a retrospective review of patients who had undergone posterolateral spinal fusion for isthmic spondylolisthesis observed significantly decreased fusion and clinical success rates in patients who continued to use NSAIDs for more than 3 months postoperatively, when compared with those who did not. This adverse effect of ketorolac was not dose-related [64]. The negative effects of NSAIDs probably result from the inhibition of the inflammatory response, which constitutes the first step in fracture repair, and from the block of the synthesis of prostaglandin E(2), which control the expression of both bone morphogenetic protein 2 and 7 [65].

1.6 Comorbidities Associated with Poor Neurologic Recovery After Surgery

The effects of preexisting medical disorders on the neurologic outcome after cervical spine surgery have not been analyzed in detail, to our knowledge. The only medical condition whose detrimental effect on neurologic recovery is sufficiently supported by published studies is diabetes mellitus.

Diabetes mellitus, one of the most frequent preexisting comorbidity, can affect the peripheral nerves and the microvascular system. Diabetic neuropathy, angiopathy, or both, may influence the result of lumbar spine surgery [26, 66, 67]. Simpson et al. compared the long-term clinical outcomes after posterior decompressive procedures for either lumbar disk degeneration or spinal stenosis between diabetic and nondiabetic patients [26]. After a mean follow-up of 5 years for diabetics and 7 years for nondiabetics, all patients were asked about a series of symptoms, i.e., recurring or persisting pain in the back or the lower extremity, paresthesias, weakness, and functional impairment, each graded as none, mild, moderate, or severe by the interviewer. On the basis of this evaluation, only 39% of diabetic patients were reported to have an excellent or good clinical result, compared with 95% of nondiabetic patients. Kawaguchi et al. evaluated the neurologic outcome after cervical laminoplasty in 18 diabetic and 34 nondiabetic patients [68]. The Japanese Orthopedic Association (JOA) score for the severity of cervical myelopathy was recorded before surgery and after a mean of 3 years in diabetic and 4.7 years in nondiabetic patients. A similar improvement in the total JOA score was observed in the two groups; however, in sensory function of the lower extremities, the postoperative score in the group with diabetes mellitus was significantly lower than in the control group. Moreover, a negative correlation was found between the recovery rate and the preoperative HbA_1 values.

Two possible reasons leading to poorer neurologic outcomes in diabetic patients should be considered. First, the possible coexistence of sensory diabetic polyneuropathy or polyradiculopathy must always be considered in the evaluation of diabetic patients who have symptoms thought to be secondary to spinal disease. Indeed, symptoms due to these conditions would not be affected by surgery. The appropriate use of electromyographic studies can help to distinguish diabetic neuropathy from radiculopathy due to compression [69]. Second, there may be microvascular changes in the spinal nerve roots of patients who have diabetes mellitus, and it is possible that compressed spinal nerve roots in these patients do not recover after decompressive procedures in the same way as do the normal roots. Studies aimed to verify the changes in the spinal cord, spinal nerve roots, and peripheral nerves in diabetic patients have described infarcts in the proximal part of the nerve trunks, demyelination and atrophy of the nerve fibers associated with patchy fibrous tissue replacement, and softening of the posterior columns in the cord [70, 71].

Core Messages

Risks factors for complications related to medical conditions

1. Risk factors for major perioperative complications

Age, cardiovascular diseases, pulmonary diseases, hypertension, diabetes, congestive heart failure, alcohol/drug abuse, psychological disorders, chronic musculoskeletal disorders

2. Risk factors for perioperative cardiac events

Class II and Class III of the Cardiac Risk Index, Age >70 years, Q-wave on ECG, angina, ventricular ectopy, diabetes

3. Risk factors for postoperative infections

Malnutrition, diabetes, pulmonary diseases, smoking, immunocompromised hosts, obesity, extended prehospitalization, high blood loss (>1,000 ml), prolonged operative time

4. Comorbidities complicating spinal fusion

Local factors (mechanical environment, fusion site preparation, blood supply, bone graft source, and quantity), patient-related factors (osteoporosis, diabetes, nutritional status, smoke, chemotherapeutic, corticosteroids, NSAID drugs)

5. Comorbidities associated with poor neurologic recovery after surgery

Diabetic neuropathy

Modifiable risk factors should be eliminated or corrected before elective surgery

Elective surgery

Main therapeutic targets to reach before surgery:

- Diabetes: keep $HbA_1 < 7\%$ (optimal 6.2%) and/or fasting blood glucose <150 mg/dL (optimal <126)
- Cardiovascular diseases: optimal management of fluids and compensation of anemia
- Pulmonary diseases: assure $pO_2 > 60$ and/or $pCO_2 < 50$
- Hypertension: adjust therapy to obtain PAS < 150 mmHg and/or PAD < 90 mmHg
- Smoking/alcohol/drug abuse: quit!

Emergency surgery

- Diabetes: compensation by IV Insulin (GKI) to maintain blood glucose between 150 and 200 mg/dL during the first 3–5 days postsurgery. Resume preoperative therapy as soon as possible
- Cardiovascular diseases: optimal management of fluids and compensation of anemia. Continuous cardiologic consultation
- Pulmonary diseases: optimal airways and ventilation management during and after surgery
- Correction of anemia: transfusions if Hgb < 9 g/dL

References

1. Wang MCD, Chan L, Maiman DJ et al (2007) Complications and mortality associated with cervical spine surgery for degenerative disease in the United States. Spine 32: 342–347
2. Zeidman SM, Ducker TB, Raycroft J (1997) Trends and complications in cervical spine surgery: 1989–1993. J Spinal Disord 10:523–526

3. Bertalanffy H, Eggert HR (1989) Complications of anterior cervical discectomy without fusion in 450 consecutive patients. Acta Neurochir (Wien) 99:41–50
4. Romano PS, Campa DR, Rainwater JA (1997) Elective cervical discectomy in California: postoperative in-hospital complications and their risk factors. Spine 22:2677–2692
5. Harris OA, Runnels JB, Matz PG (2001) Clinical factors associated with unexpected critical care management and prolonged hospitalization after elective cervical spine surgery. Crit Care Med 29:1898–1902
6. Emery SE, Smith MD, Bohlman HH (1991) Upper-airway obstruction after multilevel cervical corpectomy for myelopathy. J Bone Joint Surg Am 73:544–551
7. Johnson VE, Huang JH, Pilcher WH (2007) Special cases: mechanical ventilation of neurosurgical patients. Crit Care Clin 23:275–290
8. Mangano DT (1990) Perioperative cardiac morbidity. Anesthesiology 72:153–184
9. Eagle KA, Brundage BH, Chaitman BR, Ewy GA, Fleischer LA, Hertzer NR, Leppo JA, Ryan T, Schlant RC, III Spencer JA, Spittell WH Jr, Twiss RD, Ritchie JL, Cheitlin MD, Gardner TJ, Garson A Jr, Lewis RP, Gibbons RJ, O'Rourke RA, Ryan TJ (1996) Guidelines for perioperative cardiovascular evaluation for noncardiac surgery: report of the American College of Cardiology/American Heart Association Task Force on Practice Guidelines. Circulation 93: 1278–1317
10. Mangano DT, Goldman L (1995) Preoperative assessment of patients with known or suspected coronary disease. N Engl J Med 333:1750–1756
11. Goldman L, Caldera DL, Nussbaum SR et al (1977) Multifactorial index of cardiac risk in noncardiac surgical procedures. N Engl J Med 297:845–850
12. Detsky AS, Abrams HB, McLaughlin JR et al (1986) Predicting cardiac complications in patients undergoing non-cardiac surgery. J Gen Intern Med 1:211–219
13. Palda VA, Detsky AS (1997) Perioperative assessment and management of risk from coronary artery disease. Ann Intern Med 127:313–328
14. American College of Physicians (1997) Guidelines for assessing and managing the perioperative risk from coronary artery disease associated with major noncardiac surgery. Ann Intern Med 127:309–312
15. Eagle KA, Coley CM, Newell JB et al (1989) Combining clinical and thallium data optimizes preoperative assessment of cardiac risk before major vascular surgery. Ann Intern Med 110:859–866
16. Poldermans D, Arnese M, Fioretti P et al (1995) Improved cardiac risk stratification in major vascular surgery with dobutamine-atropine stress echocardiography. J Am Coll Cardiol 26:648–653
17. Abbey DM, Turner DM, Warson JS et al (1995) Treatment of postoperative wound infections following spinal fusion with instrumentation. J Spinal Disord 8:278–283
18. Glassman SD, Dimar JR, Puno RM et al (1996) Salvage of instrumental lumbar fusions complicated by surgical wound infection. Spine 21:2163–2169
19. Keller RB, Pappas AM (1972) Infection after spinal fusion using internal fixation instrumentation. Orthop Clin North Am 3:99–111
20. Roberts FJ, Walsh A, Wing P et al (1998) The influence of surveillance methods on surgical wound infection rates in a tertiary care spinal surgery service. Spine 23: 366–370
21. Weinstein MA, McCabe JP, Cammisa FP Jr (2000) Postoperative spinal wound infection: a review of 2, 391 consecutive index procedures. J Spinal Disord 13:422–426
22. Massie JB, Heller JG, Abitbol JJ et al (1992) Postoperative posterior spinal wound infections. Clin Orthop Relat Res 284:99–108
23. Levi AD, Dickman CA, Sonntag VK (1997) Management of postoperative infections after spinal instrumentation. J Neurosurg 86:975–980
24. Capen DA, Calderone RR, Green A (1996) Perioperative risk factors for wound infections after lower back fusions. Orthop Clin North Am 27:83–86
25. Hu SS, Fontaine F, Kelly B et al (1998) Nutritional depletion in staged spinal reconstructive surgery.The effect of total parenteral nutrition. Spine 23:1401–1405
26. Simpson JM, Silveri CP, Balderston RA et al (1993) The results of operations on the lumbar spine in patients who have diabetes mellitus. J Bone Joint Surg Am 75: 1823–1829
27. Thelander U, Larsson S (1992) Quantitation of C-reactive protein levels and erythrocyte sedimentation rate after spinal surgery. Spine 17:400–404
28. Klein JD, Garfin SR (1996) Nutritional status in the patient with spinal infection. Orthop Clin North Am 27:33–36
29. Fang A, Hu SS, Endres N, Bradford DS (2005) Risk factors for infection after spinal surgery. Spine 30:1460–1465
30. Savitz MH, Malis LI, Meyers BR (1974) Prophylactic antibiotics in neurosurgery. Surg Neurol 2:95–100
31. Savitz MH, Malis LI (1976) Prophylactic clindamycin for neurosurgical patients. NY State J Med 76:64–67
32. Malis LI (1979) Prevention of neurosurgical infection by intraoperative antibiotics. Neurosurgery 5:339–343
33. Savitz MH, Katz SS (1981) Rationale for prophylactic antibiotics and neurosurgery. Neurosurgery 9:142–144
34. Beiner JM, Grauer J, Kwon BK, Vaccaro AR (2003) Postoperative wound infections of the spine. Neurosurg Focus 15:1–5
35. Gepstein R, Eismont FJ (1989) Postoperative spine infections. In: Garfin SR (ed) Complications of Spine Surgery. Williams & Wilkins, Baltimore, pp 302–322
36. DePalma AF, Rothman RH (1968) The nature of pseudarthrosis. Clin Orthop Relat Res 59:113–118
37. Steinmann JC, Herkowitz HN (1992) Pseudarthrosis of the spine. Clin Orthop Relat Res 284:80–90
38. Gruber R, Koch H, Doll BA et al (2006) Fracture healing in the elderly patient. Exp Gerontol 41:1080–1093
39. Lu C, Miclau T, Hu D et al (2005) Cellular basis for age-related changes in fracture repair. J Orthop Res 23: 1300–1307
40. Robinson CM, Court-Brown CM, McQueen MM et al (2004) Estimating the risk of nonunion following nonoperative treatment of a clavicular fracture. J Bone Joint Surg Am 86:1359–1365
41. Parker MJ (1994) Prediction of fracture union after internal fixation of intracapsular femoral neck fractures. Injury 25: B3–B6
42. Bruder SP, Fink DJ, Caplan AI (1994) Mesenchymal stem cells in bone development, bone repair, and skeletal regeneration therapy. J Cell Biochem 56:283–294

43. Pfeilschifter J, Diel I, Scheppach B et al (1998) Concentration of transforming growth factor beta in human bone tissue: relationship to age, menopause, bone turnover, and bone volume. J Bone Miner Res 13:716–730
44. Walsh WR, Sherman P, Howlett CR et al (1997) Fracture healing in a rat osteopenia model. Clin Orthop Relat Res 342: 218–227
45. Cozen L (1972) Does diabetes delay fracture healing? Clin Orthop Relat Res 82:134–140
46. Loder RT (1988) The influence of diabetes mellitus on the healing of closed fractures. Clin Orthop Relat Res 232: 210–216
47. Bibbo C, Lin SS, Beam HA, Behrens FF (2001) Complications of ankle fractures in diabetic patients. Orthop Clin North Am 32:113–133
48. Sarisözen B, Durak K, Dinçer G et al (2002) The effects of vitamins E and C on fracture healing in rats. J Int Med Res 30:309–313
49. Einhorn TA, Bonnarens F, Burstein AH (1986) The contributions of dietary protein and mineral to the healing of experimental fractures. A biomechanical study. J Bone Joint Surg Am 68:1389–1395
50. Blumenthal SL, Baker J, Dossett A et al (1988) The role of anterior lumbar fusion for internal disc disruption. Spine 13:566–569
51. Brown CW, Orme TJ, Richardson HD (1986) The rate of pseudarthrosis (surgical nonunion) in patients who are smokers and patients who are nonsmokers: a comparison study. Spine 11:942–943
52. Silcox DH 3rd, Daftari T, Boden SD et al (1995) The effect of nicotine on spinal fusion. Spine 20:1549–1553
53. Porter SE, Hanley EN Jr (2001) The musculoskeletal effects of smoking. J Am Acad Orthop Surg 9:9–17
54. Skott M, Andreassen TT, Ulrich-Vinther M et al (2006) Tobacco extract but not nicotine impairs the mechanical strength of fracture healing in rats. J Orthop Res 24:1472–1479
55. Burchardt H, Glowczewskie FP Jr, Enneking WF (1983) The effect of adriamycin and methotrexate on the repair of segmental cortical autografts in dogs. J Bone Joint Surg Am 65:103–108
56. Friedlaender GE, Tross RB, Doganis AC et al (1984) Effects of chemotherapeutic agents on bone. I. Short-term methotrexate and doxorubicin (adriamycin) treatment in a rat model. J Bone Joint Surg Am 66:602–607
57. Hahn TJ (1978) Corticosteroid-induced osteopenia. Arch Intern Med 138:882–885
58. Jowsey J, Riggs BL (1970) Bone formation in hypercortisonism. Acta Endocrinol (Copenh) 63:21–28
59. Høgevold HE, Grøgaard B, Reikerås O (1992) Effects of short-term treatment with corticosteroids and indomethacin on bone healing. A mechanical study of osteotomies in rats. Acta Orthop Scand 63:607–611
60. Solheim E, Pinholt EM, Bang G et al (1992) Inhibition of heterotopic osteogenesis in rats by a new bioerodible system for local delivery of indomethacin. J Bone Joint Surg Am 74:705–712
61. Lebwohl NH, Starr JK, Milne EL et al (1994) Inhibitory effect of ibuprofen on spinal fusion in rabbits. American Academy of Orthopaedic Surgeons annual meeting; 278 Abstract
62. Dimar JR 2nd, Ante WA, Zhang YP et al (1996) The effects of nonsteroidal anti-inflammatory drugs on posterior spinal fusions in the rat. Spine 21:1870–1876
63. Glassman SD, Rose SM, Dimar JR et al (1998) The effect of postoperative nonsteroidal anti-inflammatory drug administration on spinal fusion. Spine 23:834–838
64. Deguchi M, Rapoff AJ, Zdeblick TA (1998) Posterolateral fusion for isthmic spondylolisthesis in adults: a study of fusion rate and clinical results. J Spinal Disord 11:459–464
65. Hiltunen A, Aro HT, Vuorio E (1993) Regulation of extracellular matrix genes during fracture healing in mice. Clin Orthop Relat Res 297:23–27
66. Arai H, Takahashi K, Yamagata M et al (1997) Surgical results of lumbar spinal canal stenosis in diabetic patients. Presented at the annual meeting of the International Society for the Study of the Lumbar Spine, Singapore, June 3
67. Cinotti G, Postacchini F, Weinstein JN (1994) Lumbar spinal stenosis and diabetes. Outcome of surgical decompression. J Bone Joint Surg Br 76:215–219
68. Kawaguchi Y, Matsui H, Ishihara H et al (2000) Surgical outcome of cervical expansive laminoplasty in patients with diabetes mellitus. Spine 25:551–555
69. Hirsh LF (1984) Diabetic polyradiculopathy simulating lumbar disc disease. Report of four cases. J Neurosurg 60: 183–186
70. Raff MC, Asbury AK (1968) Ischemic mononeuropathy and mononeuropathy multiplex in diabetes mellitus. N Engl J Med 279:17–21
71. Gydell K, Skanse B (1956) A rare type of femoral-sciatic neuropathy in diabetes mellitus. Acta Med Scand 155: 463–468

Hematologic Issues in Cervical Spine Surgery

2

Giuseppe Avvisati, Ombretta Annibali, Elisabetta Cerchiara, Marianna De Muro, Rosa Greco, Francesco Marchesi, Carolina Nobile, Odoardo Olimpieri, Azzurra Romeo, and Maria Cristina Tirindelli

Contents

G. Avvisati (✉)
Hematology, University Campus Bio-Medico,
Via Àlvaro del Portillo, 21, 00128 Rome, Italy
e-mail: g.avvisati@unicampus.it

2.1 Changes in Blood Cell Count Parameters

2.1.1 *Anemia*

Anemia is defined as a reduction of hemoglobin (Hb) levels of <13 g/dL for a man and <12 g/dL for a woman. It is very frequent among hospitalized patients and can be a serious problem in patients who undergo cervical spine surgery. Anemia can be classified as:

- Mild (Hb: >10 g/dL)
- Moderate (Hb : 8–10 g/dL)
- Severe (Hb : 6–8 g/dL)
- Very severe (Hb: <6 g/dL)

To identify the causes of anemia, we can use functional and morphologic criteria. However, from a practical point of view, the morphologic criteria are preferred and require the reticulocytes absolute number and the mean corpuscular volume (MCV), respectively. The flowchart for identifying the causes of anemia using morphologic criteria is reported in Fig .2.1.

2.1.1.1 Approach to the Anemic Patient

Soon after a diagnosis of anemia has been made, the next step is to take an accurate clinical history and perform a physical examination to evaluate the signs and symptoms of anemia. These signs and symptoms may be: (a) *directly related to anemia*, and therefore, may present in all patients, independently from the cause of anemia, such as pallor, anorexia, fatigue, roaring in the ears, tachycardia, heart murmur, arrhythmia; until when

L. Denaro et al. (eds.), *Pitfalls in Cervical Spine Surgery*,
DOI: 10.1007/978-3-540-85019-9_2, © Springer-Verlag Berlin Heidelberg 2010

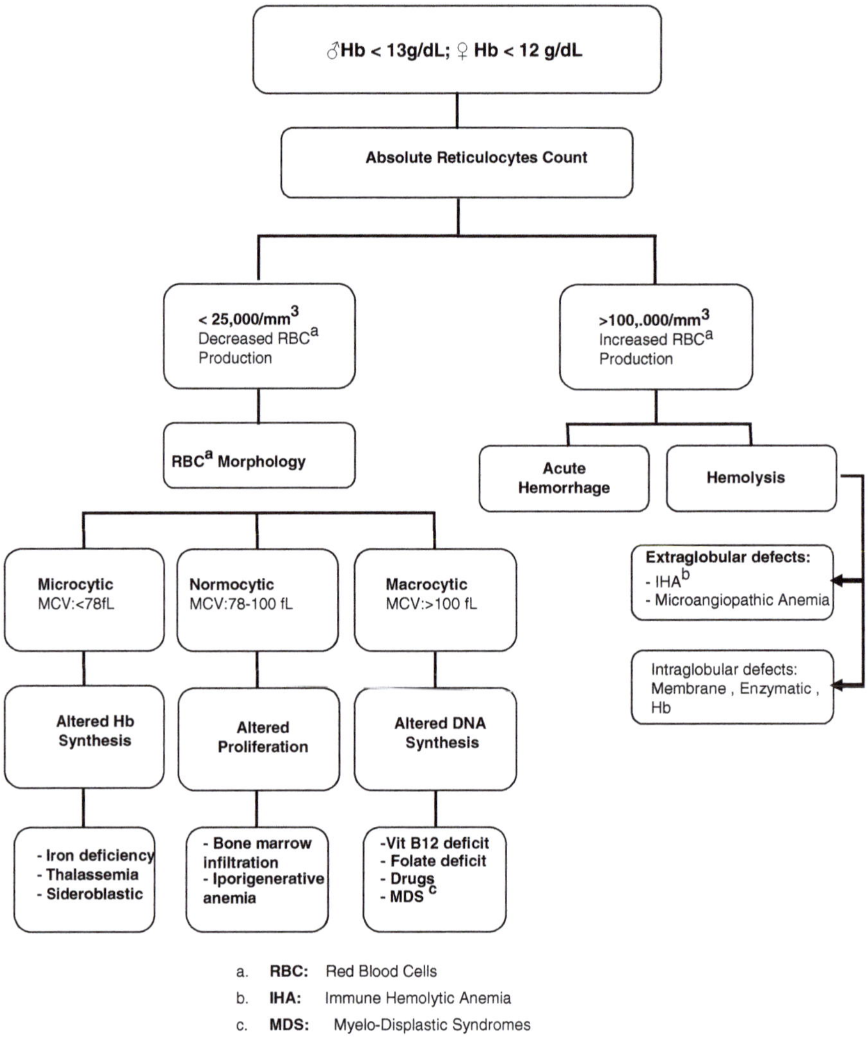

Fig. 2.1 Flow chart for identifying the causes of anemia by morphologic criteria

the Hb levels are <8 g/dL, patients may present rest dyspnea, congestive heart failure, angina, lethargy, mental confusion, mood alterations; or (b) *determined by acute bleeding*, such as easy fatigability, lassitude, muscle cramps, postural dizziness, lethargy, lipotimia, syncope, persistent hypotension, shock, and death.

Apart from these general signs and symptoms, there are others that are specific and can be related to a particular type of anemia. In fact, the presence of alopecia, glossitis, angular cheilitis, stomatitis with aftoid lesions, dysphagia, fragility of nails, and koilonychia is suggestive of iron depletion. The presence of glossitis, dysphagia, possibly associated with neurological changes (ataxia, polyneuropathy), is evocative of folate and/or Vitamin B12 deficit [1].

For a better evaluation of the anemia, it is also important to perform the following laboratory tests: absolute reticulocytes count, peripheral blood smear morphologic examination, serum total and direct biluribin, LDH, ferritin, folate and Vitamin B12 serum levels, and soluble transferrin receptor (sTfR). This last test is useful to differentiate between iron-deficiency anemia and anemia of chronic disorders when serum ferritin levels are normal or high; high sTfR levels are indicative of iron depletion [2].

In the presence of reduced levels of serum ferritin, folate, or Vitamin B12, a replacement therapy with these nutritional elements is indicated. In case of anemia with low absolute reticulocytes count associated with leukopenia/leukocytosis and/or thrombocytopenia/

thrombocytosis, it is very important to seek the hematologist's advice before any surgical intervention, because the cause of anemia may influence the possibility to perform a surgical procedure such as in the case of a diagnosis of acute leukemia.

Moreover, anemia may also be a postoperative complication, related to blood loss during surgery. Therefore, a low hemoglobin level observed before cervical spine surgery requires investigation, and must be corrected to prevent more severe postoperative anemia, which can expose the patient to cardiovascular complications, delay healing of the tissue, and blood transfusions, with an increased risk of transfusion-related adverse events. Once the anemia has been corrected, we can reduce the exposure to homologous blood using autologous blood transfusions or acute normovolemic hemodilution.

2.1.1.2 Anemia's Decalogue for the Surgeon

(a). The management of anemia should be tailored to the cause and severity of anemia.

(b). Blood transfusion therapy is indicated generally only in case of severe (Hb:6–8 g/dL) or very severe (Hb <6 g/dL) anemia not related to iron, folate, or Vitamin B12 deficiency.

(c). In the presence of reduced levels of serum ferritin, folate, or Vitamin B12, replacement therapy with these nutritional elements is indicated.

(d). In anemia caused by iron, folate, or Vitamin B12 deficiency, blood transfusions therapy may be required to avoid more severe complications, when symptoms or hemodynamic instability and/or co-morbidities are present.

(e). To correct iron-deficiency (low serum ferritin levels) anemia, slow intravenous infusion (1 vial diluted in 250 mL of saline solution 0.9%, infused in 1 h) or oral iron can be used.

(f). The choice between intravenous and oral iron depends on the surgical urgency.

(g). Erythropoietin (EPO) therapy may be useful in case of moderate anemia (Hb: 8–10 g/dL) in the absence of co-morbidities.

(h). In the presence of severe co-morbidities, such as cardiac or pulmonary disease, blood transfusion therapy is mostly indicated to correct anemia.

(i). If surgery can be postponed, intravenous iron therapy combined with EPO therapy may increase the Hb to levels that allow preoperative autologous blood collection (even in those patients with anemia of chronic diseases), thus reducing the use of homologous blood transfusions.

(j). In case of anemia with low absolute reticulocytes count associated with leukopenia/leukocytosis and/or thrombocytopenia/thrombocytosis, one should seek the hematologist's advice before any surgical intervention.

2.1.2 *Polycythemia*

The diagnosis of polycythemia may be suspected in patients with abnormally high hematocrit (Hct), Hb concentration, and/or red blood cells (RBC) count even though RBC value is least often used to suggest this diagnosis, as patients with thalassemia minor may have an elevated RBC count, but a normal or reduced Hct or Hb, due to the presence of microcytic, poorly hemoglobinized, hypochromic red cells [3]. These three measurements (Hct, Hb, and RBC) are concentrations, and therefore, dependent on the plasma volume as well as the RBC mass. Hence, it is necessary to differentiate the relative (or apparent) and unapparent polycythemia from absolute polycythemia.

- *Relative polycythemia* is a condition in which there is a reduction in the plasmatic volume with a relative increase in RBC mass. As a consequence, Hct, Hb concentration, and RBC count are apparently increased. It can be caused by dehydration, diuretic drugs, alcohol, obesity, and hypertension.
- *Unapparent polycythemia* is a condition in which the RBC mass and plasma volume are equally increased; hence, Hb and Hct remain normal. In this case, erythrocytosis can only be detected via blood volume and genetic studies.
- Absolute polycythemia is a condition in which there is a true (absolute) increase in RBC mass. It can be primary or secondary.
- Primary polycythemia: depending on an effective hyper-production of RBC mass caused by an intrinsic bone-marrow alteration, it is determined by an acquired or inherited DNA mutation leading to an abnormal RBC production; it includes the *polycythemia vera* (PV) and the rare familial variants.
- Secondary polycythemia: caused by elevated EPO synthesis, responsible for the increased RBC

production by bone marrow. It is most often due to an EPO response to hypoxia, but can also result from increased EPO secretion by congenital or acquired causes such as: presence of a congenital oxygen high-affinity Hb or a tumor (kidney, liver, little brain (cerebellum), adrenal glands, lung, uterus).

2.1.2.1 Polycythemia and Cervical Spinal Surgery

If a patient has an increased Hct value (>52% in men and >48% in women) and an increased Hb concentration (>18 g/dL and >16 g/dL, respectively), it is absolutely important to diagnose whether or not these altered values are due to a PV or are the consequence of a relative or secondary polycythemia. The prognosis and management are different depending on the diagnosis. Therefore, orthopedic surgeons before surgery should ask for a hematologist's consultation. The hematologist, through an accurate history, physical examination, and some laboratory tests, will determine the etiology of polycythemia and evaluate the presence of an *increased risk of arterial and/or venous thrombotic events or bleeding,* and the type of the prophylactic therapy needed to avoid these complications.

2.1.2.2 Tips for the Orthopedic Surgeon in the Presence of a PV

If a patient with PV needs cervical spinal surgery, the orthopedic surgeon must ask the hematologist about how to prevent the possible thromboembolic (TE) or hemorrhagic complications.

Although these patients always receive low-dose aspirin (75–100 mg/day) as prophylaxis for arterial thrombosis, its use cannot be recommended to reduce the TE risk following elective spinal surgery [4].

However, as its use can predispose the patient to an increased risk of bleeding during surgery, aspirin should be discontinued at least 1 week before surgery to avoid bleeding complications. As for TE complications, their incidence during elective spinal surgery is unknown; however, recent guidelines recommend that in case of additional risk factors (advanced age, cancers, neurological deficit, previous TE events, or anterior surgery access), TE prophylaxis should be performed. Therefore, because the patients with PV have a neoplastic disease and very often might have suffered from a previous TE episode, they should receive antithrombotic prophylaxis for spinal surgery.

2.1.3 Reduction in the White Blood Cell Count

In adults, a reduction in the white blood cells (WBC) count of <4,000/μL is defined as leukopenia. Its etiology may be related to disorders of production or distribution and turnover of the leukocytes, and to the use of some drugs or infectious diseases. Therefore, before a cervical spinal surgery intervention, the causes of leucopenia should be carefully investigated. However, from a practical view point, only *absolute neutropenia* (neutrophiles <1,500/μl) and *absolute lymphopenia* (lymphocytes <1,000/μl) will be described.

2.1.3.1 Absolute Neutropenia

Absolute neutropenia (neutrophiles <1,500/μL) can predispose the patient to severe infective diseases. Neutrophiles play a pivotal role in the defense of the human body against infections. Therefore, the risk for acute or chronic infections must be evaluated before listing neutropenic patients for surgery. Also, bacterial, viral, parasitic, and rickettsial infections may be responsible for this condition. The main causes of absolute neutropenia are: *acquired* (infectious diseases, drugs, immune and autoimmune disorders, severe folate and Vitamin B12 deficiency, hypersplenism, hematologic malignancies) or *congenital* (very rare and occurring in childhood) [5]. Furthermore, the absolute neutrophil count (ANC) is used to define the severity of neutropenia as follows:

- *Mild*: *ANC <1,500/μL and >1,000/μL*
- *Moderate*: *ANC <1,000/μL and >500/μL*
- *Severe*: *ANC <500/μL*
- *Very severe*: *ANC <100/μL*

Only those patients with severe or very severe neutropenia are considered at high risk for infections by opportunistic or nonopportunistic microbial agents. Moreover, in a patient who is a candidate for surgery, unexplained neutropenia, associated with anemia and/or thrombocytopenia, must be carefully investigated by a trained hematologist before surgery is performed to exclude the presence of hematologic malignancies.

2.1.3.2 Absolute Lymphocytopenia

A condition of absolute lymphocytopenia (lymphocytes <1,000/μL) may be caused by: drugs (i.e., glucocorticoids, some anti-metabolites chemotherapy, and immune-suppressor drugs), some infectious diseases (i.e., HIV infection in AIDS phase, HBV, HCV, TBC, typhus fever, sepsis, pneumonia), radiotherapy, sarcoidosis, autoimmune disorders, chronic renal failure, some hematologic malignancies (i.e., Hodgkin's lymphoma in advanced phase of disease), and some rare congenital immune disorders [6]. To avoid complications, the cause of lymphocytopenia should be determined before surgery is performed.

2.1.4 Increase in White Blood Cell Count

- An increase in WBC of >10,000/μL is defined as leukocytosis, and may have many causes, which should be carefully investigated before any surgical intervention. Moreover, some pathologic conditions are responsible for an absolute increase in a single type (neutrophiles, lymphocytes, monocytes eosinophiles, basophiles) of WBC associated or not associated with leukocytosis. Therefore, the first step in the diagnostic process of this condition is to define which type of WBC is increased; as a consequence, in adults, depending on the type of WBC increased, we can observe the following conditions:
- *Absolute neutrophilia*: *neutrophiles >7,500/μL*
- *Absolute lymphocytosis*: *lymphocytes >4,000/μL*
- *Absolute monocytosis*: *monocytes >1,000/μL*
- *Absolute eosinophilia*: *eosinophiles >500/μL*
- *Absolute basophilia*: *basophiles >200/μL (very rare)*

Frequently, however, there is only a relative increase in a subtype of WBC, determining an alteration in the leukocytes formula, without an increase in the absolute number of some types of WBC. These conditions are defined as *"relative"* increase (i.e., in case of a WBC count of 4,270/μL with 20% of monocytes, despite the percentage of monocytes being high, its absolute number is <1,000/μL; thus, we can conclude the condition as "relative monocytosis").

2.1.4.1 Absolute Neutrophilia

The presence of an absolute neutrophilia (*neutrophiles >7,500/μL*) arises from various clinical conditions such as infections, chronic inflammation, neoplasia or a hematological malignancy, or a fracture. Moreover, transient neutrophilia is normal in the postoperative period, caused by the response of the human body to the surgical stress. Persistent neutrophilia may be associated with a surgery-related infective complication. An increase in the absolute number of neutrophiles before surgery can be a good reason for a hematologic consultation.

2.1.4.2 Absolute Lymphocytosis

An increase in the absolute number of lymphocytes (*lymphocytes >4,000/μL*) may be caused by hematologic malignancies or by viral, certain bacterial, or parasitic infections. Moreover, vasculitis, inflammatory bowel diseases, emergency medical conditions, acute trauma, and hypersensitivity reactions (drug-induced or related to acute serum sickness) may cause absolute lymphocytosis. A trained hematologist can easily verify its pathogenesis.

2.1.4.3 Absolute Eosinophilia and Absolute Monocytosis

These conditions are less frequent than absolute neutrophilia and lymphocytosis; therefore, we will not describe these conditions.

2.1.5 Changes in Platelet Count

2.1.5.1 Abnormal Increase in Platelet Count

The normal platelet count ranges from 150,000 to 450,000/μL, and a platelet count >500,000/μL is defined as thrombocytosis [7].

However, <10% of isolated thrombocytosis reflects a hematological disorder. Therefore, most cases of thrombocytosis occur within a systemic disorder, *secondary or reactive thrombocytosis* [8], such as those occurring because of:

- Recent trauma or surgery
- Prior surgical removal of the spleen
- Local or systemic complaints suggesting infection or inflammation
- Iron deficiency
- Pregnancy
- Malignancy

A *primary thrombocytosis* may be due to a myeloproliferative disorder, and when isolated, is generally pathognomonic of *essential thrombocythemia* (ET).

Therefore, in the presence of a pathologic increase in platelet count, it is very important to exclude that *thrombocytosis* is a reactive process. Once a reactive process has been excluded, the next step is to accurately classify whether or not the thrombocytosis is a result of a myeloproliferative disorder such as ET, chronic myelogenous leukemia (CML), idiopathic myelofibrosis (IMF), PV, myelodysplastic syndrome (MDS), and acute myeloid leukemia (AML) [9]. Thus, patients in whom a reactive process cannot be identified, require a hematological consult and a bone marrow examination with reticulin staining and cytogenetic studies to better define the myeloproliferative disorder responsible for thrombocytosis.

Patients with primary thrombocytosis as well as those with thrombocytosis secondary to malignancy require a correct TE prophylaxis because the risk of TE episodes range from 10 to 25% and is not related to the number of platelets [10].

2.1.5.2 Abnormal Decrease in Platelet Count

A platelet number <150,000/μL defines thrombocytopenia, and may predispose to excessive bleeding [7]. However, bleeding during surgery because of a reduction in the number of platelets does not generally occur until the platelet count is <50,000/μL, and clinical or spontaneous bleeding does not occur until the platelet count is <10,000–20,000/μL [11]. Once thrombocytopenia has been reported, it should be confirmed by repeated testing and examination of the peripheral blood smear to exclude cases of pseudothrombocytopenia. In the presence of a confirmed result of thrombocytopenia, the initial step is to perform a comprehensive history and physical examination to understand the cause of it.

Drugs are a common cause of thrombocytopenia. The spectrum of drugs reported to cause thrombocytopenia is broadening and changing progressively. A complete list and analysis of all published reports of drug-induced thrombocytopenia is available on the internet (http://w3.ouhsc.edu/platelets). Patients with thrombocytopenia may be asymptomatic, and thrombocytopenia may be first detected on a routine complete blood count (CBC). The most common symptomatic presentation of thrombocytopenia is bleeding, characteristically mucosal and cutaneous. Following confirmation of thrombocytopenia, to diagnose its cause, it is better to consult a hematologist.

In thrombocytopenic patients at risk of, or complaining of, severe hemorrhagic complications, the guidelines of The Italian Society of Haemostasis and Thrombosis, may be applied [12], which is summarized as follows:

- *Prophylaxis of hemorrhagic events during surgery*:
- High hemorrhagic risk and surgery procedures at high risk of hemorrhage impossible to control by local hemostatic measures: 1 unit/10 kg of body weight of random donor platelets or 1 U of platelets pheresis
- Low hemorrhagic risk and surgery procedures at high risk of hemorrhages: desmopressin if not contraindicated (i.e., previous thrombosis or thromboembolism, severe arteriopathy)
- Low hemorrhagic risk and minor surgery: local hemostasis
- *Treatment of hemorrhagic episodes:*
- *Major* hemorrhagic event: 1 unit/10 kg of body weight of random donor platelets or 1 U of platelets pheresis
- *Minor* hemorrhagic event: local hemostasis

2.1.6 How a Cervical Spine Surgeon should Manage Patients with Changes in Blood Cell Count

In the presence of changes in the blood cell count, surgeons should recognize these alterations and seek a consultation with a trained hematologist, who, by means of laboratory and instrumental tests, will recognize the cause responsible for the changes observed in the blood cell count. In the meantime, the hematologist will provide the surgeon with correct suggestions about the possibility of performing the surgical intervention immediately or after the solution of the problem responsible for the changes in the blood cell count.

2.2 Patients with Monoclonal Gammopathy [13]

A monoclonal gammopathy (paraproteinemia or dysproteinemia) is defined as the presence of immunologically homogeneous protein commonly referred to as a paraprotein or monoclonal protein (M-protein, where the "M" stands for monoclonal) in serum or urine, produced by a single clone of plasma cells. The routinely recommended method for the detection and quantification of an M-protein in serum or concentrated urine is the agarose gel electrophoresis, an inexpensive and easy to perform screening procedure.

Before cervical spine surgery, serum protein electrophoresis should be considered in any patient with:

- Elevated erythrocyte sedimentation rate
- Elevated serum viscosity
- Unexplained anemia
- Back pain, weakness, or fatigue
- Osteopenia
- Osteolytic lesions
- Spontaneous fractures
- Renal insufficiency with a bland urine sediment
- Heavy proteinuria in a patient over the age of 40 years
- Hypercalcemia
- Hypergammaglobulinemia
- Immunoglobulin deficiency
- Bence Jones proteinuria
- Unexplained peripheral neuropathy

However, an M-protein can be present in a number of different disorders, including B-cell and plasma-cell proliferations. The most common of these are listed in Table 2.1.

Table 2.1 Disorders associated with the presence of a monoclonal gammopathy

Plasma cell disorders
Monoclonal gammopathy of undetermined significance (MGUS)
Biclonal gammopathy of undetermined significance
Idiopathic Bence Jones proteinuria
POEMS syndrome, Osteosclerotic myeloma
Castleman's disease
AL (light chain) amyloidosis
Solitary plasmacytoma
Multiple myeloma (MM)
Smoldering MM
B-cell lymphoproliferative disorders
Non-Hodgkin's lymphoma
Chronic lymphocytic leukemia
Lymphoplasmacytic lymphoma (Waldenstrom macroglobulinemia)
Posttransplant monoclonal gammopathies
Connective-tissue disorders
Systemic lupus erythematosus
Rheumatoid arthritis
Sjogren syndrome
Scleroderma
Psoriatic arthritis
Associated with infections
Hepatitis C virus infection
HIV/AIDS
Dermatologic disorders
Miscellaneous disorders
Cryoglobulinemia
Cryofibrinogenemia
Chronic myelogemous leukemia
Acquired von Willebrand disease
Myelodysplastic syndrome

The most common causes of monoclonal gammopathy are: MGUS and MM

2.2.1 Monoclonal Gammopathy of Undetermined Significance (MGUS)

MGUS is found in approximately 1–2% of the patients. The incidence is generally higher in patients over 70 years. In well-performed epidemiologic studies, the prevalence of MGUS in subjects ≥50, ≥70, and ≥85 years of age was 3.2, 5.3, and 7.5%, respectively. Differentiation of a patient with MGUS from the one with multiple myeloma (MM) may sometimes be difficult at the time of initial presentation. By definition, the diagnosis of MGUS requires the absence of anemia, hypercalcemia, renal failure, and lytic bone lesions related to the plasma cell proliferative disorder. However, the mere presence of clinical findings such as anemia, hypercalcemia, renal failure, or lytic bone lesions in conjunction with an M-protein does not automatically indicate MM or related malignancy, as these abnormalities may be due to other unrelated coexisting diseases (see Table 2. 2.1). To differentiate MGUS from a related plasma-cell malignancy, patients should have a CBC, serum creatinine, serum calcium, and a complete radiographic bone survey of the skeleton, including all long bones. Patients who exhibit abnormalities with respect to the above-mentioned tests should undergo additional tests to determine the etiology of the abnormalities, and whether they are indeed related to a plasma-cell proliferative disorder.

2.2.2 Multiple Myeloma

MM is caused by the malignant proliferation of plasma cells in the bone marrow producing an M-protein. Plasma cells frequently invade the adjacent bone, producing skeletal destruction that results in pathological fractures and bone pain. Other symptoms of this disease are anemia, hypercalcemia, and impairment of renal function. An M-protein in the serum or urine is present in 97% of these patients.

In particular, a serum M-protein is observed in 80% of the patients at diagnosis, while immune-fixation reveals an M-protein in over 90%. An IgG M-protein is found in about 50% of the patients, while 20% have an IgA M-protein, and monoclonal light chain alone (light-chain myeloma) is found in almost 20% of the patients. M-protein (Bence Jones protein) in urine is observed in approximately 75% of the patients.

The most critical criterion for symptomatic or treatable disease is the evidence of organ or tissue impairment (end-organ damage) manifested by anemia, hypercalcemia, lytic bone lesions, renal insufficiency, hyperviscosity, amyloidosis, or recurrent infections. Most patients with MM are symptomatic. However, it is possible that during screening tests for unrelated disorders, patients without any symptoms attributable to myeloma may be diagnosed as having MM (asymptomatic myeloma). Other patients may demonstrate local symptoms owing to plasmacytoma. Solitary plasmacytoma is rare. The diagnosis requires histologic evidence of a monoclonal plasma cell infiltrate in the lesion, absence of other lesions, and lack of marrow plasmacytosis elsewhere.

2.3 Preoperative Evaluation of the Hemorrhagic Risk

Besides thrombocytopenia, a quantitative defect of platelet number (see above), thrombocytopathy, a qualitative (abnormal function) defect of platelets, as well as the alterations in the coagulation parameters (prothrombin time = PT, activated partial thromboplastin time = aPTT, and fibrinogen) may increase the hemorrhagic risk in cervical spine surgery.

2.3.1 Abnormal Hemostatic and Coagulation Parameters

A good knowledge of the basic principles of the hemostatic system is mandatory in cervical spine surgery, as unexpected bleedings or thrombosis episodes can rapidly become life-threatening emergencies in the intraoperative and postoperative period.

The reason of this extreme susceptibility to coagulation-related complications can be found in the vascular anatomy of the cervical district [14]. The vertebral and basilar arteries provide up to 20% of the total cerebral blood flow, and are the principal affluent to the arterial circulation system of the cerebellum and brainstem. Any alteration that involves the vertebrobasilar circulation can cause irreversible ischemic damages to vital structures.

The incidence of severe hemostatic alterations after cervical surgery is difficult to assess, overly depending on the patient's conditions and comorbidities, but it has been estimated in 1:20,000 patients subjected to cervical manipulation, even though more stringent studies have documented the incidence rates as high as 1:4,500.

To prevent ischemic injuries from arterial occlusions, the vertebrobasilar system is rich in collateral vessels that can rapidly redirect the blood flow to the hypoperfused zone. Nonetheless, any collateral system has intrinsic limits, and cannot overcome large flow interruptions. Other possible elements involved in thrombotic alterations are blood flow interruptions during surgery, and possible endothelial damages following manipulation. Several studies showed that arterial blood flows can be stopped during surgery for up to 3 h without thrombotic complications, provided that an adequate antithrombotic prophylaxis had been performed. Nonetheless, the characteristic flow intermittency in vertebrobasilar artery during spinal surgery can be an additional stimulus for thrombus formation, and can lead to another hemostatic issue, namely, the endothelial damage.

Given these characteristics, the evaluation of thrombo-hemorrhagic risk factors for every single patient should be accurate and exhaustive, from history taken at the bedside to preoperative laboratory screening tests. Only an adequate familiarity with the coagulation system can provide a safe approach to such challenging surgery.

2.3.1.1 Qualitative Platelets Defects (Thrombocytopathies)

Platelets are important for primary hemostasis. Physiologically, when platelets are exposed to damaged endothelium, they adhere to the exposed basement membrane collagen and change their shape from smooth disks to spheres with pseudopodia. Subsequently, they secrete the contents of their granules, a process referred to as the release reaction. Finally, additional platelets aggregate on those platelets that have adhered to the vessel wall. As a result, the primary hemostatic plug is formed and bleeding is arrested.

Platelet abnormalities can be classified into quantitative (abnormal in number, see Sect. 2.1.5.1) and qualitative defects (abnormal in function). Qualitative platelets defects (thrombocytopathies) can either be inherited or more commonly acquired (secondary to disease, drugs, etc.) (Table 2.2). Typically, patients with platelet disorders have mucocutaneous bleeding of variable severity and excessive hemorrhage after surgery or trauma.

Inherited qualitative platelets disorders constitute a large group of diseases involving a wide range of genetic defects that can lead to bleeding symptoms of varying severity. They are associated with abnormalities of platelet glycoproteins (resulting in, e.g., Bernard–Soulier Syndrome and Glanzmann Thrombasthenia), platelet granules, and signal transduction and secretion. Congenital disorders generally increase the risks for excessive bleeding after significant hemostatic challenges (e.g., surgery, major dental procedures, trauma). Typically, abnormal bleeding occurs with a rapid onset [15].

Table 2.2 Acquired platelets disorders

Drugs affecting platelets function
Nonsteroidal anti-inflammatory drugs (Aspirin, ibuprofen, indomethacin,etc.)
Thienopyridines (ticlopidine, clopidogrel)
GpIIb–IIIa receptor antagonists (Abciximab, eptifibatide, tirofiban)
Drugs that increase plateletcAMP or cGMP levels (Prostacyclin, iloprost, nitric oxide, theophylline)
β-Lactam antibiotics (Penicillins, cephalosporins)
Anticoagulants and fibrinolytic agents (Heparin, streptokinase, tPA, urokinase)
Cardiovascular drugs (Nitrates, calcium channel blockers, quinidine)
Volume expanders (Dextran, hydroxyethyl starch)
Psychotropic agents and anesthetics (Antidepressants, phenothiazines)
Oncologic drugs
Foods and food additives (Fish oil, cumin, ginkgo biloba, etc.)
Hematologic disorders associated with abnormal plateletsfunction:
Chronic myeloproliferative disorders
Leukemias and myelodysplastic syndromes
Monoclonal Gammopathies
Acquired von Willebrand disease
Systemic disorders associated with abnormal platelets function:
Uremia
Antiplatelet antibodies
Cardiopulmonary bypass
Liver diseases
Disseminated intravascular coagulation

Acquired qualitative platelets disorders are more frequent in clinical practice. Platelet function may be adversely affected by drugs and by hematologic and nonhematologic disorders. As the use of aspirin and other nonsteroidal anti-inflammatory drugs is pervasive in current medical practice, acquired platelet dysfunction is much more frequent than inherited dysfunctions (Table 2.2) [16].

Drug-induced qualitative platelet dysfunction is clearly the most common cause of acquired thrombocytopathies. The list of medications or dietary supplements associated with platelet dysfunction is long and growing (Table 2.2). These include aspirin and other nonsteroidal anti-inflammatory drugs, ticlopidine, clopidogrel, antibiotics, cardiovascular drugs, psychotropic drugs, and dietary items, such as herbal supplements, among others. In a healthy individual, drug-induced platelet dysfunction is usually of no clinical significance. However, in patients with coagulation disorders, uremia, or thrombocytopenia, and in patients who are undergoing surgery or anticoagulation therapy, impairment of platelet function by drugs may lead to serious bleeding [16].

Aspirin is the most notable drug in this regard because of its frequent use, its irreversible effect on platelet prostaglandin synthesis, and its documented effect on hemostatic competency [17]. The inhibition of platelet release reaction occurs within 15–30 min after ingestion with aspirin doses as low as 40–80 mg, and persists as long as the affected platelet survives (8–10 days). Thus, a single small dose of aspirin impairs the release reaction for up to 96 h [18]. Other *nonsteroidal anti-inflammatory drugs* (such as ibuprofen, indomethacin) reversibly inhibit platelet prostaglandin synthesis and usually have little effect on hemostasis [19]. The antiplatelet effect of a number of drugs has proved useful in preventing arterial thrombosis, but excessive bleeding can complicate their use. In addition to aspirin, these drugs include *ticlopidine* and *clopidogrel* [20]. Their effect on platelet aggregation may be seen within 24–48 h of the first dose, but does not reach a maximum for 4–6 days. The effect on platelet function may last for 4–10 days after the drugs have been discontinued. A number of other drugs and a number of foods and food additives may affect platelet function, but these effects do not appear to be clinically significant.

Hematologic diseases associated with abnormal platelet function include marrow processes in which platelets may be intrinsically abnormal, such as the clonal myeloid diseases, dysproteinemias in which abnormal plasma proteins can impair platelet function, and acquired forms of von Willebrand disease. Of the systemic diseases, renal failure is most prominently associated with abnormal platelet function because of retention of platelet inhibitory compounds. Platelet function may be abnormal in the presence of antiplatelet antibodies, following cardiopulmonary bypass, in association with liver disease, or in disseminated intravascular coagulation [16].

2.3.1.2 Coagulopathies

These alterations require accurate preoperative evaluation [21]. The most important part of an accurate preoperative evaluation of possible coagulation alterations is history taking. In this process, one should always consider that frequently normal people consider their bleeding to be excessive. In dubious cases, further help can be obtained by physical examination and laboratory tests.

Physical examination is important in assessing the possible coagulation problems, and the physician should have a particular focus on skin and mucosal hemorrhagic manifestations, such as small red focal areas (<2 mm) that do not disappear with finger pressure (petechiae). Petechiae are more commonly found on sites subjected to shear and pressure stresses (under belt skin or periorbitary regions, especially after crying or intense coughing); when they merge into larger areas, they are called purpura (<1 cm) or ecchymoses (>1 cm), and are frequently associated with platelets disorders. Primary coagulation disorders are, however, more frequently associated with large and spontaneous bruises, painful hemarthroses, and intracavitary blood effusions.

Every patient should, therefore, be asked about:

- Past bleeding episodes associated with surgical procedures (e.g., appendectomy, circumcision, tonsillectomy, or dental extractions).
- Spontaneous bruises formation and/or petechial lesions.
- History of frequent nosebleeds (if confined to a single nostril, a hematologic systemic disease is improbable; if bilateral and recurrent in absence of major trauma, also consider hereditary hemorrhagic teleangiectasias or von Willebrand disease).
- Presence of recurrent hemorrhagic and/or thrombotic episodes in family members.
- Excessive bleeding during childbearing or menstrual cycles.
- Recurrent episodes of gingival hemorrhage in the absence of local alterations.
- Excessive bleeding from minor cuts, with particular regard to the time to stop and the need for direct pressure or tissue paper.
- Even a single episode of hemarthrose is worth for further investigations for hemophilia, especially in infants and children.
- Comorbidities such as epatic diseases, alterations in nutrient absorption, alcohol assumption history, or vitamin deficiencies.
- Very important is the presence of renal failure or liver diseases.
- Drug assumption (with particular attention to nonsteroidal anti-inflammatories, oral anticoagulants such as warfarin and acenocoumarol, herbal remedies, and other medications available without prescription); NB: oral anticoagulants should be suspended at least 4 days before surgery and an adequate prophylaxis with low molecular weight heparin (LMWH) should be started at the same time; clopidogrel should be discontinued 14 days before any major surgical procedure, aspirin and

lysine acetylsalicylate administration should be interrupted at least 7 days before surgery, whereas Clopidogrel and Ticlopidine should be interrupted 4–6 days prior to surgery.

2.3.1.3 The laboratory Interface

As pointed out earlier, laboratory tests can be extremely helpful in assessing possible coagulation disorders that can put at risk the patient's life during cervical surgery [22]; notwithstanding, the need for routine preoperative testing is controversial. While coagulation tests can in fact detect many asymptomatic disorders that may cause surgical bleedings, many studies bring into question their positive predictive value for perioperative hemorrhagic complications.

Coagulation test can be divided into routine tests and secondary tests.

Routine Tests

Prothrombin Time (PT)

PT analyzes the "extrinsic and common pathway factors," and it is particularly sensible in detecting alterations of factors VII, X, V, thrombin, and fibrinogen.

The main causes of PT alterations are:

- Sampling errors
- Anticoagulant therapy
- Factor VII, X, V, thrombin, or fibrinogen deficiencies (*it is also mandatory* to *test the hepatic function)*
- Coagulation-acquired inhibitors (antibody against factor VII, X, V, thrombin, or fibrinogen), antibodies, anti-phospholipids
- MM paraprotein

Activated partial thromboplastin time (aPTT)

The aPTT test evaluates the intrinsic pathway (composed by factor XII, XI, VIII, and IX) together with the common pathway. Abnormalities in aPTT are caused by:

- Sampling errors
- Heparin or anticoagulant therapy
- Factor XII, XI, IX, VIII, X, V, thrombin, or fibrinogen deficiencies (*NB: consider hemophilia; testing the hepatic function is also mandatory)*
- Coagulation-acquired inhibitors (antibody against factor XII, XI, IX, VIII, X, V, thrombin, or fibrinogen), antibodies, anti-phospholipids
- Von Willebrand disease
- MM paraprotein

Second-Line Tests

Second-line tests are special assays to further discriminate the first-line tests' abnormalities, and should always be requested under the advice of an expert hematologist. The most commonly performed second-line tests are single-factor concentration assays, used to characterize and evaluate the deficiency of single coagulation factors, such as factor VIII and factor IX in hemophila A and B, respectively. dRVVT and KCT-SCT, specific aPTT-derived tests performed with low concentrations of phospholipids, are useful in detecting Lupus Anticoagulant. Moreover, two second-line tests could be useful to evaluate the presence of heparin in blood samples: thrombin time (TT) and reptilase time (RT). TT measures the clotting time after the addition of thrombin to plasma. It is prolonged only in the presence of heparin, MM paraprotein, and hypofibrinogenemia. In the presence of a prolonged TT, an RT test should be performed. RT is not sensitive to heparin, and hence, in the presence of an abnormal TT and a normal RT, the alteration is due to heparin in the tested sample.

As pointed out earlier, correct evaluation of the hemorrhagic risk is mandatory in every patient who is a candidate for cervical spine surgery, because it will reduce the risk of hemorrhagic complications that can rapidly become life-threatening emergencies in intra- and postoperative periods.

2.4 Preoperative Evaluation of the Thromboembolic Risk

The vertebral and basilar arteries provide up to 20% of the total cerebral blood flow, and are the principal affluent to the arterial circulation system of cerebellum and brainstem. Any alteration that involves the vertebrobasilar circulation can cause irreversible ischemic damages to vital structures. Therefore, a correct evaluation, before surgery, of the TE risk in these patients may result in a sharp decrease in the ischemic risk [3].

The term *Thrombophilia* is now used to describe a predisposition to an increased risk of thromboembolism.

Thromboembolism is a multifactorial disorder produced by congenital abnormalities of anticoagulant or procoagulant factors combined with acquired pathological conditions [23]. The patients-related risk factors for venous thromboembolism (VTE) are summarized in Table 2.3.

A correct approach to the evaluation of TE risk should start with a full history dealing with previous TE episodes suffered by the patients or their relatives. *Only in the presence of a positive personal or familiar history for thromboembolism, we should perform laboratory tests to identify congenital or acquired causes of thrombophilia* [24]. Moreover, in the evaluation of the TE risk, we also have to consider those pathologies frequently associated with an elevated risk of deep vein thrombosis (DVT) or pulmonary embolism (PE) [25], such as cancer, autoimmune disorders, inflammatory bowel disease, hematologic malignancies, older age, previous history of thromboembolism, and recurrent fetal loss (see Table 2.3).

Table 2.3 Patient-related risk factors for VTE

Inherited
Factor V Leiden
Prothrombin 20210 mutation
Protein C deficiency
Protein S deficiency
Antithrombin III deficiency
Acquired
Active heart or respiratory failure
Acute medical illness
Age over 60 years
Antiphospholipid antibodies
Autoimmune disorders
Cancer and Chemotherapy
Central venous catheter in situ
Continuous travelformore than 3 h approximately 4 weeks before or after surgery
Hyperhomocystenemia
Immobility (Paralysis or limb in plaster)
Inflammatory bowel disease
Monoclonal gammopathy
Myeloproliferative diseases
Nephrotic syndrome
Obesity (body mass index≥30 kg/m^2)
Paroxismal nocturnal hemoglobinuria
Personal or family history of venous thromboembolism
Pregnancy and puerperium
Recent myocardial infarction or stroke
Severe infection
Tobacco usage
Trauma: Hip Fracture, Acute spinal injury
Use of oral contraceptive or hormonal replacement therapy
Varicose veins associated with phlebitis

Table 2.4 Risk of thromboembolism in cervical spine surgery according to patient-, disease-, and surgery-related variables

Risk	Hereditary factors	Acquired factors
Low	Heterozygous factor V_{Leiden} Heterozygous prothrombin 20210	Oral contraceptives Pregnancy Elevated Factor VIII
Moderate	Heterozygous ATIII, Protein C or Protein S deficiency	Surgery for malignancy Sepsis Prolonged immobilization Antiphospholipid antibodies Myeloproliferative disorders PNH[a]
High	Homozygous factor V_{Leiden} Homozygous prothrombin 20210	Associated total hip and knee replacement Hip fracture Anterior or anterior-posterior combined surgical approach
Very high	Homozygous or double heterozygous ATIII, protein C or protein S deficiency	Mucin-secreting adenocarcinoma

[a]Paroxismal nocturnal hemoglobinuria

In presence of one or more of the abovementioned risk factors, a correct program of thromboprophylaxis should be applied (see paragraph X5 below), even though the thrombotic risk is dependent on the type and duration of the surgery. Moreover, the need for a thrombophilic screening should always be suggested by an expert in thromboembolism. Depending on the laboratory results obtained and on the associated pathologic conditions, it is possible to identify which is the risk for the development of thromboembolism in patients (Table 2.4) who are candidates for cervical spine surgery.

2.5 Thromboprophylaxis in Cervical Spine Surgery

During the last 15–20 years, spine surgery has changed radically, developing into a well-defined area of specialist surgery. As a consequence, some attention is now being given to DVT and PE events in spinal surgery. The incidence of DVT during spine surgery is not well documented, because only case reports or retrospective studies are reported. Patients at greatest risk for VTE are those undergoing major lower extremity orthopedic surgery, and those who have experienced major trauma or spinal cord injury (SCI). However, while thromboprophylaxis guidelines are well known for general orthopedic surgery, especially in elective hip, knee, and trauma procedures, the optimal prophylaxis against the risk of DVT and PE for patients undergoing cranial or spinal procedures remains controversial [26]. Given the paucity of data, it is not possible to give firm recommendations about thromboprophylaxis in spine surgery patients. Moreover, some patients may not require any specific thromboprophylaxis. The risk of VTE appears to be low when any of the following methods of thromboprophylaxis is used: postoperative LDUH (Low Dose Unfractionated Heparin) or LMWH, or intraoperative and then postoperative GCS (Graduated Compression Stockings), and/or IPC (Intermittent Pneumatic Compression). For spine surgery patients with additional VTE risk factors, such as a neurologic deficit or prolonged immobility, advanced age, malignancy, previous VTE, or an anterior surgical approach, thromboprophylaxis with one of the above-mentioned options is recommended. Spine surgery includes many surgical procedures for a variety of pathologies, and involves a highly heterogeneous class of patients. Therefore, a careful analysis in terms of TE risks is required in each individual case (Tables 2.3 and 2.4). Three main variables need consideration:

1. *Patient-related variables*, such as age, gender (oral contraceptive use or hormonal substitutive therapy), bed rest, obesity and concomitant pathologies (hypertension, diabetes, varicose veins), genetic thrombophilic factors (see Table 2.3)
2. *Disease-related variables*, such as trauma, tumor, deformity, degenerative pathology, and finally
3. *Surgery-related variables*, such as anterior, posterior, or combined approach (the higher risk of PE after combined anterior–posterior spinal fusions indicates that retraction and manipulation of the great vessels may lead to stasis or intimal damage that can predispose to clot formation), positioning, instrumentation, operating time, and location (cervical, thoracic, lumbar spine) [27].

As there is no unique risk factor, and spinal surgery is so varied, it is therefore not possible to suggest a standardized thromboprophylaxis for spinal surgery, as can be done for hip and knee surgery. In Tables 2.5 and 2.6, we report the regimens to prevent VTE in elective spine surgery and acute SCI, respectively, suggested by The Eighth ACCP Conference on Antithrombotic and Thrombolytic Therapy, held in 2008 [28].

Table 2.5 Thromboprophylaxis in elective spine surgery (Summarized from ref [28])

No risk factors for VTE(see Tables 2.3 and 2.4) Early and persistent mobilization, not routinely use of specific thromboprophylaxis Presence of some risk factors[a](see Tables 2.3 and 2.4) One of the following thromboprophylaxis is recommended *Additional risk factors for VTE*(see Tables 2.3 and 2.4) Intra and postoperative mechanical prophylaxis with intermittent pneumatic compression (IPC) ± graduated compression stockings (GCS) or Postoperative LDUH or LMWH *Multiple risk factors for VTE*(see Tables 2.3 and 2.4) Intra and postoperative mechanical prophylaxis with IPC ± GCS associatedwithpostoperative LMWH or LDUH
Patients with ruptured cranial or spinal vascular malformations (e.g., brain aneurysms) should not be offered pharmacological prophylaxis until the lesion has been secured.

[a]Advanced age, malignancy, presence of a neurologic deficit, previous VTE, or an anterior surgical approach

Table 2.6 Thromboprophylaxis in patients with acute spinal cord injury (SCI) (Summarized from ref [28])

In all patients with acute SCI, routine thromboprophylaxis is recommended
Once primary hemostasis is evident,start thromboprophylaxis with LMWH, alternatives include the combined use of IPC and either LDUH or LWMH
In case anticoagulant thromboprophylaxis is contraindicated because of high bleeding risk early after injury,optimal use of IPC and/or GCS is recommended.When the high bleeding risk decreases, add pharmacologic thromboprophylaxis to the mechanical thromboprophylaxis
In patients with an incomplete SCI associated with the evidence of a spinal hematoma on CT or MRI, use mechanical thromboprophylaxis instead of anticoagulant thromboprophylaxis, at least for the first few days after injury
Following acute SCI, do not use LDUH alone
Do not use an IVC (intravenous caval) filter for thromboprophylaxis
Following acute SCI, for patients undergoing rehabilitation, continue LMWH thromboprophylaxis or use an oral vitamin K antagonist (INR target, 2.5; range, 2.0–3.0)

Core Messages

- Before performing a cervical spine surgery procedure, changes in blood cell count parameters as well as changes in the serum protein electrophoresis profile should be critically evaluated by an expert hematologist.
- Any risk factors for bleeding or thromboembolism should also be carefully evaluated to reduce hemorrhagic or thromboemblic complications that may complicate this type of surgery and become rapidly life-threatening emergencies during intra- and postoperative periods.
- It is very important to verify the presence of: Disorders associated with the presence of a monoclonal gammopathy (Table *2.1*), Acquired platelets disorders (Table *2.2*), Patient-related risk factors for VTE (Table 2.3), and the Risk of Thromboembolism according to patient-, disease-, and surgery-related variables (Table 2.4) to better define the type of thromboprophylaxis in elective spine surgery (Table 2.5) or in patients with acute SCI (Table 2.6).
- The management of anemia should be tailored to the cause (Fig. 2.1) and severity of anemia.

References

1. Marks PW, Glader B (2005) Approach to anemia in the adult and child. In: Hoffman R, Benz AI jr, Shattil SJ, Furie B, Cohen HJ, Silberstein LE, McGlave P (eds) Hematology, basic principles and practice, 4th edn. Elsevier, Churchill Livingstone, Amsterdam, New York
2. Weiss G, Goodnough LT (2005) Anemia of chronic disease. N Engl J Med 352:1011–1023
3. Bergqvist D (2007) Risk of venous thromboembolism in patients undergoing cancer surgery and options for thromboprophylaxis. J Surg Oncol 95:167–174
4. Ruggeri M, Rodeghiero F, Tosetto A et al; Gruppo Italiano Malattie Ematologiche dell'Adulto (GIMEMA) Chronic Myeloproliferative Diseases Working Party (2008) Postsurgery outcomes in patients with polycythemia vera and essential thrombocythemia: a retrospective survey. Blood 111:666–671
5. Palmblad JE, Von dem Borne AE (2002) Idiopathic, immune, infectious and idiosyncratic neutropenias. Semin Hematol 39:113–120
6. Kipps TJ (1995) Lymphocytosis and Lymphocytopenia. In. Beutler E, Lichtman MA, Coller BS, Kipps DJ (eds) Williams hematology. Mc Graw Hill, New York
7. Buckley MF, James JW, Brown DE et al (2000) A novel approach to the assessment of variations in the human platelet count. Thromb Haemost 83:480–484
8. Schafer AI (2004) Thrombocytosis. N Engl J Med 350: 1211–1219
9. Messinezy M, Westwood N, Sawyer B et al (1994) Primary thrombocythaemia: a composite approach to diagnosis. Clin Lab Haematol 16:139–148
10. Vannucchi AM, Barbui T (2007) Thrombocytosis and thrombosis. Hematology Am Soc Hematol Educ Program 363–370
11. George JN, Woolf SH, Raskob GE et al (1996) Idiopathic thrombocytopenic purpura: a practice guideline developed by explicit methods for the American Society of Hematology. Blood 88:3–40
12. http://www.siset.org/lineeguida/LG4.pdf (Last revision 4 June 2007)
13. International Myeloma Working Group (2003) The International Myeloma Working Group criteria for the classification of monoclonal gammopathies, multiple myeloma and related disorders: a report of the International Myeloma Working Group. Br J Haematol 121:749–757
14. Lord RS (1973) Vertebrobasilar ischaemia and the extracranial arteries. Med J Aust 7:32–37
15. Hayward CPM, Rao AK, Cattaneo M (2006) Congenital platelet disorders: overview of their mechanisms, diagnostic evaluation and treatment. Haemophilia 12:128–136
16. Shen Y-M, Frenkel E (2007) Acquired platelet dysfunction. Hematol Oncol Clin N Am 21:647–661
17. Patrono C (1994) Aspirin as an antiplatelet drug. N Engl J Med 330:1287–1293
18. Hirsh J, Dalen JE, Fuster V et al (1995) Aspirin and other platelet-active drugs. The relationship among dose, effectiveness, and side effects. Chest 108:247–257
19. Antman EM, Benett JS, Daugherty A et al (2007) Use of nonsteroidal antiinflammatory drugs: an update for clinicians: a scientific statement from the American Heart Association. Circulation 115:1634–1642
20. Jacobson AK (2004) Platelet ADP receptor antagonists: ticlopidine and clopidogrel. Best Pract Res Clin Haematol 17:55–64
21. Reding MT (2005) Hematologic problems in the surgical patient: bleeding and thrombosis. In: Hoffman R, Benz AI jr, Shattil SJ, Furie B, Cohen HJ, Silberstein LE, McGlave P (eds) Hematology, basic principles and practice, 4th edn. Elsevier, Churchill Livingstone, Amsterdam, New York
22. Kitchen S, Makris M (2005) Laboratory tests of hemostasis. In: O'Shaughnessy D, Makris M, Lillicrap D (eds) Practical hemostasis and thrombosis. Blackwell, USA
23. Ageno W, Squizzato A, Garcia D et al (2006) Epidemiology and risk factors of venous thromboembolism. Semin Thromb Hemost 32:651–658
24. Mazzolai L, Duchosal MA (2007) Hereditary thrombophilia and venous thromboembolism: critical evaluation of the clinical implications of screening. Eur J Vasc Endovasc Surg 34:483–488
25. Simioni P, Tormene D, Spiezia L (2006) Inherited thrombophilia and venous thromboembolism. Semin Thromb Hemost 32:700–708
26. Epstein NE (2005) A review of the risk and benefits of differing prophylaxis regimens for the treatment of deep venous

thrombosis and pulmonary embolism in neurosurgery. Surg Neurol 64:295–302

27. Brambilla S, Ruosi C, La Maida GA et al (2004) Prevention of venous thromboembolism in spinal surgery. Eur Spine J Feb; 13(1):1–8
28. Geerts WH, Bergqvist D, Pineo GF, Heit JA et al (2008) Prevention of venous thromboembolism: American college of chest physicians evidence-based clinical practice guidelines (8th edn). Chest 133:381S–453S

Complications in Surgical Management of Cervical Spinal Metastases

3

Giuseppe Tonini, Bruno Vincenzi, Chiara Spoto, and Daniele Santini

Contents

G. Tonini (✉)
Department of Medical Oncology, University Campus Bio-Medico, Via Alvaro del Portillo 200, 00128 Rome, Italy
e-mail: b.vincenzi@unicampus.it

3.1 Spinal Metastases: Introduction

3.1.1 Epidemiology

Bone is the third most frequent metastatic site. The vertebral column is the most common site for bone metastases, with an incidence of 30–70% in patients with stage IV cancer [1]. Among patients with cancer, in 12–20%, the initial clinical presentation is spinal column metastases [2]. Furthermore, metastases are the most frequent spinal column cancer in the United States, with approximately 18,000 new cases diagnosed annually. Multiple lesions at noncontiguous levels occur in 10–40% of the cases. Breast, lung, and prostate cancers have been the most common malignancies with secondary spine involvement [3]. These are followed by renal cancer, gastrointestinal cancer, thyroid cancer, sarcoma, and the lympophoreticular malignances: lymphoma and multiple myeloma. Metastases from prostate cancer, breast cancer, melanoma, and lung cancer commonly cause spinal metastases in 90.5, 74.3, 54.5, and 44.9% of patients, respectively.

3.1.2 Anatomical Localization and Pathophysiology

Spinal metastases can occur at three main sites: extradural, intradural extramedullary (IDEM), and intramedullary (IM). More than 98% of spinal metastases are extradural, because the dura mater provides a relative barrier for metastatic disease; IDEM and IM disease account for less than 1% of spinal metastatic disease. Both IDEM and IM disease most commonly originate from drop metastases in patients with either

L. Denaro et al. (eds.), *Pitfalls in Cervical Spine Surgery*,
DOI: 10.1007/978-3-540-85019-9_3, © Springer-Verlag Berlin Heidelberg 2010

primary or metastatic brain disease. Extradural metastases occur through three mechanisms [4]:

- Direct local extension into the extradural space
- Retrograde spread through the valveless extradural venous channels of the spine (Batson plexus)
- Arterial emboli with subsequent spread through cortical veins

Eighty percent of spinal metastases involve vertebral bodies rather than the posterior vertebral elements. Metastases occur most frequently in the lumbar spine followed by the thoracic and then the cervical spine. However, thoracic lesions (70%) are most often *symptomatic* because of the smaller space available for the spinal cord in this region, followed by lumbar (20%) and cervical (10%) lesions. The cervical spine is the least frequent site of spread of spinal metastatic involvement (20% of all metastatic spinal tumors). Cervical spine involvement by metastatic cancer differs in presentation and management from the other spinal locations, and depends on whether the atlantoaxial or subaxial regions are involved. The most likely primary tumors to metastasize to the cervical spine are from the breast, prostate, and lung. Multiple myeloma, although by definition is not a metastatic tumor, also may present with cervical spine involvement.

3.1.3 Presentation

The presentation of bony metastases includes bony pain, pathologic fracture, radiculopathy, myelopathy, and progressive deformity. Spinal cord compression can occur from fracture, tumor invasion, or progressive osteoblastic remodeling. Approximately 85% of metastases causing spinal instability and neurologic compromise arise anteriorly from the vertebral body [5]. Symptomatic spinal cord compression occurs in 8.5–20% of patients with vertebral column metastases [6]. Of patients with spinal cord compression, 90% present with pain and 47% with neurologic symptoms. Sensory loss occurs in 70–80%, paraparesis or paraplegia in more than 60%, and bowel and/or bladder difficulty in 14–77%. Only 11–34% of patients presenting with spinal cord compression are ambulatory at diagnosis. In addition, radiculopathy secondary to posterior element involvement and subsequent nerve root impingement can also occur. Simple neurologic grading scales allow clinicians to assess clinical outcome [7, 8] (Table 3.1).

Table 3.1 Ambulatory neurologic grading scales

Score	Grade	Description
Frankel Score	A	No motor or sensory function
	B	Preserved sensation only, no motor function
	C	Nonambulatory, wheelchair bound, some motor function
	D	Ambulatory,but with neurological symptoms
	E	Normal neurological functions
Tomita Scale	I	Able to walk without support
	II	Able to walk with support
	III	Unable to walk
	IV	Paraplegia
Cooper Scale	0	Intact
	1	Walks independently but not normally
	2	Walks with cane or walker
	3	Stands,but is not ambulatory
	4	Slight movement,but cannot walk or stand
	5	No movement
Brice and McKissock Scale	I	Mild weakness, but able to walk
	II	Moderate weakness, able to move legs, but not against gravity
	III	Severe weakness, slight residual motor and sensory function
	IV	No motor, sensory, or sphincter function below the level of the lesion

The syndrome of cervical spine metastatic disease [9] may present with a wide spread of clinical signs and symptoms. Not uncommonly, asymptomatic pathologic lesions are detected on screening for an unrelated problem. Rao et al. [10] identified 11% of patients presenting with cervical lesions, who were asymptomatic and were identified only through routine screening studies. Symptoms may range from local nonmechanical and referred pain to mechanical pain from pathologic fracture or instability to neurologic manifestations of nerve root and spinal cord compression. The average age range of patients with a diagnosis of cervical spine metastases is from 58 to 61 years with no sex predominance [11]. Pain is the predominant symptom in most patients with metastatic disease of the cervical spine with localized, unremitting discomfort reported in 89–93%. The nonmechanical pain attributable to tumor infiltration is often described as a progressively worsening symptom not related to the activities and present at night when sleep interruption is common. Pain may be uni- or bilateral, with referred pain to the trapezial and shoulder area. Local mechanical pain present with discomfort exacerbated by motion and relieved with rest or relative immobilization, indicating pathologic instability. A sudden onset of pain with minimal trauma or applied force to the neck may indicate a pathologic fracture. Deformity associated with acute pathologic fracture is rare. Deformity in the lower cervical spine is usually a slowly developing angulation from anterior and middle vertebral body collapse. Destruction of the C2 spinous process with detachment of the insertion of the paraspinal musculature may lead to a progressive feeling of head heaviness and inability to hold the head upright without assistance. Neurologic dysfunction is estimated to occur in 5–10% of patients with metastatic spine disease and may present with variable intensity and rapidity of onset. Although uncommon, cervical radiculopathy may result from tumor metastasis into the epidural space in the foramen, or develop secondary to retropulsion of weakened bony fragments from invasion of tumor tissue. Patients describe a burning, dysesthetic-type pain radiating in a specific dermatomal pattern suggestive of nerve root involvement. Weakness, sensory and reflex deficits may also accompany the primary symptom of pain.

Spinal cord compression with symptoms and signs of *myelopathy* may also develop and become a presenting feature of cervical metastatic disease. Spinal cord compression is more common in the subaxial cervical area as opposed to the atlantoaxial region secondary to differential space available for the dural sac at these levels. Motor deficits are often the presenting features, most likely from the anterior epidural space being invaded by tumor from the vertebral body. Long tract signs including lower extremity spasticity, difficulty with ambulation, myelopathic hand syndrome [12], and intrinsic hand muscle atrophy may be seen. Sphincter disturbance is usually a late finding of spinal cord compression and indicates a poor prognosis for eventual recovery of function.

3.1.4 Management: Past and Present

Management for spinal metastases is largely palliative. Only rarely, usually in patients with renal cell carcinoma, can cure be the goal if the spine is the only known site of metastasis [13]. Treatment can involve chemotherapy, radiation therapy, and surgery. Spinal tumors with spinal cord compression historically had been managed with decompressive laminectomy in an attempt to alleviate neural compression before the availability of spinal instrumentation. This procedure, however, cannot provide efficient decompression for vertebral tumor ventral to the spinal cord [14]. In the case of compromised anterior spinal stability by vertebral tumor, laminectomy will produce posterior spinal instability resulting in circumferential instability, aggravating the clinical symptoms. Furthermore, significant wound complications were associated with laminectomies. Subsequently, radiation therapy has become the most common treatment, with surgery reserved for salvage or adjuvant therapy. Radiotherapy often is the primary treatment in the majority of patients. Frequently, the total dose is 30 Gy in ten fractions. After radiotherapy, 20% of patients improve neurologically, 30% stabilize, and 50% deteriorate. Young et al., in 1980, reported that the outcome of 16 patients with spinal metastases who received laminectomy and radiation was no better than 13 patients treated with radiotherapy alone. In the 1980s, another type of surgical procedure was developed for the treatment of MESCC (metastatic epidural spinal cord compression). The tumor was removed and immediate circumferential decompression was achieved usually through an anterior approach. When needed, intraoperative reconstruction of the spine allowed immediate stabilization. Several uncontrolled surgical series [15] reported that direct decompressive surgery, with or without postoperative radiotherapy, was superior to radiation alone. To determine the value of surgery in the management of MESCC, Patchell et al. [16] undertook a randomized trial comparing the efficacy of direct decompressive surgery plus postoperative radiotherapy with that of radiotherapy alone. This prospective trial showed that patients with MESCC undergoing direct decompressive surgery plus postoperative radiotherapy retain the ability to walk for longer, and regain this ability more often than those treated with radiotherapy alone. Surgery allows most patients to remain ambulatory for the remainder of their lives, whereas patients treated with radiation alone spend a substantial proportion of their remaining time paraplegic. Surgical treatment also results in increased survival time. Therefore, patients in the surgery group were less susceptible to infections, blood clots, and other problems that result in the death of paraplegic patients. Surgical treatment also reduces the need for corticosteroids and opioid pain relief (Table 3.2).

Currently, the use of one approach or a combination of approaches allows the surgeon to excise the tumor, reconstruct the spinal column, and place the internal

Table 3.2 Direct decompressive surgery plus radiation therapy vs. radiation therapy alone for metastatic epidural spinal cord compression at median of 93–102 days

Outcomes	Surgery and radiation therapy	Radiation therapy alone
Ability to walk	84%	57%
Maintenance of continence	156	17
Maintenance of muscle strength	566	72
Maintenance of functional ability	566	72
Survival time	126	100

fixation devices to achieve immediate stabilization. This last change in treatment of spinal metastases is probably best illustrated by Byrne's two review articles. In a review article of early 1990s, radiotherapy alone had become the primary definitive treatment for most patients with spinal metastases. In his most recent article, published in 2004, Byrne reviewed the remarkable advances in the past few years in spinal imaging, radiosurgery, minimally invasive procedures, such as vertebroplasty and kyphoplasty, and open spinal surgery with reconstruction through instrumentation. As these advances provide more opportunities to treat patients with vertebral metastases, radiotherapy is no longer considered as the universal first-choice treatment [17, 18].

3.1.5 Surgical Indications and Approaches

Traditionally, the *indications* for open surgery include [19]:

- Spinal instability or collapse by bone destruction
- Progressive neurologic deficit secondary to neural compression
- Fracture-dislocation of the spine
- Radioresistant tumor that is enlarging (e.g., melanoma, sarcoma)
- Good performance status before spinal cord compression
- The need for an open biopsy
- Intractable pain unresponsive to nonsurgical treatment measures, such as radiation therapy, chemotherapy, or hormonal therapy
- Direct tumor extension from primary lesion, such as Pancoast tumor, invading the vertebra

Even if a patient satisfies one or more of the above-mentioned indications, the type and goals of surgery must be determined by the patient's ability to tolerate the procedure, and more importantly, by their estimated life expectancy. Emergency surgery is mandated in rapidly progressive or advanced paraplegia or tetraplegia. Severe and irreversible spinal cord injury will result without prompt decompression of the thecal sac and nerve roots. Surgical decompression is not likely to reverse a complete paralysis with a duration greater than 24 h. MRI is the optimal imaging modality.

Many *surgical strategies* are used to treat spinal metastatic disease. Currently, technical advances allow resection of tumors at all levels of the spinal column. Options differ regarding timing, surgical approach, and reconstruction. The approach depends on the location of the tumor and the surgical goal.

In general, the *goals* of surgery are as follows:

(1) To correct and prevent any further deformity by stabilizing the spine
(2) Decompressing the neural structures (spinal cord and nerves)
(3) Obtaining a diagnosis if the primary is unknown
(4) Preventing local recurrence

The *locations* of tumors usually dictate the surgical approach. The ideal indication for using the anterior approach is when the lesion involves one or two adjacent vertebral bodies. If metastatic lesions involve the circumferential structure as well as the combination of anterior and posterior approaches, one stage or separated stages can be used to achieve radical excision of the tumor. However, these procedures should be performed with the patient's general condition in mind. For patients with more than two adjacent vertebral lesions with intractable pain and failure of analgesics, limited posterior approach for pain relief and ease of nursing may be considered. Issues regarding surgical indications and management differ for upper and lower cervical lesions and certainly by tumor type, number of sites involved, location within the vertebra, and the presence or absence of other spinal, or extraspinal sites of involvement.

3.2 Surgery-Related Prognosis in Bone Metastatic Patients

Survivorship after surgical management of symptomatic spinal metastases has been well documented. Harrington reported survivorship of 84% at 6 months, 77% at 1 year,

51% at 2 years, and 45% at 3 years [20]. Bauer reported survivorship of 67% at 3 months and only 23% at 1 year [21]. Survival was closely related to the tumor burden. No patient who had a visceral or brain metastasis was alive at 12 months, compared with 32% of those who had skeletal metastases only. The mean postoperative survival of patients with symptomatic spinal metastases ranges from 10 to 16.5 months [22–26]. Recently, Patil et al. [27] published a retrospective study reporting inpatient mortality, complications, and outcomes after surgery for spinal metastasis from 1993 to 2002 on a national level. They demonstrated:

- The significant negative effect of postoperative complications on mortality and resource utilization (a single postoperative complication increased the mean length of stay (LOS) by 7 days and the mortality rate by 11%).
- The negative prognostic value of preoperative comorbidity on patient's outcomes (one comorbidity increased the risk of in-hospital death by almost fourfold),
- Complications are more likely in older patients and in patients with two or more comorbidities.

In conclusion, the survivorship after surgery management of spinal metastases is rising, thanks to technological advances, but also because of a more adequate presurgical quantification of risks and patient selection.

3.2.1 Surgery-Related Complications

The surgical management of a patient with metastatic spine disease necessitates an understanding of the medical risks and comorbidities associated with this disease process; this is especially important because surgical intervention is palliative, and complications must be minimized for surgical benefit to outweigh the risks. Surgical intervention for metastatic spinal disease represents a complex undertaking in a population with an increased risk of complications: elderly, debilitated patients with impaired immune function, poor nutritional status, and low bone marrow reserve are at a much higher risk of mortality and morbidity, regardless of the surgical approach.

Complications can be classified as:

(1) Surgical (e.g., bleeding, wound infections, cerebrospinal fluid (CSF) fistulas)
(2) Hardware-related (broken, misplaced, migrated)
(3) Medical (e.g., pneumonia)
(4) Neurologic (i.e., new deficit)

3.2.1.1 Surgical Complications

Perhaps, the most feared complication of spine tumor surgery is uncontrolled *bleeding*, which can result from tumor hypervascularity, dilated epidural venous plexus, soft-tissues' paraspinal blood vessels, and even uninvolved bone. Massive hemorrhage is a relatively rare event, but surgical planning often can obviate significant bleeding that may result in poor neurologic outcomes, incomplete spinal cord decompression, inability to provide adequate spinal fixation, or death. The most important preoperative considerations are the vascularity of the tumor and abnormal coagulation parameters.

- *Vascularity of the tumor*

It is important to consider preoperative embolization for hypervascular tumors. Many tumor histologies have been identified that typically have large segmental feeding vessels resulting in hypervascularity. These tumors, including renal cell carcinoma and follicular thyroid carcinoma, may benefit from preoperative embolization (Table 3.3).

Embolization for hypervascular tumors makes surgery safer and potentially provides for better epidural and paraspinal tumor decompression. Guzman et al.

Table 3.3 Classification of tumors according to grade of vascularization

Hypervascular tumors	Hypervascular tumors (no benefit from preoperative embolization)	Non vascular tumors
Renal cell carcinoma Follicular thyroid carcinoma Neuroendocrine tumor Paraganglioma Hepatocellular carcinoma Leiomyosarcoma Angiosarcoma	Multiple myeloma Melanoma	Colon carcinoma Non small cell lung carcinoma Breast carcinoma Sarcomas (e.g., osteogenic)

[28] reported perioperative and postoperative outcomes after embolization for hypervascular tumors; completely embolized tumors had an average blood loss of 1,900 mL, whereas unembolized tumors had an average blood loss of 5,500 mL. Despite complete embolization, resection of hypervascular tumors still may result in significant bleeding, not from the tumor, but from dilated epidural veins. On angiogram, hypervascular tumors often have a significant degree of arteriovenous shunting, which may account for this increased venous bleeding [29].

- *Abnormal coagulation parameters*

Preoperative assessment of coagulation indices is important to prevent intraoperative bleeding. Numerous factors cause thrombocytopenia, platelet dysfunction, or an elevated international normalized ratio (INR). It is important to ascertain the etiology of abnormal coagulation indices to determine whether they are potentially correctable. Commonly, thrombocytopenia results from chemotherapy or radiation-induced bone marrow suppression. Common medications, such as Sulfametoxazole+Trimetoprim, used as prophylaxis to prevent pneumocystic pneumonia in patients being treated with steroids, also can result in thrombocytopenia. Heparin may cause heparin-induced thrombocytopenia, an immune reaction against heparin–platelet complex IV factors. An elevated INR in cancer patients most commonly results from malnutrition and vitamin K deficiency. Patients may take warfarin (Coumadin) to treat a deep venous thrombosis or pulmonary embolism.

Patients undergoing resection of metastatic spine tumors are at increased risk for *infection and wound dehiscence*. Factor associated with wound infection include postoperative incontinence, posterior approach, surgery for tumor resection, and morbid obesity [30]. Risk factors include spinal implants, high-dose corticosteroids, malnutrition, neutropenia, and recent external-beam radiation [31]. Preoperatively, little can be done to ameliorate these risks. High-dose steroids should be administered for neurologic protection in patients with high-grade spinal cord compression without consideration for postoperative infections. However, some preoperative interventions may be helpful. Neutropenia, particularly an absolute neutrophil count of less than 1, seems to carry a higher risk of infection. Recovery of the absolute neutrophil count often can be achieved using filgrastim (Neupogen), a human granulocyte colony-stimulating factor. The second potentially correctable risk factor for wound complications is the timing of radiation. Preoperative conventional external-beam radiation therapy given within 6 weeks of surgery seems to increase the risk of wound dehiscence or infection. This increased risk may be related to the ongoing effects of radiation over this period. With the evolution of conformal photon radiation therapy, such as Intensity Modulated Radiation Therapy (IMRT), the acute radiation effects to the soft tissue may be significantly lessened, allowing one to operate safely in the early postradiation period. After surgery, external-beam radiation therapy or IMRT can be given 2 weeks after surgery without significant risk to the wound. Resection and reconstruction of epidural tumors can result in *dural tears*. Most of these are diagnosed intraoperatively and primarily repaired with sutures. Large tears that cannot be sutured are repaired with dural patch grafts using DuraGuard (Promedics), which is the treated bovine pericardium and sews watertight. *Pneumocephalus* from spinal CSF leak is a rare complication typically associated with an apical pneumothorax, most commonly seen in resection of superior sulcus tumors. As CSF extravasates into the chest, pleural air is drawn into the intracranial space. Often patients have headache or cognitive changes several days to weeks after surgery. If the pneumothorax has resolved, discontinuing chest tube suction may resolve the pneumocephalus by decreasing the CSF leak. If there is an unresolved pneumothorax, the CSF leak needs to be closed primarily in the spine [32].

3.2.1.2 Hardware-Related Complications

Spinal stabilization is used in most spine tumor cases, especially given that facetectomies and pedicle osteotomies are often used to expose epidural tumors. Structural grafts and instrumentation are indicated in patients with spinal instability, resulting from pathologic fractures or from the necessary bone resection for effective tumor removal. Bone quality for tumor patients is often compromised from prior radiation and osteoporosis. Little can be done to improve bone quality before operations.

For anterior reconstruction in the cervical spine, the authors most commonly have used fibula allografts, polyetheretherketone carbon fiber, or titanium cages, because they give excellent structural support and enable deformity reduction.

3.2.1.3 Medical Complications

Medical comorbidities that have an impact on surgery are assessed preoperatively to optimize the outcomes. Many patients have pulmonary compromise from preexisting chronic obstructive pulmonary disease, prior chest surgery, and chemotherapy. Pulmonary function tests are performed to determine the suitability for surgery. Patients with metastatic disease are often at high risk for developing *deep venous thrombosis or pulmonary embolism* as a result of immobilization from paresis or deconditioning and hypercoagulability related to the primary cancer. In the perioperative period, deep venous thrombosis prophylaxis consists of pneumatic compression boots and subcutaneous heparin (5,000 mg twice daily) or low-molecular-weight heparin (enoxaparin 40 mg twice per day), which can be administered once daily. A high index of suspicion needs to be maintained in patients admitted with swollen, painful lower extremities or with significant risk factors. These patients routinely undergo preoperative lower extremity Doppler ultrasound. Patients who have a newly diagnosed deep venous thrombosis or who are being treated with anticoagulants or a known deep venous thrombosis should receive a percutaneous vena cava filter. Although patients have a filter, they still require complete anticoagulation postoperatively. Patients with metastatic tumor to the spine have a high probability of local tumor recurrence. Klekamp and Samii [33] reported a series of 106 patients with spinal metastases who underwent surgery and adjuvant radiation or chemotherapy. Recurrence rates were 60% at 6 months, 69% at 1 year, and 96% at 4 years. High-dose conformal radiation therapy may improve local tumor control, but aggressive tumors, such as hormone-refractory prostate, lung, and colon carcinoma, may recur in the early postoperative period. Recurrent pain after resection and instrumentation indicates tumor recurrence, fixation failure, or both. When patients present with a change in pain or new neurologic symptoms, plain spinal radiographs and MRI are obtained.

3.2.1.4 Complications Rates of Spinal Surgery and Minimally Invasive Spinal Surgery

A number of studies have assessed the outcomes of surgery with respect to pain relief, neurological recovery, survival, and complications (Table 3.4). For example, in the series of 80 patients reported by Sundaresan et al. [34], 16 patients suffered from surgical complications such as wound breakdowns and hematomas, four had hardware complications, two had medical complications, one had a neurologic complication, and one died owing to respiratory failure. Gokaslan et al. [35] performed transthoracic vertebrectomies in 72 patients. Complications, ranging from minor atelectasis to pulmonary embolism, occurred in 21 patients, with a 30-day mortality rate of 3%. Patil et al. reported an in-hospital mortality rate of 5.6% and a complication rate of 21.9%. The most common complications were pulmonary (6.7%) and postoperative hemorrhages or hematomas (5.9%). In an attempt to reduce surgical morbidity and decrease recovery time, a minimally invasive spinal surgery (MISS) is rapidly flourishing. Minimally invasive spinal procedures are endoscopic techniques, percutaneous vertebroplasty, and kyphoplasty. Ultraminimal/noninvasive spinal radiosurgery is another prospective. One area that has received much attention recently is the use of endoscopes in the resection of metastatic tumors in the thoracic spine: the three phases of the surgery – vertebrectomy, reconstruction, and stabilization – can be performed entirely by endoscopic techniques [36]. Vertebroplasty, the injection of methylmethacrylate into the compression fracture, and kyphoplasty, the injection of methylmethacrylate into a balloon inflated in the vertebral body, are increasingly performed in patients with epidural metastatic lesions with good pain relief. Most of these procedures are performed under biplane fluoroscopy. However, they can be used as intraoperative adjuvants to bolster fusions or to treat painful levels without epidural compression. Kyphoplasty in selected patients can lead to restoration of vertebral body height. More than 80% of patients experience significant pain relief, leading to greater mobilization [37]. Percutaneous vertebroplasty (PV), first described in 1987 [29], is a minimally invasive approach and an alternative to open surgery for restoring stability to the spine. For osteoporotic fractures, complete relief of symptoms and restoration of mobility within 24 h of the procedure have been reported for 90% of patients [38]. In the treatment of osteolytic bone metastases, the results have been similarly encouraging [39]. PV may be applicable to patients with pain due to instability who may not be suitable for invasive spinal surgery due to medical comorbidities, multilevel disease, or having a profound neurological deficit. Complication rates of PV have been reported to be 1.3% in osteoporosis and 10% in metastatic disease [40]. These include cement entering the nerve root

Table 3.4 Literature review of results of circumferential spinal cord decompression in patients with metastasis

Authors year	No of patients	Pain (% improved)	Mortality (%)	Morbidity (%)	Other complications	
Harrigton (1984)	52	NA	11.5	17.3	Hardware	5
					Surgical	2
					Neurological	1
					Medical	2
Fidler (1986)	18	NA	5.6	NA		
Harrington [28]	77	NA	6.5	18	Hardware	5
					Surgical	5
					Neurological	1
					Medical	3
Kostuik (1988)	100	81	0	21	Hardware	10
					Surgical	3
					Neurological	4
					Medical	4
Moore (1989)	26	71	31	7.7	Surgical	2
Sundaresan (1991)	54	90	5.5	15	Hardware	1
					Surgical	2
					Neurological	1
					Medical	4
Hammerberg (1992)	56	91	3.6	16.7	Surgical	6
					Hardware	3
Cooper et al. (1993)	33	97	3	42	Surgical	1
					Neurological	2
					Medical	11
Akeyson (1996)	25	80	0	44	Surgical	7
					Hardware	4
Sundaresan (1996)	110	90	5	48	Hardware	11
					Surgical	45
					Neurological	2
					Medical	10
Gokaslan (1998)	72	92	3	43	Surgical	10
					Neurological	6
					Medical	15
Weigel (1999)	76	89	7	24	Hardware	4
					Surgical	6
					Neurological	4
					Medical	4
Wise (1999)	80	NA	2.5	36	Hardware	2
					Surgical	9
					Neurological	2
					Medical	16
Bilsky (2000)	25	100	12	32	Surgical	1
					Neurological	2
					Medical	5
Hatrick (2000)	42	90	0	19	Hardware	2
					Surgical	3
					Neurological	3
Fourney (2001)	100	87	0	65	Hardware	3
					Surgical	21
					Neurological	3
					Medical	19

(*continued*)

Table 3.4 (continued)

Authors year	No of patients	Pain (% improved)	Mortality (%)	Morbidity (%)	Other complications	
Sundaresan (2002)	80	95	1.3	29	Hardware	4
					Surgical	16
					Neurological	1
					Medical	2
Finkelstein (2003)	987	NA	9(1month)	NA	Medical/surgical	87
					Wound infection	108
					Hardware	86
					DVP	55
					UTI	212
Patil (2007)	26233	NA	5.6	NA	Surgical	1960
					Neurological	158
					Medical	3731

Modified from Klimo et al. [15]

foramen or spinal canal resulting in radiculopathy or spinal cord compression. Systemic complications include embolic events due to marrow fat, tumor fragments, or cement entering the circulation. Complications are minimized by the use of biplanar flouroscopy, "live" imaging during injection, the addition of increased concentration of barium to facilitate visualization, intraosseous venogram, limiting the volume of fill, gentle and slow injection, and the use of viscous cement.

3.2.2 Presurgical Quantification of Risk and Patient Selection

The risk of developing complications is dependent on both the characteristics of the operation and the preoperative medical status of the patient. For this reason, an accurate preoperative evaluation is very important in decision-making and outcomes obtained. Patient selection is critical for a good surgical outcome. Extensive surgery is rarely justified in patients with limited survival, and several authors have attempted to identify clinical predictors of survival in cases of metastatic disease. The factors to be considered in the selection of patient for surgery may include:

- The extent of tumor
- The type of tumor
- Presence of solitary or multiple lesions
- Spinal stability
- Neurologic status
- Patient's general health status
- Patient's age
- Expected length of survival
- The relative sensitivity of the tumor to radiotherapy and chemotherapy

A few authors specifically focus on patient survival, patient diagnosis, and surgical procedure selection. The significance of the *primary cancer type* on survival is well established. After the detection of spine involvement by bone scan, Tatsui et al. reported a 1-year survival of 0 and 22% for gastric and pulmonary cancers and 78 and 83% for breast and prostate primaries, respectively [41]. By knowing that the average survival time in different tumors is variable, with the longest time noted in breast, prostate, and kidney cancers ranging from 1.5 to 2 years [25, 42], if a patient is predicted to survive for more than 3–6 months, surgery may be indicated. Patients with lung cancer and metastatic lesions survive fewer than 6 months; melanoma metastatic to the spine has the shortest median survival of 4 months: palliation should be the goal of treatment, and symptom treatment should be individualized. Spinal surgery is recommended only in very exceptional cases. In a population-based study, Finkelstein et al. used Cox multivariate regression to model survival as a function of potential predictor variables in a cohort of 987 patients. They also quantified postoperative complication rates and identified the significant risk factors associated with poor survival and outcome [43]. Primary cancers of the lung, melanoma, and upper gastrointestinal tract had the poorest survivorship with median survival of 87, 69.5, and 56 days, respectively. The median survival was longest in patients with lymphoma (706 days) and myeloma (591 days). Intermediate survivorship of 223 and 346 days were found for prostate and breast cancer primaries, respectively. There was an overall 1- and 3-month mortality rate of 9 and 29%, respectively. *Increasing age* (1.04 relative risk per year) and primary lung cancer were significant risk factors for death within 30 days of surgery. For overall survival, each year of advancing age had a 1% increased risk of death. Lung primary had a 2.65 relative risk of mortality within 30 days. Weigel et al. [25] corroborated these findings, reporting that patients 60 years of age or younger survived statistically longer than those older than 60 years of age, while tumor location was not statistically significant. The effect of a *preoperative neurological deficit* on survivorship has been evaluated by a number of authors. In a multicenter study by Argenson et al., patients with a preoperative deficit had significantly lower mean survival at 1 and 3 years after surgery [44]. Patients with preoperative neurological deficits are 19% more likely to die when compared with those without deficits. Furthermore, patients with preoperative neurological deficits were 71% more likely to get a postoperative infection, due to the administration of preoperative radiation. Sioutos et al. [24] found that patients who were preoperatively ambulatory, and those in whom the disease involved only one vertebra, survived statistically longer than patients who were nonambulatory and those with multilevel disease. The overall extent of the disease, age, and tumor location (i.e., anterior or posterior elements of the spine) were not predictive. Not surprisingly, patients with metastatic renal carcinoma survived the longest, whereas those with breast carcinoma experienced longer life spans than individuals with lung metastases. In contrast to the findings of Sioutos et al., Weigel et al. did not find preoperative neurological function to be an important factor in survival. Other preoperative parameters have been analyzed. Yamashita et al. [45] reported longer survival in patients with spinal or pelvic lesions when compared with those with appendicular lesions or both. Other authors have similarly found increased infection rates and poorer outcomes following surgery in the presence of *preoperative irradiation* [46].

3.2.2.1 Classifications: Prediction of Life Expectancy and Optimal Treatment Selection

Some authors have proposed classification schemes as a guide for the treatment of patients with metastatic disease. Harrington [19] divided patients with spinal metastases into five categories based on the extent of neurologic compromise and bone destruction.

- Patients in Class I have no significant neurologic involvement
- Patients in Class II have involvement of bone without collapse or instability and minimal neurologic involvement
- Patients in Class III have major neurologic impairment without significant involvement of the bone
- Patients in Class IV have vertebral collapse with pain attributable to mechanical causes or instability, but without significant neurologic compromise
- Patients in Class V have vertebral collapse or instability with major neurologic impairment

Patients in Classes I and II generally obtain pain relief with chemotherapy or hormonal manipulation. If these are unsuccessful, then local radiation is recommended. Patients in Class III usually respond to radiotherapy alone. If neurologic compromise is acute, then the addition of steroid treatment should be considered. Surgical treatment is considered for patients in Class IV and Class V. A specific classification system applied to the management of cervical metastatic tumors has been proposed by Raycroft et al. [47]. Their classification scheme was based on the location and extent of the lesion, and neurologic status of the patient. Three categories were described including localized painful tumor involvement without neurologic compromise confined to the anterior column only, bony and neurologic involvement with spinal cord compression, and diffuse bony involvement including the anterior and posterior columns without significant neurologic compromise. The main purpose of this classification was to determine the type of surgical treatment appropriate for each category after failure of conservative treatment. Tokuhashi et al. developed an index to predict the survivability after surgery for spinal metastases [48]. There were six clinical parameters:

- General condition (Karnofsky index)
- Number of extraspinal bone metastases
- Number of metastases in the vertebral body
- Metastases to the major internal organs
- Primary site of the cancer
- Severity of spinal cord palsy

Each parameter was given a score of 0–2. Although no individual parameter was predictive, the summed scores correlated with the survival periods (Table 3.5).

The authors applied this system to 64 patients and reported that patients with a total score of 9 or higher survived an average of 12 months or more; those with 8 points or less survived 12 months or less; and those with 5 points or less survived 3 months or less. Based

Table 3.5 Prognostic scoring system of Tokuhashi et al. for preoperative evaluation of a patient with metastases to the spine

	Finding	Points
Karnofsky performance scale	Good (80–100)	2
	Moderate (50–70)	1
	Poor (10–40)	0
Number of extraspinal bone metastases	0	2
	1 or 2	1
	≥3	0
Number of metastases to vertebral bodies	1	2
	2	1
	≥3	0
Metastases to major organs	None	2
	Resectable	1
	Unresectable	0
Primary site for the tumor	Lung or stomach	0
	Kidney, liver, uterus, other, or unidentified	1
	Thyroid, prostate, breast, rectum	2
Spinal cord palsy	None	2
	Incomplete (Frankel C or D)	1
	Complete (Frankel A or B)	0

on this information, they recommended that patients with a score of 9 points or greater should have an excisional procedure, whereas a palliative operation is indicated for patients scoring 5 points or less. No recommendations were made for patients with a total score of 6–8 points. The Tokuhashi system would be a valuable tool in preoperative discussion and decision-making, and its value has been confirmed by other authors. Enkaoua et al. [49], found it predictive of survival after surgery in patients with most metastatic tumors of the spine. In 1999, Zimmermann et al. [50] reported that the Tokuhashi score is a useful tool for prognosis estimation in patients with spinal metastases. In 2000, Oberndorfer et al. [51] followed 38 patients with different primary tumors and showed a decrease in the Tokuhashi score 3 months after various therapies from 0.8 to 2.4 points. In 2001, Tomita et al. noted that the scoring system of Tokuhashi et al. would not reflect all the different treatment options of spinal surgery, especially not the more radical surgical procedures for successful local tumor control in spinal metastases. Tomita and other authors supposed a better survival according to a more radical (excisional) treatment in patients with spinal metastases and an intermediate or good prognosis. Therefore, Tomita et al. [52] presented their own prognostic scoring to provide a

Table 3.6 Scoring system of Tomita et al. for metastases to the vertebral spine

Parameter	Findings	Points
Growth rate	Slow growth rate[a]	1
	Moderate (intermediate) growth rate[b]	2
	High (rapid) growth rate[c]	4
Visceral metastases	None	0
	Treatable	2
	Untreatable	3
Pattern of bone metastases	Solitary or isolated	1
	Multiple	2
Total score	*Management*	
2 or 3	Long-term control with wide or marginal tumor excision	
4 or 5	Local control with marginal or intralesional excision	
6 or 7	Palliative surgery for short-term tumor control	
8–10	Supportive care for terminal illness	

[a]A slow growth rate is usually associated with cancer of the breast, prostate, and thyroid

[b]A moderate growth rate is usually associated with cancer of the kidney and endometrium

[c]A rapid growth is usually associated with cancer of the lung, liver, colon, and stomach

treatment strategy for patients with spinal metastases. An appropriate surgical procedure is selected based on a score derived by assessing three prognostic factors. The three factors are as follows:

- Grade of malignancy (slow growth, 1 point; moderate growth, 2 points; rapid growth, 4 points)
- Visceral metastases (no metastasis, 0 points; treatable, 2 points; untreatable, 4 points)
- Bone metastases (solitary or isolated, 1 point; multiple, 2 points)

Summation of these three factors gives a prognostic score between 2 and 10 points. For patients with a score of 2–3 points, the treatment goal is long-term local control and a wide or marginal excision is recommended. For a score of 4–5 points, marginal or intralesional excision is recommended for middle-term local control. For a score of 6–7 points, the treatment goal is short-term palliation and palliative surgery is recommended. Finally, a score of 8–10 points indicates nonoperative supportive care. In their series of 61 patients, successful local control was achieved in 43(83%) of 52 surgically treated patients (Table 3.6).

Bauer and Wedin [53] reported five positive criteria for survival: absence of visceral metastases, absence of pathological fracture, solitary skeletal metastasis, a primary tumor of the breast or kidney and lymphoma or myeloma, but not lung cancer. In 2000 and 2005, Tokuhashi revised his own score System [54, 55] following critical announcements of different authors. He introduced a modified assignment of points for the primary tumors. This parameter now ranges from 0 to 5 points, leading to a possible total sum of 15 points. The treatment suggestion varied from nonoperative/palliative treatment for patients with 8 or less points (predicted survival prognosis less than 6 months) or patients with multiple vertebral metastases, to excisional procedures in patients with 12 or more points (predicted survival 1 year or longer) or patients with a total score of 9–11 points (predicted survival of 6 months or more) and with metastasis in a single vertebra.

Ulmar et al. [56] retrospectively studied 217 consecutive patients surgically treated for vertebral metastases. They calculated the original and modified Tokuhashi score, and evaluated the predictive value for the individual life expectancy. They confirmed that the original and modified Tokuhashi score assure a significant predictive value, but recommended using a modified version of the score according to their own treatment algorithm: they performed an additional ventral instrumentation in patients with a predicted survival of at least 12 months to provide sufficient system stability; in a worse prognosis, they used only a dorsal stabilization combined with a decompression. The scoring system of Tokuhashi et al. and Tomita et al. were based on retrospective analysis, and these studies analyzed only the surgically-treated patients. In 2005, Katagiri et al. [57] published a new scoring system based on the results of a prospective study conducted on patient with skeletal metastases treated surgically or nonsurgically between 1992 and 1999. They identified five significant prognostic factors for survival, namely, the site of the primary lesion, the performance status (Eastern Cooperative Oncology Group status 3 or 4), the presence of visceral or cerebral metastases, any previous chemotherapy, and multiple skeletal metastases. In their discussions, the authors concluded that, with this new practical prognostic scoring system, life expectancy may be predicted more accurately, and thus, the optimal treatment better selected (Table 3.7).

Table 3.7 Scoring system of Katagiri et al. for predicting survival in patients with metastases to the spinal column

Parameter		Finding	Points
Primary lesion			
Rapid growth		Hepatocellular carcinoma, gastric carcinoma, lung carcinoma	3
Slow growth		Breast carcinoma, prostate carcinoma, multiple myeloma, malignant lymphoma, thyroid carcinoma	0
Moderate growth		Other carcinoma and sarcoma	2
Visceral or cerebral metastases			2
Previous chemotherapy			1
Performance status (ECOG) 3 or 4			
Multiple skeletal metastases			1
Score	*Group*	*Probability of 1-year survival (%)*	*Management*
≤2	A	89	Excisional spinal surgery
3–5	B	49	Anterior or posterior instrumentation procedure if radiotherapy is not expected to be effective
6–8	C	11	Supportive care

Core Messages

Complications in surgical management of cervical spinal metastases

- As the dura mater provides a relative barrier for metastatic disease, extramedullary and intramedullary disease account for less than 1% of spinal metastatic disease.
- The presentation of bony metastases includes bony pain, pathologic fracture, radiculopathy, myelopathy, and progressive deformity.
- Spinal cord compression can occur from fracture, tumor invasion, or progressive osteoblastic remodeling.
- Simple neurologic grading scales allow clinicians to assess clinical outcome, including Frankel Score, Tomita Scale, Cooper Scale, Brice and McKissock Scale.
- Deformity associated with acute pathologic fracture is rare. Deformity in the lower cervical spine is usually a slowly developing angulation from anterior and middle vertebral body collapse. Destruction of the C2 spinous process with detachment of the insertion of the paraspinal musculature may lead to a progressive feeling of head heaviness and inability to hold the head upright without assistance.
- Long tract signs including lower extremity spasticity, difficulty with ambulation, myelopathic hand syndrome, and intrinsic hand muscle atrophy may be seen. Sphincter disturbance is usually a late finding of spinal cord compression and indicates a poor prognosis for eventual recovery of function.
- Management for spinal metastases is largely palliative. Only rarely, usually in patients with renal cell carcinoma, can cure be the goal if the spine is the only known site of metastasis. Treatment can involve chemotherapy, radiation therapy, and surgery.
- Traditionally, the indications for surgery include: spinal instability or collapse by bone destruction; progressive neurologic deficit secondary to neural compression; fracture-dislocation of the spine; radioresistant tumor that is enlarging (e.g., melanoma, sarcoma); good performance status before spinal cord compression; the need for an open biopsy; intractable pain unresponsive to nonsurgical treatment measures, such as radiation therapy, chemotherapy, or hormonal therapy; and direct tumor extension from primary lesion, such as Pancoast tumor, invading the vertebra.
- Emergency surgery is mandated in rapidly progressive or advanced paraplegia or tetraplegia. Severe and irreversible spinal cord injury will result without prompt decompression of the thecal sac and nerve roots.
- *Goals* of surgery are to correct and prevent any further deformity by stabilizing the spine; decompressing neural structures (spinal cord and nerves); receiving a diagnosis if the primary is unknown; and preventing local recurrence.
- One of the most feared complications of spine tumor surgery is uncontrolled bleeding, which can result from tumor hypervascularity, dilated epidural venous plexus, soft tissues' paraspinal blood vessels, and even uninvolved bone. Massive hemorrhage is a relatively rare event, but surgical planning often can obviate significant bleeding that may result in poor neurologic outcomes, incomplete spinal cord decompression, inability to provide adequate spinal fixation, or death.
- Embolization for hypervascular tumors makes surgery safer and potentially provides for better epidural and paraspinal tumor decompression. Despite complete embolization, resection of hypervascular tumors may still result in significant bleeding, not from the tumor, but from the dilated epidural veins. On angiogram, hypervascular tumors often have a significant degree of arteriovenous shunting, which may account for this increased venous bleeding.
- Patients undergoing resection of metastatic spine tumors are at increased risk for infection and wound dehiscence. Factors associated with wound infection include postoperative incontinence, posterior approach, surgery for tumor resection, and morbid obesity. Risk factors include spinal implants, high-dose corticosteroids, malnutrition, neutropenia, and recent external-beam radiation.

- Medical comorbidities that have an impact on surgery are assessed preoperatively to optimize outcomes.
- Many patients have pulmonary compromise from pre-existing chronic obstructive pulmonary disease, prior chest surgery, and chemotherapy. Pulmonary function tests are performed to determine the suitability for surgery.
- Patients with metastatic disease are often at high risk for developing a deep venous thrombosis or pulmonary embolism as a result of immobilization from paresis or deconditioning and hypercoagulability related to the primary cancer.

References

1. Wong DA, Fornasier VL, MacNab I (1990) Spinal metastases: the obvious, the occult, and the impostors. Spine 15:1–4
2. Schick U, Marquardt G, Lorenz R (2001) Intradural and extradural spinal metastases. Neurosurg Rev 24:1–5
3. Jacobs WB, Perrin RG (2001) Evaluation and treatment of spinal metastases: an overview. Neurosurg Focus 11:1–11
4. Arguello F, Baggs RB, Duerst RE et al (1990) Pathogenesis of vertebral metastasis and epidural spinal cord compression. Cancer 65:98–106
5. Constans JP, de Devitis E, Conzelli R et al (1983) Spinal metastases with neurological manifestations. Review of 600 cases. J Neurosurg 59:111–118
6. Schaberg J, Gainor BJ (1985) A profile of metastatic carcinoma of the spine. Spine 10:19–20
7. Brice J, McKissock W (1965) Surgical treatment of malignant extradural spinal tumours. BMJ 1:1341–1344
8. Karnofsky DA, Burchenal JH (1949) Clinical evaluation of chemotherapeutic agents in cancer. In: Macleod CM (ed) Evaluation of chemotherapeutic agents. Columbia University Press, New York, pp 199–205
9. Jenis LG, Dunn EJ, An HS (1999) Metastatic disease of the cervical spine. Clin Orthop 359:89–103
10. Rao S, Babini K, Schldhauer T et al (1992) Metastatic malignancy of the cervical spine. A nonoperative history. Spine 17:407–412
11. Atanasiu J, Badatcgeff F, Pidhorz L (1993) Metastatic lesions of the cervical spine. Spine 18:1279–1284
12. Ono K, Ebara T, Fuji K et al (1987) Myelopathy hand – new clinical signs of cervical cord damage. J Bone Joint Surg 69B:215–219
13. Boriani S, Biagini R, De Iure F et al (1996) EN bloc resections of bone tumors of the thoracolumbar spine. A preliminary report on 29 patients. Spine 21:1927–1931
14. Post YRF, EM KGA (1980) Treatment of spinal epidural metastases. Randomized prospective comparison of laminectomy and radiotherapy. J Neurosurg 53:741–748
15. Klimo P, Thompson CJ, Kestle JRW et al (2005) A meta-analysis of surgery versus conventional radiotherapy for the treatment of metastatic spinal epidural disease. Neuro Oncol 7:64–76
16. Patchell RA, Tibbs PA, Regine WF et al (2005) Direct decompressive surgical resection in the treatment of spinal cord compression caused by metastatic cancer: a randomized trial. Lancet 366:643–648
17. Byrne TN (1992) Spinal cord compression from epidural metastases. N Engl J Med 327:614–619
18. Byrne TN (2004) Metastatic epidural cord compression. Curr Neurol Neurosci Rep 4:191–195
19. Harrington KD (1986) Metastatic disease of the spine. J Bone Joint Surg 68A:1110–1115
20. Harrington KD (1988) Anterior decompression and stabilization of the spine as treatment for vertebral collapse and spinal cord compression from metastatic malignancy. Clin Orthop 233:177–197
21. Bauer HC (1997) Posterior decompression and stabilization for spinal metastases. Analysis of sixty-seven consecutivecpatients. J Bone Joint Surg Am 79:514–522
22. Hirabayashi H, Ebara S, Kinoshita T et al (2003) Clinical outcome and survival after palliative surgery for spinal metastases: palliative surgery in spinal metastases. Cancer 97:476–484
23. Ibrahim A, Crockard A, Antonietti P et al (2008) Does spinal surgery improve the quality of life for those with extradural (spinal) osseous metastases? An international multicenter prospective observational study of 223 patients. Invited submission from the joint section meeting on disorders of the spine and peripheral nerves. J Neurosurg Spine 8(3):271–278
24. Sioutos PJ, Arbit E, Meshulam CF et al (1995) Spinal metastases from solid tumors: analysis of factors affecting survival. Cancer 76:1453–1459
25. Weigel B, Maghsudi M, Neumann C et al (1999) Surgical management of symptomatic spinal metastases: postoperative outcome and quality of life. Spine 24:2240–2246
26. Wise JJ, Fischgrund JS, Herkowitz HN et al (1999) Complications, survival rates and risk factors of surgery for metastatic disease of the spine. Spine 24(18):1943–1951
27. Patil CG, Lad SP, Santarelli J et al (2007) National inpatient complications and outcomes after surgery for spinal metastasis from 1993–2002. Cancer 110:625–630
28. Guzman R, Dubach-Schwizer S, Heini P et al (2005) Preoperative transarterial embolization of vertebral metastases. Eur Spine J 14:263–268
29. Prabhu VC, Bilsky MH, Jambhekar K et al (2003) Results of preoperative embolization for metastatic spinal neoplasms. J Neurosurg 98(2 Suppl):156–164
30. Olsen MA, Maysfield J, Lauryssen C et al (2003) Risk factors for surgical site infection in spinal surgery. J Neurosurg 98:149–155
31. McPhee IB, Williams RP, Swanson CE (1998) Factors influencing wound healing after surgery for metastatic disease of the spine. Spine 23:726–733
32. Hentschel SJ, Rhines LD, Wong FC et al (2004) Subarachnoid-pleural fistula after resection of thoracic tumors. J Neurosurg 100:332–336

33. Klekamp J, Samii M (1998) Surgical results for spinal metastases. Acta Neurochir 140(9):957–967
34. Sundaresan N, Rothman A, Manhart K et al (2002) Surgery for solitary metastases of the spine. Rationale and results of treatment. Spine 27:1802–1806
35. Gokaslan ZL, York JE, Walsh GL et al (1998) Transthoracic vertebrestomy for metastatic spinal tumors. J Neurosurg 89:599–609
36. McLain RF (2001) Spinal cord decompression: an endoscopically assisted approach for metastatic tumors. Spinal Cord 39:482–487
37. Fourney DR, Schomer DF, Nader R et al (2003) Percutaneous vertebroplasty and kyphoplasty for painful vertebral body fractures in cancer patients. J Neurosurg 98(1 suppl):21–30
38. Deramond H, Depriester C, Galibert P et al (1998) Percutaneous vertebroplasty with polymethylmethacrylate. Technique indications, and results. Radiol Clin North Am 36:533
39. Alvarez L, Perez-Higueras A, Quinones D et al (2003) Vertebroplasty in the treatment of vertebral tumors: postprocedural outcome and quality of life. Eur Spine J 12:356–360
40. Chiras J, Depriester C, Weill A et al (1997) Percutaneous vertebral surgery. Techniques and indications. J Neuroradiol 24:45–59
41. Tatsui H, Onomura T, Morishita S et al (1996) Survival rates of patients with metastatic spinal cancer after scintigraphic detection of abnormal radioactive accumulation. Spine 21(8):2143–2148
42. Sundaresan N, Scher H, DiGiacinto GV et al (1986) Surgical treatment of spinal cord compression in kidney cancer. J Clin Oncol 4:1851–1856
43. Finkelstein JA, Zaveri G, Wai E et al (2003) A population based study of surgery for spinal metastases survival rates and complications. J Bone Joint Surg (Br) 85B:1045–1050
44. Argenson C, Cordonnier D, Enkaoua E et al (1997) Place de la chirugie dans la traitment des metastases du rachis. SOF.C.O.T. Reunion Annuelle, Novembre 1996. Rev Chir Orthop 83(Suppl):109–174
45. Yamashita K, Denno K, Ueda T et al (1993) Prognostic significance of bone metastases in patients with metastatic prostate cancer. Cancer 71:1297–1302
46. Ghogawala Z, Mansfield F, Borges L (2001) Spinal radiation before surgical decompression adversely affects outcomes of surgery for symptomatic metastatic spinal cord compression. Spine 26:818–824
47. Raycroft J, Hockmann R, Southwick W (1978) Metastatic tumors involving the cervical vertebrae: surgical palliation. J Bone Joint Surg 60A:763–768
48. Tomita K, Kawahara N, Kobayashi T et al (2001) Surgical strategy for spinal metastases. Spine 26:298–306
49. Enkaoua EA, Doursounian L, Chatellier G et al (1997) Vertebral metastases: a critical appreciation of the pre-operative prognostic Tokuhashi score in a series of 71 cases. Spine 22(19):2293–2298
50. Zimmermann JS, Grop MW, Riegel T (1999) Spinales Kompressionssyndrom. Zum Thema: Onkologische Nolfalle. Onkologe 5:1054–1061
51. Obemdorfer S, Grisold W (2000) Letter to the editor. Spine 25:653–654
52. Tomita K, Kawahara N, Kobayashi T et al (2001) Surgical strategy for spinal metastases. Spine (Phila Pa 1976). Feb1; 26(3):298–306
53. Bauer HC, Wedin R (1995) Survival after surgery for spinal and extremity metastases. Acta Orthop Scand 66(1):J3–J6
54. Tokuhashi Y (2000) Letter to the editor. Spine 25:654
55. Tokuhashi Y, Matsuzaki H, Toriyama S et al (1990) Scoring system for pre-operative evaluation of metastatic spine tumor prognosis. Spine 15:1110–1113
56. Ulmar B, Huch K, Naumann U et al (2007) Evaluation of the Tokuhashi prognosis score and its modifications in 217 patients with vertebral metastases. EJSO 33:914–919
57. Katagiri H, Takahashi M, Wakai K et al (2005) Prognostic factors and a scoring system for patients with skeletal metastasis. J Bone Joint Surg 87:698–703

4 Systematic Approach to the Patient to Minimize Errors of Diagnosis and Surgical Indications

Umile Giuseppe Longo, Luca Denaro, and Vincenzo Denaro

Contents

U. G. Longo (✉)
Department of Orthopedic and Trauma Surgery, Campus Biomedico University, Via Alvaro del Portillo 200, 00128 Rome, Italy
e-mail: g.longo@unicampus.it

4.1 Introduction

Neck pain is an important cause of disability, leading to approximately 1.9 million physician visits annually in the United States [1]. The diagnosis of the pathology responsible for neck pain can be often challenging [2]. Neck pain can arise from pathologies of the cervical spine, as well as from brachial plexus, shoulder, or peripheral nerves, and a systematic approach to the patient is of crucial importance to avoid errors of diagnosis and to plan the optimal management [3]. Orthopedists must never forget that they are managing patients (person with problems), and not "cases", "admissions", or "diseases" [4]. This remains a key point in this era of high technology in clinical medicine. Critical to patient's safety in cervical spinal surgery is ensuring that the correct patient, proper surgical site, and the extent of the pathologic lesion are all properly and precisely identified preoperatively, and confirmed by the appropriate investigations [2]. Correct clinical evaluation and adequate preoperative planning contribute to minimize complications and improve outcome [5–8]. Complete preoperative evaluation involves history-taking, clinical examination, and, depending on the clinical suspicion, radiographs, magnetic resonance imaging (MRI), computed tomography (CT), bone scan, electromyography (EMG), and somatosensory-evoked potentials (SEPs) and motor-evoked potentials (MEPs) [9]. Clinical presentation and the severity of signs and symptoms must also be considered prior to surgery, as well as age, general health of the patient, and comorbidities (diabetes mellitus, hypertension, cardiovascular disease, obesity, asthma, chronic obstructive pulmonary disease, coagulopathy, osteoporosis) (see Chap. 1) [10].

L. Denaro et al. (eds.), *Pitfalls in Cervical Spine Surgery*,
DOI: 10.1007/978-3-540-85019-9_4, © Springer-Verlag Berlin Heidelberg 2010

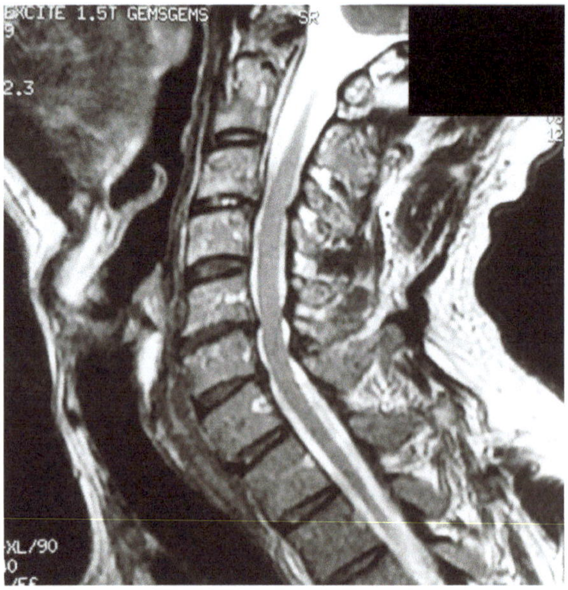

Fig. 4.1 A 58-year-old woman was referred to our center for surgical management of degenerative spinal stenosis. MRI showed multiple C3-C4, C5-C6, C7-C8 discal protrusions. Clinical symptoms and signs were unremarkable, and electrodiagnostic studies confirmed the absence of pathologies. The patient was successfully managed conservatively. 'Treat the patients, not the MRI'!

Recent decades witnessed spectacular advances that have resulted not only in the improvement of surgical techniques, but also in a better understanding of disease processes and more precise preoperative investigations. Increased knowledge of the normal function and disease of the cervical spine allows to better define the criteria for surgical intervention, and to more rationally select the most appropriate surgical approach in each patient [2]. The history and examination usually are sufficient to carry out the diagnosis, and the role of imaging and electrophysiology is to confirm the diagnosis [2]. In general practice, one of the most frequent errors is to attribute a pathological interpretation to MRI or CT before considering the signs and symptoms of the patient (Fig. 4.1) [11]. Many patients are visited for the first time after imaging tests have already been performed. Diagnosis formulated only on the basis of MRI or CT views, which do not take into account the history and clinical examination of the patient, may induce to operate on the imaging and not on the patient. Therefore, imaging should not deter the physician from taking a thorough history and physical examination, which remain the cornerstone of the diagnosis of neck pain (Fig. 4.2).

The medical literature provides several cases of diagnostic pitfalls in patients with cervical pain [12–14]. Classical examples of this circumstance are represented by patients with extra-spinal pathologies, in whom concomitant imaging features of cervical arthrosis leads to misdiagnosis. For example, the cancer of the apex of the lung can cause brachialgia. The symptoms may be attributed to an associated asymptomatic discal herniation, without considering the Pancoast syndrome [2]. Another example is the patient with Parsonage–Turner syndrome. The hyperthermia preceding the disease can be interpreted as influenza, and the neurologic signs can be attributed to an associated simple cervical discopathy. A further example is the patient with cervical unco-arthritis and diabetic polyneuropathy, who can complain of brachialgia without radicular signs. These are the typical cases of patients undergoing surgery with poor clinical result because of errors of diagnosis [2].

In the present chapter, we present a systematic approach to the patient in an attempt to minimize errors of diagnosis and indications.

4.2 Approach to the Patient with Neck Pain: History

The essential first step in the approach to the patient with neck pain is to understand the type of complained pain [15]. A majority of patients are anxious and afraid, and can have comorbidities and psychologic distress. Orthopedists must transmit confidence and reassurance, without being arrogant. Anxiety of the patient can be alleviated and patients may be encouraged to share all the aspects of their medical history when the orthopedist has a professional attitude. All elements of familial, social, and cultural backgrounds must be considered. The ideal patient–physician relationship is based on thorough knowledge of the patient, mutual trust, and ability to communicate [4].

The orthopedist must remember that hospitals are intimidating environments for most patients. They find themselves surrounded by numerous members of the health care team and many strange devices. They may be obliged to share a room with other patients with other clinical problems. It may not be surprising to find the patients feeling disoriented. Physicians should make an effort to understand the hospital experience from the perspective of the patient.

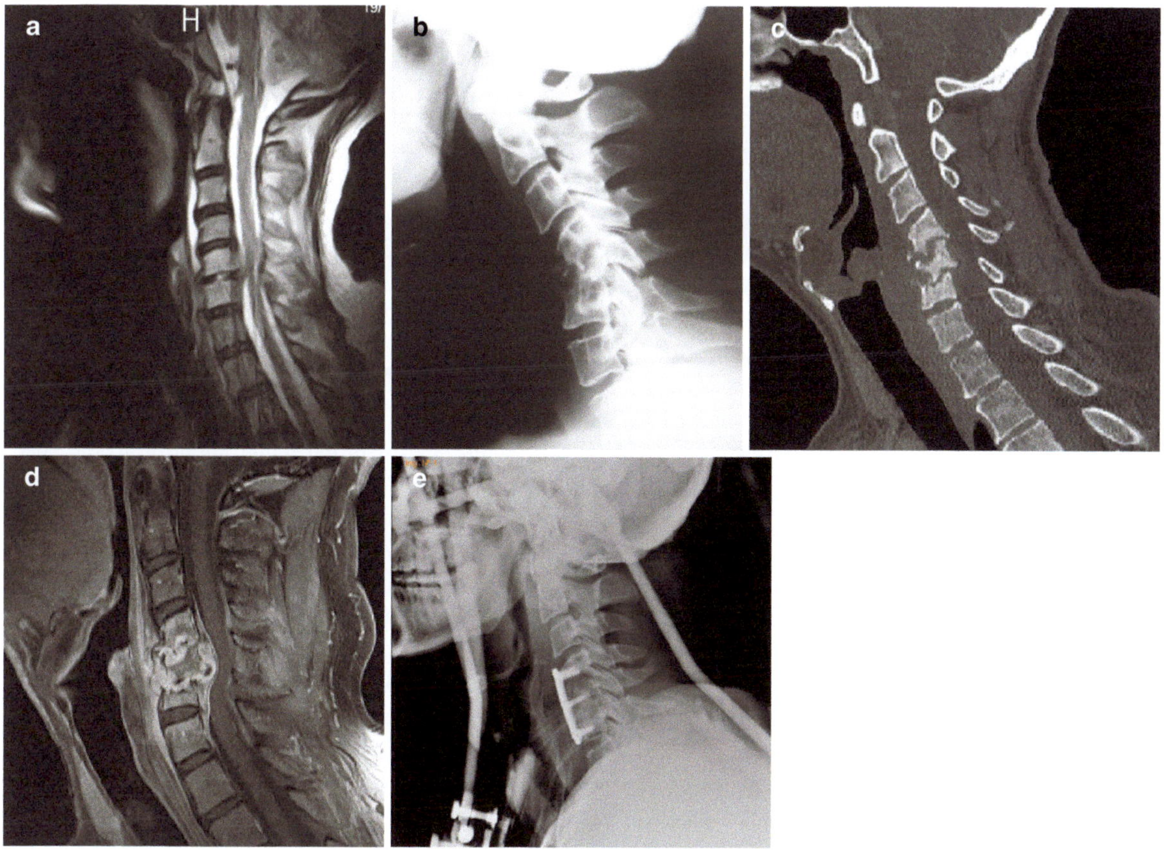

Fig. 4.2 A 60-year-old man presented to another hospital with a clinical history of rapid onset of cervical pain. MRI (**a**) was interpreted as demonstrating cervical disk prolapses. The patient was managed with corticosteroids. The patient was referred to the senior author (V.D.) for clinical evaluation of progressive paralysis of the right arm. Radiographs (**b**), CT scan (**c**), and MRI (**d**) showed structural collapse of the body of C5. The patient was immediately managed with Halo fixator, and anterior decompression and stabilization was performed 2 days after Halo application (**e**). The histopathology and microbiology confirmed a diagnosis of tuberculosis

The history should include all the facts of medical significance in the life of the patient, giving the most attention to recent events. The orthopedist should leave the patient the opportunity to tell his/her own story of the pathology without frequent interruptions. It is fundamental to give time to the history-taking process, as the patient may have the sensation that the orthopedist gives no importance to his/her symptoms, and therefore, may hold back relevant information. Sometimes, events judged irrelevant by the patient may provide the key to solve the clinical problem. A well-taken history is more than a list of symptoms. The social history can provide important insights into the types of symptoms complained by the patient. The family history can identify not only rare genetic disorders, but often reveals risk factors for common pathologies, which may influence the symptoms of the patient [16]. The process of history-taking is a unique opportunity to observe the behavior of the patient and look for features to be researched more thoroughly during the physical examination. Also, the process of history-taking provides the orthopedist the best opportunity to establish the basis for the ideal patient–physician relationship.

Past medical history should be thoroughly explored. Every risk factor for underlying diseases must be identified, as along with the history of chronic infection, history of trauma, drug use, history of tumors, associated musculoskeletal or rheumatic disorders, metabolic bone diseases, and the occupational history of the patient. Cervical symptoms include neck pain, radiculopathy, myelopathy, or a combination of them. Moreover, pain may be referred. Hence, a complete history of cardiovascular diseases (i.e., myocardial ischemia and aortic pathologies) is required [17].

Neck pain is the most common symptom of cervical spine pathologies. Pain must be defined in terms of the type of onset, distribution, frequency, constancy vs. intermittency, duration, quality, association with neurologic symptoms and signs, and localization. Important question to be posed to the patient is whether the pain is worst at rest or at night. In fact, the common presenting symptom of a tumor is persistent pain, worst at night. Other symptoms complained by the patients include head pain, paresthesias, muscular weakness, sphincter dysfunction, vascular symptoms, pseudoangina pectoris, eye and ear symptoms, and throat symptoms. Signs and symptoms of cervical spine tumors may mimic a herniated nucleus pulposus and cause localized weakness, sensory loss, and bowel or bladder dysfunction. Acute onset of pain and paraparesis can be the presentation of a pathologic fracture.

It is also important to investigate trigger maneuvers that can transiently worsen cervical pain, such as coughing, sneezing, and bearing down at stool (Valsalva Maneuver) [18].

In cervical spine pathologies, paresthesias generally follow the segmental distribution of the nerve roots. An involvement of the upper three nerve roots of the cervical plexus may be suspected when paresthesias involve face, head, and tongue. On the other hand, an involvement of the nerve roots from C5 to T1 should be considered in patients with paresthesias being located at the neck, shoulders, arm, forearms, and fingers.

Migraines with and without aura are often accompanied by tension headache-like symptoms, such as neck pain. Confusion and angina pectoris may be caused by lesion at C6 and C7, which can determine tenderness in the pericardium or scapular region, referred down the arm, and may be associated with the sensation of pressure on the chest. Irritation of the cervical sympathetic nerve supply to eye structures may cause ocular symptoms. A combination of lower and upper limb and urinary or rectal dysfunction can be symptoms of cervical myelopathy. Patients with cervical myelopathy may complain of difficulty with ambulation or handling objects.

4.3 Physical Examination

The aim of the physical examination is to identify the physical signs of disease. Neurological examination is critical in the diagnostic process. The importance of the physical examination is enhanced when it confirms functional or structural alterations suggested by the history. Sometimes, however, the physical signs may be the only evidence of pathology.

The physical examination must be carried out thoroughly and methodically. Inspection is the first step. The patient must be examined from head to toe in an objective search for any signs of disease, even though the orthopedist often directs his/her attention only to the neck, with the patient disrobing sufficiently to allow complete visualization only of the cervical region. During the process of systematic examination of the patient, the orthopedist must examine the patient fully undressed, with particular attention to the head, neck, upper thoracic spine, shoulders, arms, forearms, wrists, and hands. Diagnostic information can be obtained from the inspection of the skin: cafè-au-lait spots, erythema nodosum, subcutaneous masses, and needle marks (intravenous drug abuse), which can suggest neurofibromatosis, inflammatory diseases, neurofibroma or lymphadenopathy, and spine infections, respectively. The posture of the patient must be observed, as well as the movements, facial expression, and gait [18].

The orthopedist must inspect the position of the neck and presence of the normal cervical lordosis. Loss of the physiological position of the head may indicate the presence of paracervical muscle spasm. The presence of neck or paracervical muscle atrophy must also be addressed, as well as the evaluation of trapezial and shoulder musculature symmetry. The orthopedist must research the presence of muscle fasciculations, tenderness, atrophy or hypertrophy, and involuntary movements, such as myoclonus, tics, choreoathetosis, pill-rolling tremor of Parkinson's disease, intention tremor of cerebellar disease, or familial tremor. The anatomic positions of the hyoid bone, thyroid cartilage, and thyroid gland must also be evaluated.

The patient should be asked to walk normally, and then on the heels and toes. The patient's gait is an important part of the neurological examination, requiring a high integration of multiple systems, including strength, sensation, and coordination. Abnormalities of gait may suggest corticospinal tract disease, parkinsonism, ataxia, spasticity, posterior column or peripheral nerve disease, or apraxia.

When physical examination is performed in an inconsistent manner, the risk is to omit important signs. The physical examination must be recorded at the time it is elicited and repeated, because physical findings can change with time.

Both active and passive range of motion of the cervical spine must be evaluated. Flexion, extension, lateral flexion, and rotation are the basic movements of the neck. About one-third of the total movements of the neck occur at the upper cervical spine level (occiput-C3). Decrease in specific movements must be evaluated. Examination of the range of motion of the cervical spine should not be carried out in patients with acute head or cervical injury, because of the risk of neurologic damage to an unstable spine.

The second step is palpation. Anterior and posterior examination of the soft tissues of the neck must be performed. Palpation of the supraclavicular fossae allows the evaluation of vascular structures and pathological presence of abnormal masses. Anteriorly, the lymph node chain is located along the medial border of the sternocleidomastoid muscles, and cannot be palpated in normal conditions. Infections, metastases, or lymphoma may determine the enlargement of lymph nodes. Spasms of the scalene and sternocleidomastoid muscles must be evaluated. The carotid tubercle – C6 (Chassaignac's Tubercle) may be palpated deeper. The large tubercle is adjacent to the carotid pulse on the anterior part of the transverse process of C6 [18].

Posteriorly, with the patient sitting, the orthopedist must examine the superior nuchal ligament, greater occipital nerves, and the muscle. The orthopedist must palpate the occiput, the spinous processes from C2 to T1. The C2 and C7 spinous processes are larger than the others. Alignment of the spinous processes should be recorded.

Neuromechanical tests are extremely useful. Patients with root compression have pain and paresthesia elicited with Spurling test (head compression when it is inclined toward the side of the painful upper extremity) and with Valsalva test. Lhermitte's test (neck flection) can produce paresthesias in the back and in the extremities in patients with myelopathy. Lasegue test of the arms allow to reproduce or exacerbate neurologically based symptoms, by placing tension on the cervical nerve roots and the associated peripheral nerves [18]. The response to the test is considered abnormal when the maneuver reproduces the usual pain of the patient, radiating distal to the elbow.

Neurological examination includes reflexes status. The deep tendon reflexes, abdominal reflexes, and plantar responses must be routinely examined. Deep tendon reflex examination should include the biceps (C5, C6), brachioradialis (C5, C6), and triceps (C7, C8) reflexes in the upper limbs and the patellar or quadriceps (L3, L4) and Achilles (S1, S2) reflexes in the lower limbs. All reflexes can be lost with a spinal shock.

Gently stroking the abdominal surface near the umbilicus in a diagonal fashion with a sharp object elicits the superficial abdominal reflexes. These reflexes are absent in patients with upper motor neuron lesions. The plantar reflex is elicited by stroking the lateral surface of the sole of the foot. Patients with upper motor neuron lesions have a paradoxical extension of the toe, associated with extension of the other toes (extensor plantar response or Babinski sign). Bulbocavernosus and anal reflexes must be examined in all patients with sphincter disturbances. The cremasteric reflex consists of the ipsilateral elevation of the testicle following stroking of the medial thigh.

The motor examination includes observation of gait, as already stated, muscle appearance, tone, strength, and reflexes. Examination of strength of deltoid, biceps, triceps, wrist flexors and extensors, finger flexors and extensors, and interossei must be performed. The examiner must address the passive movement of the relaxed limbs to measure the muscle tone. Muscle strength can also be graded using a scale, which attributes 0 to the absence of movement, 1 to flicker or trace of contraction but no associated movement at a joint, 2 to movement with gravity eliminated, 3 to movement against gravity but not against resistance, 4– to movement against a mild degree of resistance, 4 to movement against moderate resistance, 4+ to movement against strong resistance, and 5 to full power.

Rapid pronation and supination of the forearm, and flexion and extension at the wrist allow the orthopedist to assess the tone at the upper limbs. On the other hand, in the lower limbs, the hands of the examiner are placed behind the knees with the patient in supine decubitus and rapidly raised. Increased tone results in an immediate lift of the heel off the surface, while normal tone results in drag of the ankles along the table surface for a variable distance before rising.

A lower motor neuron pathology may be suspected in the presence of weakness, decreased tone, hypotonia, and fasciculations. An upper motor neuron disorder may be suspected in the presence of weakness, hyperreflexia, spasticity, rigidity, or paratonia. Cogwheel rigidity is typical of Parkinson disease.

Sensory examination is performed in an attempt to exactly localize the lesion. Numbness, hyperpathia, hyperalgesia, and pain are sensory signs. The five primary sensory modalities are light touch, pain, temperature, vibration, and joint position, and must be elicited in each limb.

The Romberg maneuver (the patient stands with the feet close together and the eyes closed) is used to study proprioception. The test is positive when a loss of balance with closed eyes occurs.

It is necessary to determine the two-point discrimination (discrimination of two closely placed stimuli as separate), stereognosis (identification of an object by touch and manipulation alone), and graphesthesia (identification of numbers or letters written on the skin surface).

Coordination requires combination of intact muscle strength and kinesthetic and proprioceptive information. A modality to examine the patient's coordination is the evaluation of rapid alternating movements of the hands and the finger-to-nose and heel-knee-shin maneuvers. Vascular and dystrophic autonomic signs must also be evaluated by the examiner. Ischemic symptoms may be present varying from Raynaud phenomenon to ischemic digits. Blood pressure recordings in both arms and radial pulse palpation during Adson maneuver are also necessary to exclude a thoracic outlet syndrome.

4.4 Laboratory Studies

Laboratory investigations for neck pain have a minor role in most patients. However, they can provide helpful information in the diagnosis of specific diseases that may affect the cervical spine, including rheumatoid arthritis, hyperparathyroidism, infections, multiple myeloma, ankylosing spondylitis, and certain metastatic malignant cancers [19]. This chapter does not aim to provide a detailed description of laboratory investigations, for which the reader should refer to other publications. We wish to highlight that laboratory investigations are important in the evaluation of patients with neck pain, and should be performed only after a differential diagnosis has been formulated on the basis of definite signs and symptoms.

For example, cerebrospinal fluid (CSF) evaluation should be considered in patients with neck pain with a suspected infection or subarachnoid hemorrhage. Immunofluorescence studies are important on the CSF of patients with multiple sclerosis plaques. Judicious use of laboratory tests greatly enhances the ability of the orthopedist to make a correct diagnosis.

4.5 Imaging

A wide array of imaging modalities is available in the diagnostic process of cervical spinal pain, including radiographs, CT, MRI, and radionuclide bone scan with SPECT (single photon emission computed tomography) [20]. As stated earlier, increased availability of imaging data does not relieve the orthopedist from the responsibility of carefully observing, examining, and studying the patient.

Cervical spine radiographs include the anteroposterior (AP) view of the atlas and axis through the open mouth, the AP view of the lower five vertebrae, the lateral views in flexion, neutral position, extension, and both right and left oblique views. A swimmer's view is often performed to allow good visualization of the junction C7-T1. The cervical spine must be evaluated for alignment, congenital abnormalities, arthritis, fractures, subluxations, lytic lesions, fractures, and osteoporosis. AP view generally allows good visualization of the uncovertebral joints (joints of Luschka). Generally, the spinous processes are oriented in a vertical row at more or less equal distance [9]. Lateral view allows to evaluate the cervical lordosis and pathological narrowing of the disk space.

Pitfalls in interpretation of radiographs may arise from the presence of congenital or developmental anomalies (congenital basilar impression or odontoideum, partial absence of the posterior atlantal arch, spondylolisthesis, congenital block vertebrae) and variations of normal anatomy (vertebral bodies, articular processes, and apophyseal joints). For example, spondylolisthesis of the axis must be differentiated from hangman's fracture; the partial absence of the posterior atlantal arch may mimic a fracture.

Variations of relationships between the vertebrae should also be considered, especially in traumatic patients (Fig. 4.3).

MRI is an excellent way to visualize the spinal cord and soft tissues in relation to bony anatomy. MRI allows the evaluation of suspected spinal stenosis, congenital anomalies (i.e., Chiari malformations), syringomyelia (Fig. 4.4), myelomalacia (Fig. 4.5), spinal cord neoplasm, multiple sclerosis, and disk degeneration.

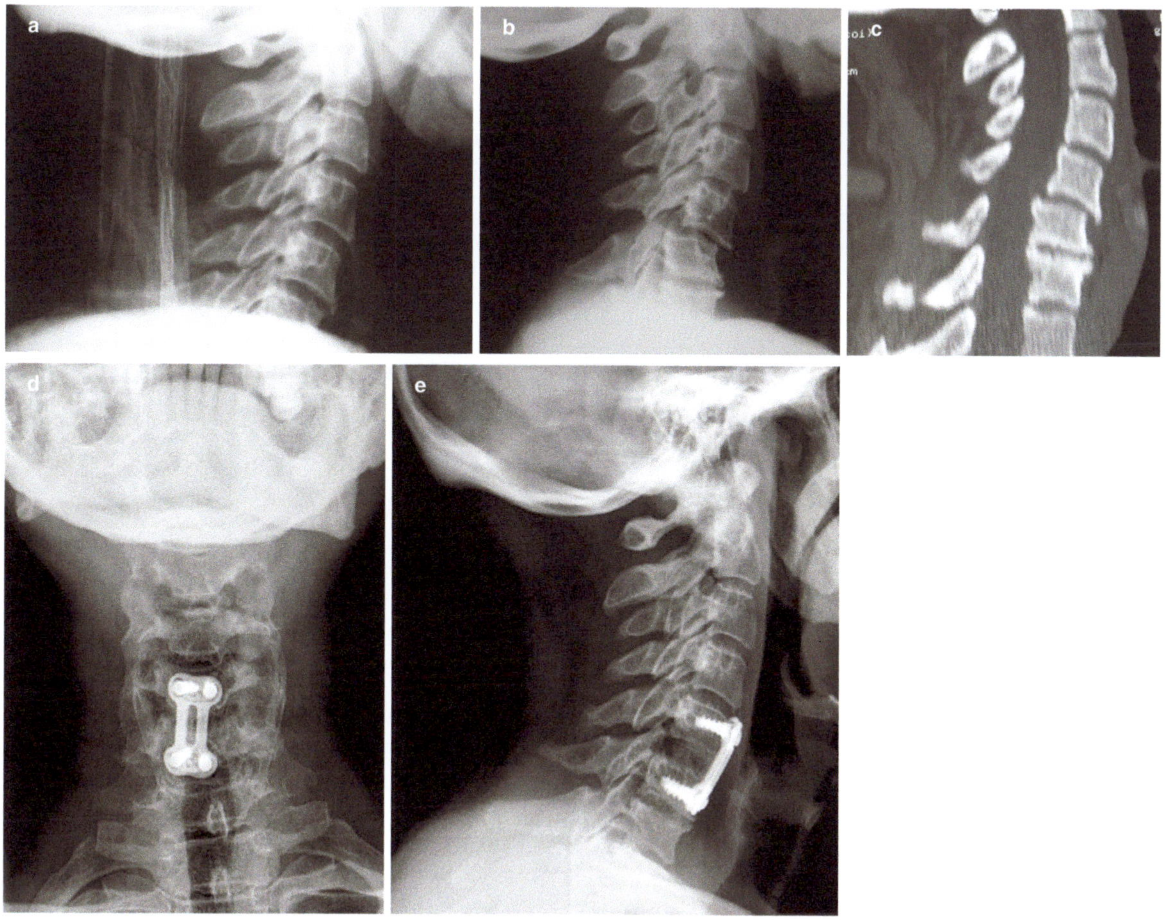

Fig. 4.3 A 67-year-old man involved in a car crash was transported to the local Accident and Emergency Department, complaining of cervical pain. Radiographs (**a**) taken with the patient supine in his bed showed no abnormalities. A soft collar was applied, and the patient was discharged. The patient was subsequently referred to the senior author (V.D.) for clinical assessment of progressive neck pain with radicular involvement of C7, 2 weeks after the accident. A lateral standing radiograph (**b**) showed a C5-C6 dislocation-fracture and fracture of the right transversal apophysis of C6, as confirmed by CT scan (**c**). The patient underwent internal fixation of the fracture. Postoperative AP (**d**) and lateral (**e**) views of the cervical spine

Patients who undergo spinal MRI should be evaluated with at least two pulse sequences, a combination of T1-, T2-, and STIR-weighted sequences.

T1-weighted images allow a contrast evaluation of bone marrow and extradural soft-tissue structures. T2-weighted images focalize on intramedullary pathology, providing a myelographic-like image of epidural impressions owing to degenerative changes. STIR-weighted images detect cord pathologies and highlight soft-tissue edema and infiltrative processes. Paramagnetic contrast media helps to diagnose intramedullary disease, and in the postoperative spine, to detect epidural inflammation and fibrosis [21].

The use of different pulse sequences and paramagnetic contrast media leads to target different anatomical structures (extradural, intradural, and intramedullary spaces). MR-myelography can be useful for the evaluation of nerve-root compression and spinal stenosis.

Myelography, originally used in conjunction with plane radiographs, is now often performed along with CT to visualize the canal.

CT is able to rapidly assess specific details of osseous injuries, spinal stenosis, and osteophytes.

MRI and CT must be considered as complementary and not competitive investigations.

Bone scintigraphy has a high sensitivity but low specificity to asses changes in the skeleton. In the pathologies of the cervical spine, it is particularly helpful to evaluate primary and metastatic tumors, vertebral compression fracture, inflammatory diseases, metabolic bone diseases, and in the assessment of bone-graft incorporation [9].

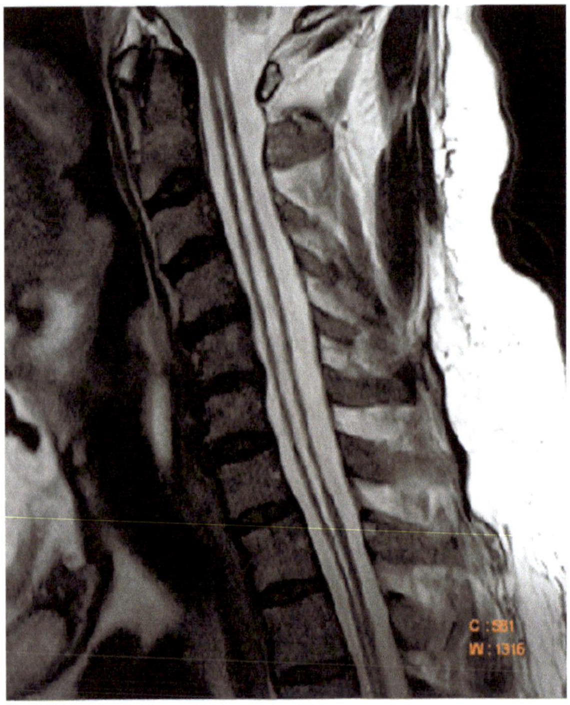

Fig. 4.4 MRI view of a 61-year-old man with syringomyelia

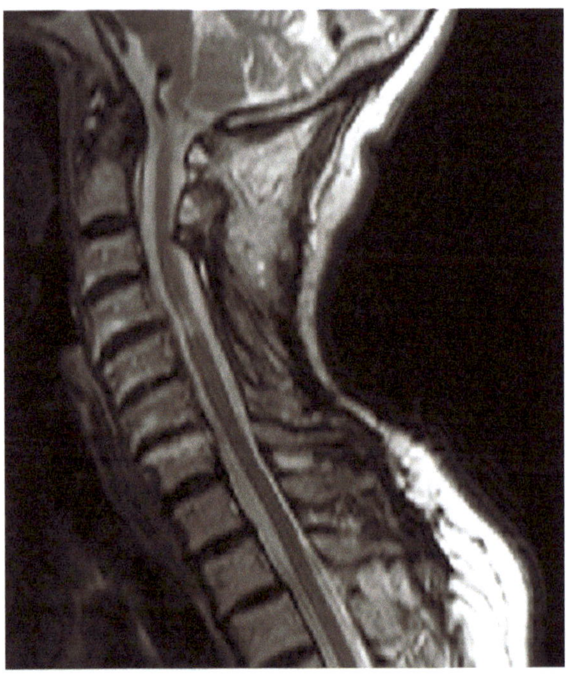

Fig. 4.5 MRI view of a 65-year-old woman with myelomalacia

4.6 Neurophysiology (Electrodiagnostic Studies)

A wide array of electrodiagnostic studies – including needle EMG, electroneurography, and evoked potentials (EPs) – is available to distinguish a lesion in the periphery from a nerve root lesion, to differentiate normal conditions from a diffuse polyneuropathy, focal entrapment neuropathy, radiculopathy, myelopathy, myopathy, and disorder of the neuromuscular junction. They should be considered as an extension of the neurologic examination [22].

Electrodiagnostic studies alone are not able to provide a diagnosis, but they can be extremely helpful in combination with clinical examination [23].

4.6.1 Electromyography

Needle EMG is a functional evaluation of the motor unit, and consists of recording the electrical activity of the muscle cell membrane. The motor unit is constituted by an anterior horn cell, its axon and neuromuscular junctions, and all the muscle fibers innervated by the axon. The number of motor units varies considerably in the average number of muscle fibers within an individual muscle (<25 in the human external rectus or platysma muscle and between 1,600 and 1,700 in the medial head of the gastrocnemius muscle).

The motor unit potential (MUP) can be recorded with a needle electrode inserted in the muscle. This represents the summated electrical activity of action potentials of all the muscle fibers constituting that motor unit. In the absence of pathologies, the relaxed muscle is electrically silent except in the end-plate region (where there are the motor axon terminal synapses on the muscle fiber). The loss of neural control determines the denervated muscles fibers to become unstable and individual muscle fiber fire in the absence of neural stimuli. Increased insertional activity, spontaneous activity, and minor motor unit recruitment are signs of denervation.

In pathologies affecting primarily the muscle fibers, the MUP will be smaller and of shorter duration. The MUP will be absent in patients with severe impairment of the anterior horn cell or its axon. MUP may be delayed in onset, unstable in appearance, or altered in shape in patients with a damage of the axon or if the myelin sheath is defective [22].

MUP can be intermittently delayed or blocked in reaching the muscle fiber in patients with pathologies of the neuromuscular junction, and in certain conditions (e.g., Lambert–Eaton syndrome, myasthenia gravis, or botulism).

EMG can be useful in any suspected peripheral nerve injury, peripheral neuropathy, radiculopathy, localized entrapment, or disease of the MUP. Chronology is important in assessing nerve injury, as Wallerian degeneration occurs within 7–10 days, and the EMG findings will vary as the axon degeneration occurs resulting in deterioration of the neuromuscular junction. EMG signs of denervation generally occur after 18–21 days.

4.6.2 *Evoked Potentials*

EPs are noninvasive measures of brain's electrical activity. An EP is an electrical potential recorded following a stimulus, as distinct from spontaneous potentials detected by electroencephalograms or electromyograms. The term EP is usually reserved for responses involving either recording from, or stimulation of, central nervous system structures [22].

4.6.2.1 Somatosensory-Evoked Potentials

Small electric cortical signals are produced by auditory, visual, and somatosensory stimuli in the neural structures along the corresponding sensory pathways. The nerves used for electrical stimulation are the posterior tibial, sural, or common peroneal nerves for lower limbs and the medial, radial, or ulnar for the upper limbs.

Several pathologies may determine delayed responses, attenuation, or loss of component waveforms. SEPs are most useful when they identify clinically unapparent abnormalities or when they confirm abnormalities that correspond to vague or equivocal signs or symptoms [22].

SEPs record responses only from the fastest conducting nerve fibers, and hence, slowing or partial conduction are hidden by normally conducting fibers. Moreover, abnormal SEPs cannot precisely localize a lesion discriminating from plexus or root localization.

SEP studies are particularly useful to investigate patients with suspected multiple sclerosis, Lyme's disease, systemic lupus erythematosus, neurosyphilis, spinocerebellar degenerations, familial spastic paraplegia, and deficiency of vitamin E or B12, among other disorders.

4.6.2.2 Motor-Evoked Potentials

MEPs are elicited by electrical or magnetic stimulation. MEPs are recorded from muscles following direct stimulation of exposed motor cortex, or magnetic or electrical transcranial stimulation of the motor cortex.

The magnetic or electrical stimuli are applied to the scalp to stimulate peripheral nerves and record the muscle action potentials.

MEPs interpretation includes the evaluation of F- and M-waves. M-wave is obtained through electrical stimulation and is the response to a supramaximal stimulus of the peripheral nerve. F-waves are the expression of the conduction time from the anterior horn cell to muscle (peripheral latency). The delay of the F-wave is a sign of proximal lesion.

4.7 General Considerations and Conclusions

Treatment should be individualized according to the demands and general conditions of the patient, and surgery should be performed only when indications are unequivocally present. Obviously, these circumstances are difficult to classify and describe [24]. Differential diagnosis can be particularly difficult, and must take into account several pathological conditions that may involve the cervical spine (Table 4.1).

The neurological signs, the duration and pattern of development of the symptoms and signs, and a full knowledge of the patient's clinical history must be ascertained before any investigation is performed. The need for specific imaging investigations such as CT and MRI is determined on the basis of the clinical findings. EMG and SEP studies may help to localize the level and type of disease process. If this stepwise progression (Fig. 4.6) is methodically followed, many causes of misdiagnoses can be avoided. This combined effort will minimize the risk of errors in diagnosis.

Table 4.1 Differential diagnosis of cervical spine pain

Hypertrophic cervical dural meningitis
Syringomyelia
Amyotrophic lateral sclerosis
Spinal muscle atrophy
Extramedullary tumors
Intramedullary tumors
Multiple sclerosis (particularly,the spinal progressive type)
Nerve entrapment syndromes (carpal tunnel and thoracic outlet)
Spastic spinal paraparesis
Neuralgic amyotrophy (Parsonage–Turner syndrome)
Funicular myelosis
Paraneoplastic myelopathy
Acute traumatic myelopathy (centro-medullary syndrome)
Friedrich syndrome
Posterior cervicosympathetic syndrome
Supraspinal (central) pathology
Cerebral tumors
Cortical atrophy
Psychoneurosis ("the great imitator")

The first step is to recognize the pathology. Once the diagnosis has been formulated, the surgeon can plan the appropriate management [5–8]. In patients with spondyloarthrosis, the surgeon can precisely define the indications to surgery, such as in patients with spinal cord compression caused by posterior osteophytes, posterolateral (uncal) osteophytes, calcification of the posterior longitudinal ligament, hypertrophy and thickening of the ligamentum flavum, and malformation of the pedicles or laminae. If myelopathy is the result of osteophytes protruding onto the anterior surface of the cord, it is appropriate to perform an anterior approach (Cloward instrumentation with or without multiple corpectomies). In such instances, it is inappropriate to limit surgery to a laminectomy without attempting to remove the anterior osteophytes that cause the compression.

However, when a patient has a wide multi level stenosis (4–5 levels), an anterior decompression to remove the cause of the stenosis, such as a multiple subtotal somatectomy [10] could be too aggressive. For this reason, in the last few years, we have preferentially performed wide laminectomies (4–5 levels), associated with a stabilization in lordosis of the operated segment. The laminectomy – with the removal of

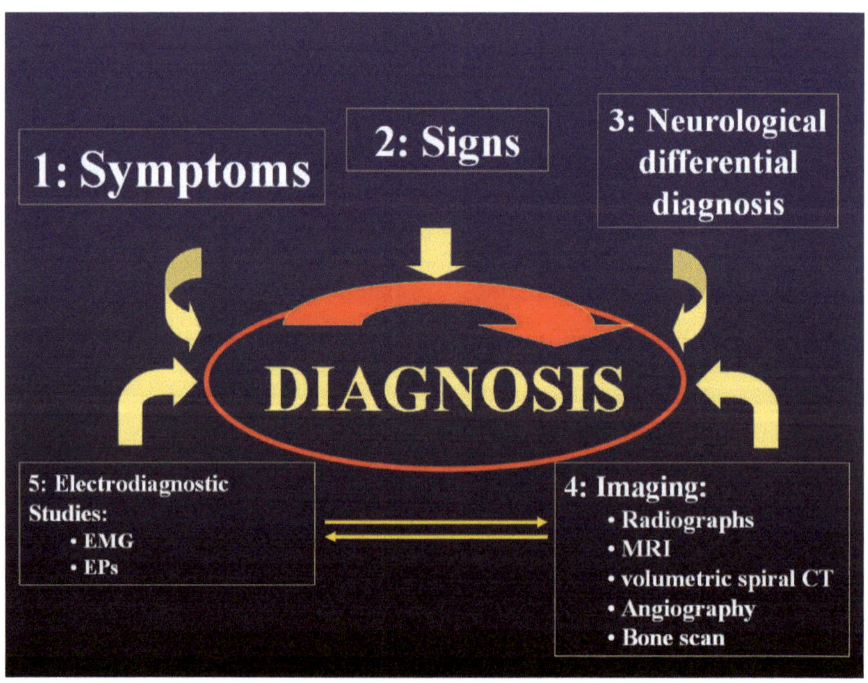

Fig. 4.6 Stepwise progression for the diagnosis of patient with neck pain

the posterior elements of the canal – determines a widening of the spinal canal. The stabilization in lordosis of the operated segment allows a back-shift of the spinal cord, so that the latter lies away from the anterior osteophytes. The fusion eliminates the movement of the operated segment [5–8].

In patients with a segmental compression (only one level) with posterior osteophytes that determine stenosis and medullary damage (with areas of myelomalacia), it is mandatory to associate the internal fixation with the removal of the osteophytes and spinal cord decompression. Internal fixation allows to eliminate any residual motion and avoids further medullary damage. As stated in Chap. 10, this is the main reason, because we do not recommend cervical disk replacement after segmental decompression.

Core Messages

- The essential first step in the approach to the patient with neck pain is to understand the type of pain complained by the patient. All aspects of familial, social, and cultural backgrounds must be considered.
- Past medical history must be thoroughly explored. Every risk factor for the underlying diseases must be identified, along with the history of chronic infection, trauma, tumors, drug use, associated musculoskeletal or rheumatic disorders, metabolic bone diseases, occupational history.
- Pain must be defined in terms of type of onset, distribution, frequency, constancy vs. intermittency, duration, quality, association with neurologic symptoms and signs, and localization. An important question to be posed to the patient is whether the pain is worst at rest or at night.
- The aim of the physical examination is to identify the physical signs of disease. Neurological examination is critical in the diagnostic process. The importance of the physical examination is enhanced when it confirms functional or structural alterations suggested by the history.
- When physical examination is performed in an inconsistent manner, the risk is to omit important signs. The physical examination must be recorded at the time it is elicited and repeated, because physical findings can change with time.
- The clinical laboratory is helpful in the diagnosis of specific diseases that may affect the cervical spine, including rheumatoid arthritis, hyperparathyroidism, infections, multiple myeloma, ankylosing spondylitis, and certain metastatic malignant cancers.
- A wide array of imaging modalities is available in the diagnostic process of cervical spinal pain, including radiographs, CT, MRI, and radionuclide bone scan with SPECT. However, accumulated laboratory and images data do not relieve the orthopedist from the responsibility of carefully observing, examining, and studying the patient.
- Bone scan is extremely helpful to determine bony involvement by neoplasm or infection.
- Several electrodiagnostic studies are available to distinguish a lesion in the periphery from a nerve root lesion, to differentiate normal conditions from a diffuse polyneuropathy, focal entrapment neuropathy, radiculopathy, myopathy, disorder of the neuromuscular junction, and anterior horn cell disease. They should be best viewed as an extension of the neurologic examination.

References

1. Cassidy JD, Côté P (2008) Is it time for a population health approach to neck pain? J Manipulative Physiol Ther 31:442–446
2. Denaro V (1991) Stenosis of the cervical spine. Springer, Berlin
3. Wilson C (2005) Rotator cuff versus cervical spine: making the diagnosis. Nurse Pract 30:44–46
4. Fauci AS, Braunwald E, Kasper DL et al (2008) Harrison's principles of internal medicine, 17th edn. McGraw-Hill, New York
5. Boni M, Cherubino P, Denaro V (1983) The surgical treatment of fractures of the cervical spine. Ital J Orthop Traumatol 9(Suppl):107–126
6. Boni M, Denaro V (1982) The cervical stenosis syndrome with a review of 83 patients treated by operation. Int Orthop 6:185–195
7. Boni M, Denaro V (1982) Surgical treatment of cervical arthrosis. Follow-up review (2–13 years) of the 1st 100 cases operated on by anterior approach. Rev Chir Orthop Reparatrice Appar Mot 68:269–280

8. Boni M, Denaro V (1980) Surgical treatment of traumatic lesions of the middle and lower cervical spine (C3–C7). Ital J Orthop Traumatol 6:305–320
9. Clark CR (2005) The cervical spine, 4th edn. The Cervical Spine Research Society, Lippincott Williams & Wilkins, Rosemont, Philadelphia
10. Boni M, Cherubino P, Denaro V et al (1984) Multiple subtotal somatectomy. Technique and evaluation of a series of 39 cases. Spine 9:358–362
11. Rao R (2002) Neck pain, cervical radiculopathy, and cervical myelopathy: pathophysiology, natural history, and clinical evaluation. J Bone Joint Surg Am 84-A: 1872–1881
12. Al-Khayat H, Al-Baker O, Groof A et al (2007) Cervical radiculopathy secondary to Hodgkin's lymphoma. Surg Neurol 67:540–543
13. Denaro L, Longo UG, Papalia R et al (2008) Eosinophilic granuloma of the pediatric cervical spine. Spine 33: E936–E941
14. Tuy BE, John TK, Uglialoro AD et al (2008) Tumoral calcinosis presenting as neck pain and mass lesion of the cervical spine. Am J Orthop 37:E191–E195
15. Binder AI (2007) Cervical spondylosis and neck pain. BMJ 10:527–531
16. Wieser ES, Wang JC (2007) Surgery for neck pain. Neurosurgery 60:S51–S56
17. Ahn NU, Ahn UM, Ipsen B et al (2007) Mechanical neck pain and cervicogenic headache. Neurosurgery 60:S21–S27
18. Reider B (2005) The orthopaedic physical examination. Saunders, Philadelphia
19. Dreyer SJ, Boden SD (2003) Laboratory evaluation in neck pain. Phys Med Rehabil Clin N Am 14:589–604
20. Mink JH, Gordon RE, Deutsch AL (2003) The cervical spine: radiologist's perspective. Phys Med Rehabil Clin N Am 14:493–548
21. Tong C, Barest G (2003) Approach to imaging the patient with neck pain. J Neuroimaging 13:5–16
22. Han JJ, Kraft GH (2003) Electrodiagnosis of neck pain. Phys Med Rehabil Clin N Am 14:549–567
23. Rao R (2003) Neck pain, cervical radiculopathy, and cervical myelopathy: pathophysiology, natural history, and clinical evaluation. Instr Course Lect 52:479–488
24. Lange U, Bastian L, Muller CW et al (2007) How to prevent overlooking cervical spine injuries: pitfalls in spinal diagnostics. Arch Orthop Trauma Surg 127:953–958

Section II

Peri-operative complications

Considerations and Anesthesiologic Complications in Spinal Surgery

5

Massimiliano Carassiti, Serena Antonelli, Demetrio Panzera, and Felice Eugenio Agrò

Contents

M. Carassiti (✉)
Department of Anesthesia, University School of Medicine
Campus Bio-Medico Via E. Longoni 83, 00155 Rome, Italy
e-mail: m.carassiti@unicampus.it

5.1 Preoperative Consideration

The preoperative evaluation of the risks in patients undergoing cervical spine surgery is important, particularly in elderly patients with co-morbidities. About 30% of the elderly patients have three or more co-morbidities, and 80% have at least one co-morbidity with increased surgical risks.

5.1.1 Age

Although the age of a patient is not a contraindication to surgery, it can be considered as a risk factor for postoperative death. Death risk is of 5% in 80-year-old patients vs. 2% in younger patients. In other types of surgery, age is not a risk factor for complications or postoperative death.

5.1.2 General Health Conditions

The Physical Status Classification of the American Society of Anesthesiologists is often used to predict the outcome of surgery on the basis of the preoperative health conditions of the patient. The percentage of death risk for different groups of patients of various ages varies little among patients in class I and II, and only slightly among those in class III and IV (Table 5.1).

5.1.3 Functional State

All complications are more frequent in inactive patients. The surgical risk is 9.7 times higher in men

L. Denaro et al. (eds.), *Pitfalls in Cervical Spine Surgery*,
DOI: 10.1007/978-3-540-85019-9_5, © Springer-Verlag Berlin Heidelberg 2010

Table 5.1 Preoperative health status

Preoperative health status	
Class	
I	Healthy
II	Light systemic disease
III	Severe not disabling systemic disease
IV	Disabling systemic diseasethatis a constant threat to life
V	Death likely in>24 h with or without human intervention

with limited preoperative activity levels, when compared with those with normal activity levels.

5.1.4 Nutrition Conditions

Preoperative nutritional support is controversial. In elderly patients who undergo total parenteral nutrition (TPN) preoperatively, the total percentage of morbidity and mortality does not decrease when compared with patients who do not receive it. Few complications have been reported in patients seriously malnourished and managed with TPN. Patients with serum albumin concentration <3.5 g/dL have a four times higher incidence of complications, with a mortality rate six times higher than patients with normal level (3.5–5 g/dL).

5.1.5 Psychological State

Social support and the desire to live are important factors to predict the outcome of a surgical procedure. These are difficult to quantify. Dementia is one of the greatest risks for a poor prognosis.

5.1.6 Cardiologic Problems

Cardiac complications are responsible for 12% of all surgical complications, and for 20% of potentially avoidable deaths. Ischemic cardiologic disease is the major factor to predict postoperative complications. To determine the cardiac risk, the index of cardiac risk by Detsky can be used (Table 5.2). Patients in class I (0–15 points) have a low cardiac risk; patients in class II (16–30 points) have an intermediate cardiac risk; and patients in class III (>31 points) have a high cardiac risk.

Table 5.2 Detsky's modified cardiac risk index

Detsky's modified cardiac risk index	
	Risk
Age>70 years	5
Myocardial infarction within 6 months	10
Myocardial infarction after 6 months	5
Canadian cardiovascular society angina classification	
Class III	10
Class IV	20
Unstable angina within 6 months	10
Alveolar pulmonary edema	
Within 1 week	10
Ever	5
Suspected critical aortic stenosis	20
Arhythmia	
Rhythm other than sinus or sinus plus atrial premature beats	5
More than five premature ventricular beats	5
Emergency operation	10
Poor general medical status (defined by Goldman risk index)	5
	120

The tolerance to physical exercise must be evaluated. The risk of postoperative cardiac complication increases if there is a rhythm other than sinus or if there are ectopic beats. A single, occasional ventricular extrasystole does not require preoperative treatment. The American College of Cardiology and the Heart Association have elaborated guidelines to help physicians to evaluate the preoperative cardiac risk and the need for further examinations and management of patients undergoing noncardiac surgery.

These guidelines are based on clinical predictive factors.

Cardiac insufficiency should be corrected as much as possible. Patients with chronic cardiac insufficiency are more likely to develop serious pulmonary edema when compared with asymptomatic patients. Digital, diuretics, vasodilators, and inhibitors of the angiotensin-converting enzyme can be used to improve cardiac performance preoperatively. The depletion of potassium from diuretics must be corrected preoperatively. Many cardiac and vasoactive drugs depress the myocardium and interact with anesthetic drugs. Cardiac drugs cannot be stopped. In particular, the sudden interruption of administration of beta-blockers can be dangerous. Hypertension must be controlled preoperatively and antihypertensive drugs should not be suspended. During anesthesia, the incidence of hypotensive phenomena is higher in patients with hypertension untreated or not adequately controlled than in those in whom pressure is well controlled.

5.1.7 Lung Disease

Lung disease greatly increases the risk of complications, and accounts for 40% of complications and 20% of deaths [1]. Lung evaluation is particularly useful in smokers and in patients with symptoms and signs of lung disease [2, 3]. Chronic obstructive pulmonary disease increases the operative risks, as patients have ineffective cough and are not able to get rid of secretions. The use of bronchodilators preoperatively can improve bronchospasm. Smokers should stop smoking before the operation. These patients are at high risk and benefit from some days of active physical therapy, which includes cupping and inspiration exercises.

5.1.8 Liver Disease

Abnormalities of liver function are a risk factor for postoperative complications. Preoperatively, only abnormalities of coagulation can be connected with the administration of Vitamin K and other blood products. The other consequences of liver disease cannot be addressed in this chapter, and may warrant referral to a hepatologist.

5.1.9 Kidney Disease

Kidney function is assessed by measuring the serum levels of nitrogen, urea, and creatinine. In older patients, the level of creatinine should be standardized for age and body weight using one of the formulas described in the literature [4]. The drug doses need to be adjusted on the basis of kidney clearance. Dehydration can be prevented by administrating fluids. If the serum levels of nitrogen, urea, and creatinine remain high, hemodialysis may reduce uremia and the high risks of surgery.

5.2 Perioperative Considerations

The endotracheal tube must be carefully anchored to the mouth. Carelessness in doing this will have repercussions, as tubes may be displaced when the patient, who was intubated while supine, is rotated and placed in the prone position. Loose endotracheal tubes for anesthesia will be easily displaced, not only during positioning of the patient once anesthetized, but also during the surgery. When this happens, surgery must be stopped immediately, and the patient must be rotated on the operating table back into the intubation position. This can be particularly dangerous in an unstable spine, which may have been rendered even more unstable by the early stages of the surgical procedure before stabilization is performed. Great care must be taken, therefore, to avoid these events that will delay or complicate the surgery.

Posterior cervical surgery may be performed in a seated position (increasing the risk of gaseous embolism [5, 6]), in the prone position (increasing the risk of ocular compression [7, 8]), or in the oblique lateral position (increasing the risk of damage to the nerves and vessels of the axilla [9]).

5.2.1 Airways Management

The optimal tracheal intubation technique for patients undergoing cervical spine surgery remains controversial. Control of the airway and intubations during cervical spine surgery may be difficult in patients with instability of the cervical spine, and in patients with deformity of the neck (i.e., rheumatoid arthritis). In the last decade, new guidelines and recommendations have improved the safety of anesthesia in patients undergoing cervical spine surgery.

New definitions have been developed:

- Difficult airway control consists of the difficulty to ventilate and/or to intubate with standard equipment
- Difficult and/or impossible intubation consists of a maneuver performed in a correct position of the head and the manipulation of the larynx, characterized by
- Difficult laryngoscopy
- The need to perform more than one attempt
- The need to have equipment and/or procedures other than standard
- Giving up and deferring

A difficult laryngoscopy means that it is difficult to visualize the vocal cords. The principal cause of complex intubating is a difficult laryngoscopy. Impossible intubation occurs in 0.05–0.35% of the anesthesiological procedures.

5.2.1.1 Direct Laryngoscopy

Direct laryngoscopy is the direct visualization of the larynx using a rigid laryngoscope to distract the structures of the upper airway. Direct laryngoscopy represents the best known and most used technique by anesthetists. It remains the "gold standard" for tracheal intubation, despite the introduction of new devices [10]. There are two main groups of laryngoscopes, depending on the shape of the blades, namely, curve and straight blades. The dimensions of the laryngoscope vary depending on the model. Some are available in different sizes to be used in relation to the weight of the patients. The laryngoscope allows to display the glottis and the vocal cords, and to introduce an endotracheal tube inside the trachea. The technique provides the alignment of the mouth-windpipe axis, putting the patient in the *sniffing* position (with the neck bent on the trunk, and the head extended on the neck).

The laryngoscope is lifted upwards and forwards, avoiding damage to the teeth. The tip is passed posterior to the epiglottis, which is lifted anteriorly. This allows visualizing the vocal cords. The tip of a curved blade is inserted into the vallecula. This technique enables the best display of the glottis. When direct laryngoscopy is not possible, the availability of some modern *devices* may be very useful to intubate.

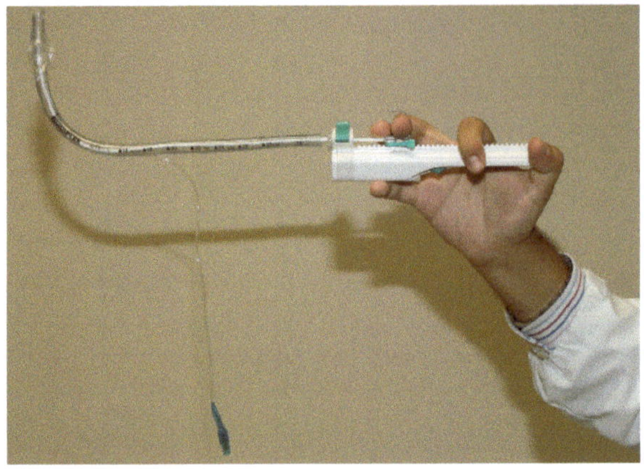

Fig. 5.1 Trachlight

5.2.1.2 Trachlight®

The Trachlight® device is composed of three parts (Fig. 5.1): a handle that allows blocking of the trachea, a flexible spindle with digital light capable to slip by adapting to the tube, and a metallic device that can be put in the spindle. The preliminary step consists of lubricating the spindle that is inserted into an endotracheal tube (TET) of appropriate diameter. Subsequently, the TET trachlight system is bent 6–9 cm from its tip, forming an angle of about 90°. The operator remains behind the patient, and holding the tongue with a gauze, pushes it forward. The head of the patient must remain neutral or slightly extended, but never in the *sniffing position*. In this way, the epiglottis remains close to the back wall of the pharynx. The light is placed on the midline, and it is possible to gently advance the device 1 or 2 cm. The operator must auscultate the chest of the patient, and check the *end-tidal* CO_2. In obese patients, the ability to detect the translighting intensity can significantly be reduced because of the thick soft tissues. Trachlight® is particularly useful in cervical spine surgery in patients with cervical instability. It allows intubating in the neutral position of the neck [11] without extending to the head with the risk of damaging the cord (Fig. 5.2).

5.2.1.3 Airtraq®

Airtraq® is a new video laryngoscope developed for the management of the airways in normal and emergency conditions. It consists of two precurved channels side-by-side. It allows avoiding maneuvers of alignment, required with direct laryngoscopy. Airtraq® can be connected to a system for the image display on an external monitor (Fig. 5.3).

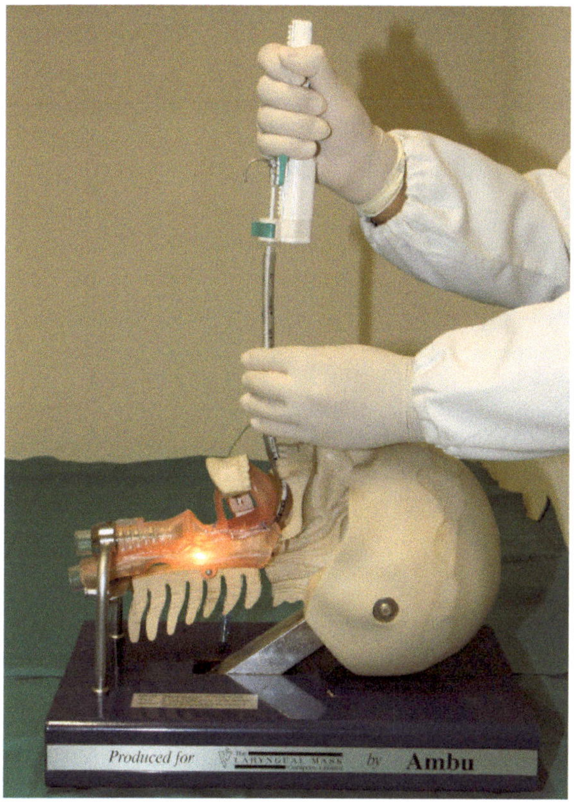

Fig. 5.2 Placement of trachlight

5.2.1.4 Glidescope®

The Glidescope® is a device, which incorporates a high-resolution digital camera located in the tip of the blade (Fig. 5.4). The glottis is displayed on a video using a high-resolution display. The blade is advanced until the tip is positioned in the vallecula. The epiglottis is elevated by lifting the blade into the vallecula, until the vocal cords are seen on the monitor (Fig. 5.5). The main advantage of the glidescope is the camera at the tip of the blade, which enables the direct vision of the glottis and epiglottis through the monitor, without the obstacle of the fleshy tissue and the tongue. Another important advantage of the Glidescope® is

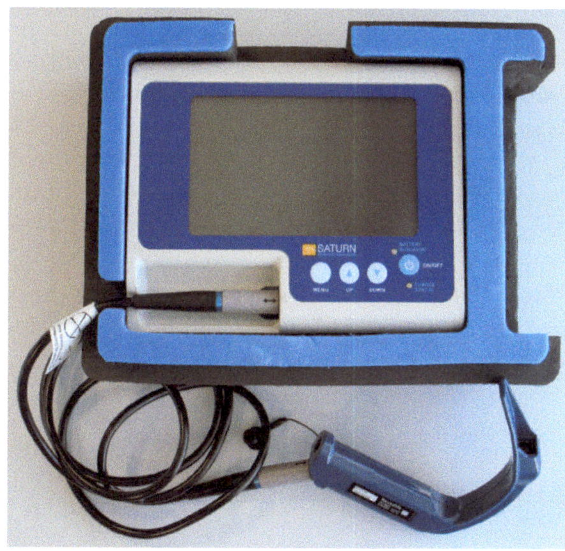

Fig. 5.4 Glidescope

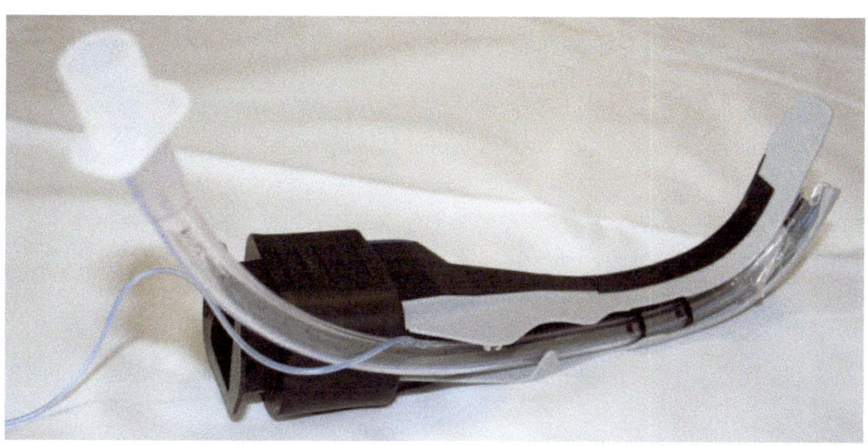

Fig. 5.3 Airtraq

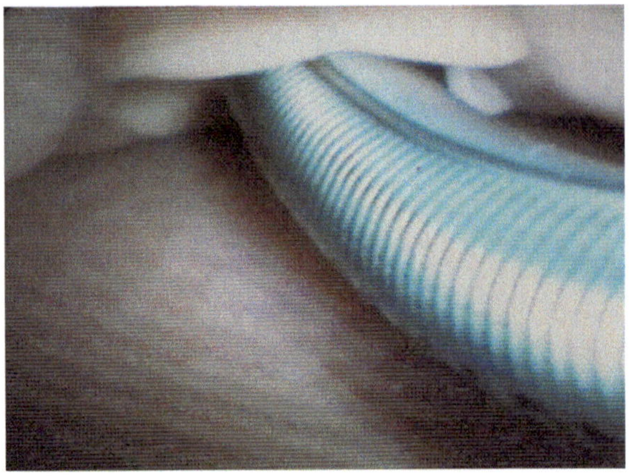

Fig. 5.5 Positioned tube vision through glidescope

that it can be used in patients with cervical instability. Moreover, the use of Glidescope® implies a time reduction in the tracheal intubation when compared with the laryngoscope. The main limitation of this new device is the difficulty in manipulating the TET through the vocal cords and simultaneously visualization of its images displayed on the monitor. These inconveniences may be minimized by using a specific stylet or Magill forceps. The glidescope represents the gold standard of the cervical spine surgery in patients in whom it is necessary to perform invasive ventilation through the oro/nasotracheal approach [10, 12].

5.2.1.5 LMA-Classic™

The Laryngeal Mask Airway-Classic (LMA-Classic™) (Fig. 5.6) is a shortened conventional silicone tube with an elliptical cuff, inflated through a pilot tube attached to the distal end. The cuff is available in a variety of sizes. The mask is inserted and the cuff is inflated until no air leak is detected.

The device is effective in maintaining a patent airway in the spontaneously breathing patients. One of the disadvantages of this device is that it is not suitable for patients at risk for regurgitation of gastric contents [13]. The LMA-Classic™ represents a significant progress, and it is useful in patients in whom it is not possible to intubate [14]. When it is really difficult to insert the device, laryngoscopy can help.

5.2.1.6 LMA-Fastrach™

The LMA-Fastrach™ (Fig. 5.7) has been developed for cardiopulmonary resuscitation and the anticipated or unexpected difficult airway. It has been designed to facilitate blind intubation without moving the head or neck, and allows continuous ventilation between the intubation attempts. In the LMA-Fastrach™, a sort of spoon handle has been added to the LMA-Classic™.

5.2.1.7 LMA-Proseal™

The LMA-Proseal™ (Fig. 5.8) is a laryngeal mask specifically designed to offer further advantages when compared with LMA-Classic™, and to extend its applications [15]. It optimizes the ventilation with positive pressure (PPV). It has the following features:

(a) A double tube that offers the first effective separation between the eating and breathing tract
(b) A double cap that provides a double-maintained pressure
(c) A new *drain tube* that has an entrance to the upper esophageal sphincter

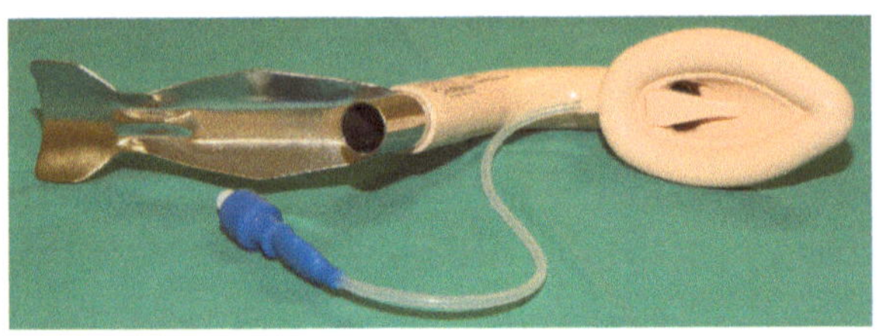

Fig. 5.7 LMA-Fastrach

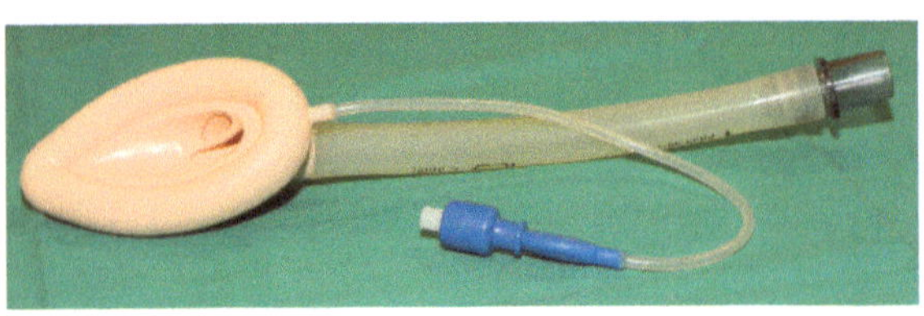

Fig. 5.6 LMA-Classic™

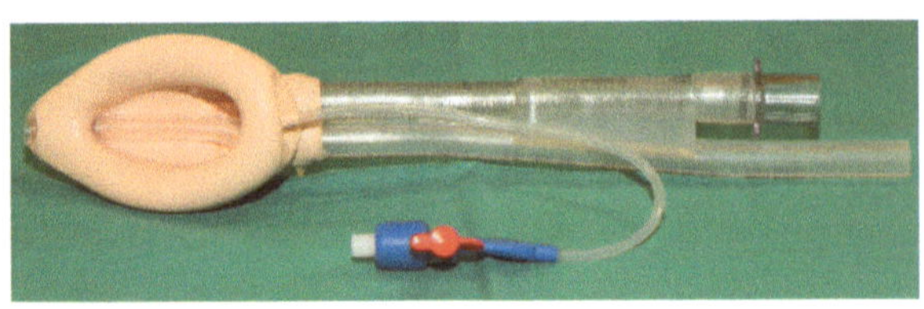

Fig. 5.8 LMA-Proseal

(d) An introducer that prevents insertion of the fingers into the mouth of the patient during insertion
(e) A double tube *design* that reduces the rotation and dislocation risk of the mask
(f) A device that stops the action of biting and which is incorporated to reduce the risk of obstruction or tube damage
(g) A cleft appropriate for the LMA-Proseal™, which allows maintaining the stability of the index finger or the thumb during the manual introduction.

5.2.1.8 Combitube

The combitube (Fig. 5.9) is a double tube that can be useful in critical conditions [16, 17]. It is very big and consists of two tubes put together with a big balloon: the blue tube should be filled with 100 mL of air, and the white one with 15 mL of air.

5.2.1.9 Cobra PLA

The cobra PLA (Fig. 5.10) is a supraglottic equipment. The initial idea was to modify the Guedel airway to accomplish mask ventilation in the most difficult airways. The first changes consisted of lengthening and widening of the distal end of the Guedel airway and placing a slot in the widened end to accommodate distal breathing hole, modifying the shape of the distal "Cobra head" portion, putting a 15 mm adapter at the proximal end, and adding a "grill" to the distal anterior surface.

5.2.1.10 Cricothyrotomy

Cricothyrotomy is a percutaneous technique required in patients who cannot be ventilated or intubated. Cricothyrotomy approach allows a safe, fast control of the airway, minimizing the risks of iatrogenic damages, including pneumothorax, pneumomediastinum, and mediastinal perforation.

Several devices are commercially available. In our clinical practice, we use the needle cricothyrotomy (Fig. 5.11).

5.2.2 *Pulmonary Ventilation in Vertebral Surgery*

Abnormalities of the physiology of lung ventilation arise from the type of decubitus. The type of mechanic ventilation in an intubated patient may have an impact on the bleeding of the operating field. The epidural venous plexus is anastomotic, and its pressure is influenced by the outflow of the circle in the inferior vena

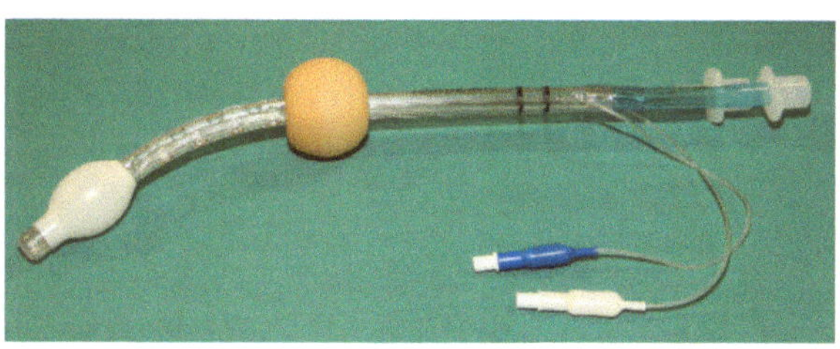

Fig. 5.9 Combitube

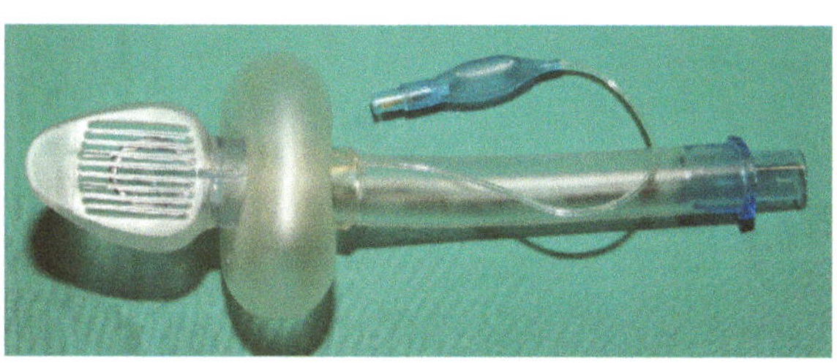

Fig. 5.10 Cobra PLA

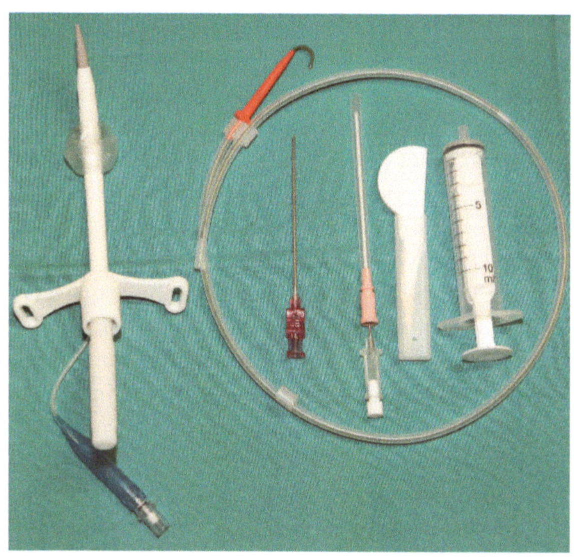

Fig. 5.11 Needle cricothyrotomy

cava. The pressure in inferior vena cava is influenced by the pressures of the abdominal wall and the diaphragm. In the prone decubitus, it is important to leave the abdomen free to facilitate normal breathing movements by a correct positioning, and have a correct myoresolution. The pressure in superior vena cava may be influenced by ventilation. The mechanic ventilation model more commonly used is: Volume Control Ventilation (VCV) and Pressure Control Ventilation (PCV).

5.2.3 Mechanic Breathing and Patient's Positioning Effects

During anesthesia in the supine position, there is a predisposition to alveolar collapse of the inferior regions of the lung. Alterations of the breathing exchanges depend on the equipment used to sustain. The prone position is sustained by lifting the anterior part of the body, to avoid compression of the abdomen.

5.2.4 Controlled Hypotension

Controlled hypotension limits intra-operative blood losses. In accurately selected patients [18], induced hypotension is a reliable and controlled technique, with low rate of risks [19]. Perfect perfusion of brain and heart must be ensured. Before a patient undergoes controlled hypotension, it is important to check his/her age and preexisting pathologies. Sedation, analgesia, and anesthesia decrease arterial pressure, cardiac output, cardiac frequency, and systemic vascular resistance. This cardio-circulatory depression can be tolerated until it does not damage the vital tissues of the brain and heart. Hypertensive episodes may occur as a consequence of hypercapnia, hypoxia, acidosis, hypervolvemia, or hypovolemia [20].

A good hypotension technique must be easy to control. It must not alter the cerebral autoregulated system, compromise the perfusion of vital organs, or use toxic substances or substances degraded into toxic metabolites. Hence, it is necessary to use short half-life drugs [21]. It is possible to modulate or induce hypotension pharmacologically by modifying the position of the patient, the ventilation, or the cardiac frequency. These mechanical maneuvers may limit the administration of toxic potential drugs.

5.2.5 Perioperative Monitoring

5.2.5.1 Breathing Monitoring (Primus/Zeus Drager®)

Breathing monitoring is the monitoring of oxygenation and inspired–expired gas. Monitoring oxygenation through a pulsimeter consists of constantly measuring the peripheral saturation of oxygen (SpO_2). It is a combination of plethysmography and spectrophotometer analysis.

5.2.5.2 Hemodynamic Monitoring

In complex spinal surgery, which can induce significant blood loss, invasive monitoring should be used. This monitoring depends mainly on the risks to which the patient is exposed, and is based on preoperative health status. In addition to electrocardiographic monitoring, it is essential to monitor bloody pressure and central venous pressure. An endo-arterial probe allows constant monitoring of the blood pressure, and facilitates the access to samples of arterial blood. The central venous catheters are important vascular access for the evaluation of the blood volume changes. The central venous catheters allow rapid fluid infusion, catheter insertion in the pulmonary artery, transvenous electrode insertion, central venous pressure monitoring (CVPM), and observation and management of gas venous embolism. The eco-guided right internal jugular vein is generally preferred to the left, given the potential risk of damaging the thoracic duct when trying to access the left internal jugular vein. Blood gas analysis must be repeated to verify the adjustment of the oxygenation of the tissues and to detect a possible metabolic acidosis. The Vigileo (Edwards®) is a new method to measure the cardiac output, based on wave analysis of the arterial pressure, which does not require calibration or thermo dilution.

5.2.5.3 Fluid Balance

Bladder catheterization should be performed in long operations. Urinary flow indicates the adequacy of kidney perfusion. Oliguria has to grab the attention on the effective perfusion of the kidney. Considering that there are possible interferences between ventilation quality and artery pressure, it is necessary to constantly follow the O_2 saturation as well as CO_2 elimination.

The use of the hemogasanalysis can guarantee an adequate control of strong ion difference and the choice of the correct fluid therapy.

5.2.5.4 Body Temperature Monitoring

It is important to constantly monitor the temperature in case of induced hypotension, as heat loss is more extensive over the dilated vessels, and the vasoconstriction that follows hypothermia could contrast the effects of the drugs used.

Core Messages

- The preoperative evaluation of the risks in patients undergoing cervical spine surgery is important, particularly in elderly patients with co-morbidities.
- The endotracheal tube must be carefully anchored to the mouth.
- When loss of endotracheal tubes occurs, surgery must be immediately stopped and the patient must be rotated on the operating table back into the intubation position. This can be particularly dangerous in an unstable spine that may have been rendered even more unstable by the early stages of the surgical procedure before stabilization is performed.
- The optimal tracheal intubation technique for patients undergoing cervical spine surgery remains controversial. Control of the airway and intubations during cervical spine surgery may be difficult in patients with instability of the cervical spine, and in patients with deformity of the neck (i.e., rheumatoid arthritis).
- Direct laryngoscopy remains the "gold standard" for tracheal intubation, despite the introduction of new devices.
- When direct laryngoscopy is not possible, the availability of some modern *devices* may be very useful to intubate.
- Cricothyrotomy is a percutaneous technique required in patients who cannot be ventilated or intubated, allowing a safe, fast control of the airway, minimizing the risks of iatrogenic damages (i.e., pneumothorax, pneumomediastinum, and mediastinal perforation).
- Abnormalities of the physiology of lung ventilation arise from the type of decubitus. The type of mechanic ventilation in an intubated patient may have an impact on the bleeding of the operating field.
- Controlled hypotension limits intra-operative blood losses. In accurately selected patients, induced hypotension is a reliable and controlled technique, with low rate of risks. Perfect perfusion of brain and heart must be ensured. Before a patient undergoes controlled hypotension, it is important to check his/her age and preexisting pathologies.

References

1. Lumb AB, Nunn IF (1991) Respiratory function and rib cage contribution to ventilation in body positions commonly used during anesthesia. Anesth Analg 73:422–426
2. Pelosi P, Croci M (1995) The prone positioning during general anesthesia minimally affects respiratory mechanics while improving functional residual capacity and increasing oxygen tension. Anesth Analg 80:955–960
3. Pelosi P, Croci M (1996) Prone positioning improves pulmonary function in obese patients during general anesthesia. Anesth Analg 83:578–583
4. Gupta R, Batra S, Chandra R, Sharma VK (2008) Compartment syndrome with acute renal failure: a rare complication of spinal surgery in knee-chest position. Spine 33(8):E272–E273
5. Moreno F, Lyons HA (1961) Effect of body posture on lung volumes. J Appl Physiol 16:27–29
6. Palmon SC, Kirsch JR (1998) The effect of the prone position on pulmonary mechanics is frame-dependent. Anesth Analg 87:1175–1180
7. Chung MS, Son JH (2006) Visual loss in one eye after spinal surgery. Korean J Ophthalmol 20(2):139–142
8. Kasodekar VB, Chen JL (2006) Monocular blindness: a complication of intraoperative positioning in posterior cervical spine surgery. Singapore Med J 47(7):631–633
9. Takahata M, Ito M, Abumi K et al (2008) Clinical results and complications of circumferential spinal cord decompression through a single posterior approach for thoracic myelopathy caused by ossification of posterior longitudinal ligament. Spine 33(11):1199–1208

10. Agrò F, Barzoi G, Montecchia F (2003) Tracheal intubation using a Macintosh laryngoscope or a glidescope in 15 patients with cervical spine immobilization. Br J Anaesth 90(5):705–706
11. Agrò F, Hung OR, Cataldo R et al (2001) Lightwand intubation using the trachlight: a brief review of current knowledge. Can J Anaesth 48(6):592–599
12. Robitaille A, Williams SR, Tremblay MH (2008) Cervical spine motion during tracheal intubation with manual in-line stabilization: direct laryngoscopy versus glidescope videolaryngoscopy. Anesth Analg 106(3):935–941
13. Agrò F, Brimacombe J, Verghese C et al (1998) Laryngeal mask airway and incidence of gastro-oesophageal reflux in paralysed patients undergoing ventilation for elective orthopaedic surgery. Br J Anaesth 81(4):537–539
14. Kihara S, Watanabe S, Brimacombe J et al (2000) Segmental cervical spine movement with the intubating laryngeal mask during manual in-line stabilization in patients with cervical pathology undergoing cervical spine surgery. Anesth Analg 91(1):195–200
15. Agrò F, Antonelli S, Mattei A (2001) The proseal LMA: preliminary data. Br J Anaesth 86(4):601–602
16. Agrò F, Barzoi G, Montecchia F (2003) The oesophageal tracheal combitube: a pilot study on airflow resistance and ventilatory pressures in 26 anaesthetised patients. Anaesthesia 58(7):722–723
17. Agrò F, Frass M, Benumof JL et al (2002) Current status of the Combitube: a review of the literature. J Clin Anesth 14(4):307–314
18. Degoute CS (2007) Controlled hypotension: a guide to drug choice. Drugs 67(7):1053–1076
19. Dutton RP (2004) Controlled hypotension for spinal surgery. Eur Spine J 13:S66–S71
20. Fenger-Eriksen C, Hartig Rasmussen C, Kappel Jensen T et al (2005) Renal effects of hypotensive anaesthesia in combination with acute normovolaemic haemodilution with hydroxyethyl starch 130/0.4 or isotonic saline. Acta Anaesthesiol Scand 49(7):969–974
21. Kadam PP, Saksena SG, Jagtap SR et al (1993) Hypotensive anaesthesia for spine surgery–nitroglycerin vs halothane. J Postgrad Med 39(1):26–28

General Complications Related to Patient Positioning

6

Luca Denaro and Vincenzo Denaro

Contents

L. Denaro (✉)
Department of Neuroscience, University of Padua,
Via Giustiniani 5, 35128 Padua, Italy
e-mail: lucadenaro@hotmail.com

6.1 Introduction

Successful surgery necessarily begins with the proper positioning of the patient [1–3], which is a key point to gain good operative exposure and to prevent the potential complications of excessive pressure on neural or vascular structures [1]. This is an important aspect of cervical spinal surgery, because of the deep and often inaccessible structures, the required accuracy for the determination of level, and the inherent risks of the positions themselves. Several complications have been reported as consequences of patient malpositioning during operative procedures to the cervical spine [4–7]. In cervical spine surgery, the supine patient position is used for anterior approaches, the prone or sitting position for posterior approaches, and the lateral or sitting approaches for circumferential approaches. Obviously, each of these positions will determine different risks.

6.2 Posterior Approach: Precautions and Recommendation

The posterior approach provides the best access to the posterior elements of the cervical spine. The most common complications of the posterior approach are associated with the patient position on the operating table, in addition to the surgical approach itself (Table 6.1). The patient is placed in the ventral decubitus (prone) position on the operating table. The sitting position with the head supported by a headrest has also been described, but the prone position is commonly preferred [8], except in patients with ankylosing spondylitis undergoing cervical osteotomy under local anesthesia, when the patient is awake. Upright position has the advantage to increase ventilation tidal volumes

L. Denaro et al. (eds.), *Pitfalls in Cervical Spine Surgery*,
DOI: 10.1007/978-3-540-85019-9_6, © Springer-Verlag Berlin Heidelberg 2010

Table 6.1 Complications of the prone position

Complications	How to avoid them: tips and tricks
Intra-operative bleeding	Maintain freedom of movement of the abdomen without compression to permit unobstructed diaphragmatic movement in respiration during surgery Use a reverse-Trendelenburg position Use local anesthetic with epinephrine starting at the spinous processes and proceeding laterally into the paravertebral tissues
Compression of the bony prominences	Use appropriate padded supports across all the bony prominences
Peripheral nerve damage	Pad all bony prominences in correspondence to the peripheral nerve and appropriately position the limbs
Fall of the lower extremities from the operative table	Fix legs and thighs to the table by straps
Movements of the head during surgery	Criss-cross tapes to position the head firmly in the headrest
Fracture of the bones of the head when using the Mayfield headrest	Do not use in patients with increased fragility of the bones of the head (tumors, osteoporosis, hemopathies), because of the risks of fracture
Venous air embolism when removing the Mayfield headrest	The head-fixating devices should be removed in the supine position monitoring for venous air embolism until all potential sites for air entry into the circulation have been occluded
Loss of endotracheal anesthetic tube	Carefully anchor endotracheal anesthetic tube to the mouth
Ocular complications	Avoid external compression on the eyes

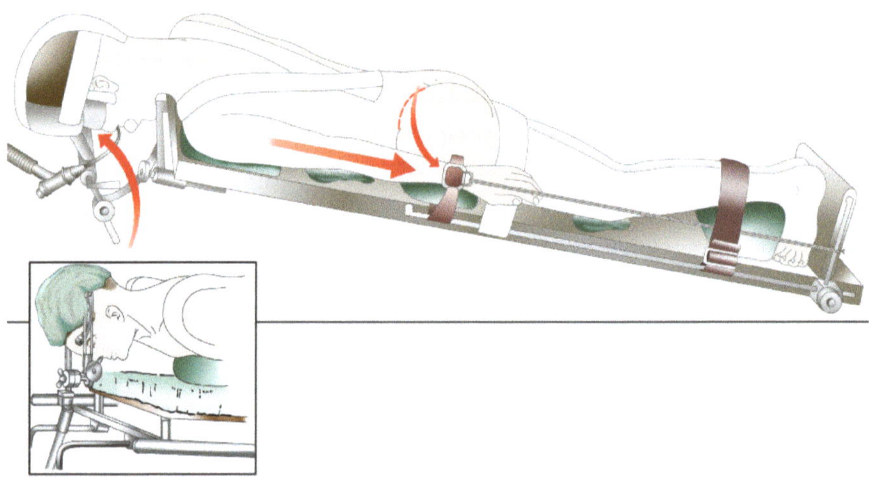

Fig. 6.1 The patient is placed on the operating table in the anti-Trendelenburg position. Supports are placed on the iliac crests, and on the sternal region to allow free movement of the abdomen. The forehead is placed on a mobile adjustable rest. The eyes are free of obstruction outside the support of the forehead. The head is held in position with tapes. Adhesive tapes apply caudal traction on the shoulders, and the arm is also under longitudinal traction

because the lungs are allowed to expand more freely than in the supine or prone positions [9].

The patient is placed on an orthopedic table using appropriate padded supports (Fig. 6.1). These are placed across the thorax and the sternum, and longitudinally across both the iliac crests to maintain freedom of movement of the abdomen without compression, and thus to permit unobstructed diaphragmatic movement in respiration during surgery. The compression of the abdomen will interfere with diaphragmatic movement during respiration [8]. Vascular outflow from the spinal cord occurs through the Batson venous plexus, a valveless epidural network that drains into the caval vena system. This plexus can become congested when the abdomen is compressed and not allowed to hang free in patients in the prone position [10]. The consequences are increased splenic venous pressure and greater intra-operative bleeding from the ensuing increased vascular pressure in the parameningeal vessels [8].

If this is combined with a limitation of diaphragmatic movement during respiration, the patient's oxygenation may also be affected [8]. This is particularly important in surgery of the thoracic and lumbar spine rather than of the cervical spine.

All bony prominences must be adequately padded. Appropriate positioning of the extremities is required, as peripheral neuropathy because of inadequate patient positioning on the operating table has been described for ulnar nerve, median nerve, and common peroneal nerve [8, 11]. However, all peripheral nerves can be theoretically involved.

The legs and thighs are well fixed to the table by straps, with the feet supported by a pillow on a fixed base. The hands are held to the side of the body by wrist bands attached to an elastic band. This places the arms in some tension so that the shoulder tips will be lowered [8]. A Tensoplast type of adhesive band passed over the shoulder is anchored to further lower the shoulder tips [8], avoiding to fix it in the region of the iliac crest, which can be the site of an eventual bone harvesting from the iliac crest. The head is placed in a horseshoe-shaped headrest that is mobile and adjustable and follows the outline of the forehead, leaving only the eyes, the nose, and the mouth accessible. Criss-crossing tapes are used to position the head firmly in the headrest. In addition, the tapes will provide tension on the skin [2]. This will also provide access for nasogastric and endotracheal tubes for anesthesia. All the above problems can be prevented using Mayfield traction, which is widely used for cervical spine surgery.

However, the Mayfield is contraindicated in patients with conditions (i.e. tumors, osteoporosis, hemopathies) that increase fragility of the bones of the head, because of the risks of fracture.

The reported complications associated with the use of the Mayfield head clamp are breakage of Mayfield headrest [12], cranial fracture [13], epidural hematoma [13], and venous air embolism [14–17]. The potential for venous air embolism exists any time the surgical wound is above the level of heart producing a subatmospheric pressure in the open veins. The head-fixating devices should be removed in the supine position to avoid venous air embolism and monitoring for venous air embolism throughout the entire intraoperative period until all potential sites for air entry into the circulation have been occluded [15].

In patients who have been in a halo traction preoperatively, the halo will be anchored to the headrest rather than the head itself [2].

The endotracheal anesthetic tubes are carefully anchored to the mouth. Carelessness in doing this will have repercussions, as tubes may be displaced when the patient, who was intubated while lying on his back, is rotated and placed in the required operative position [2]. Endotracheal tubes for anesthesia will be easily displaced, not only during positioning of the patient once anesthetized, but also during surgery. When this happens, surgery must immediately stop and the patient must be rotated on the operating table back into the intubation position. This can be particularly dangerous in an unstable spine, which may have been rendered even more unstable by the early stages of the surgical procedure before stabilization is performed [18, 19]. Great care must be taken, therefore, to avoid these events that will unnecessarily delay or complicate the surgery.

The prone position commonly used in posterior spinal procedures may produce serious injury to the cornea and to the eye. A survey by the Scoliosis Research Society showed that one eye complication occurs for every 100 spine surgeries [20]. The reported ophthalmologic complications associated with prone positioning in spine surgery are corneal abrasion (the most common ophthalmologic injury), and blindness as the result of posterior ischemic optic neuropathy, central retinal artery occlusion, or occipital cortical infarct or cortical blindness [21]. The physiopathology and the prognosis of these conditions are very different. The prone position may determine an increased intraocular pressure, particularly if excessive pressure is placed directly on the orbit. Central retinal artery occlusion is usually caused by eye compression only, while ischemic optic neuropathy is often multifactorial [22].

The patient must be positioned avoiding direct pressure around the eyes (Fig. 6.2). This complication should be avoidable using the Mayfield, rather than the headrest. This positioning must be assessed by the

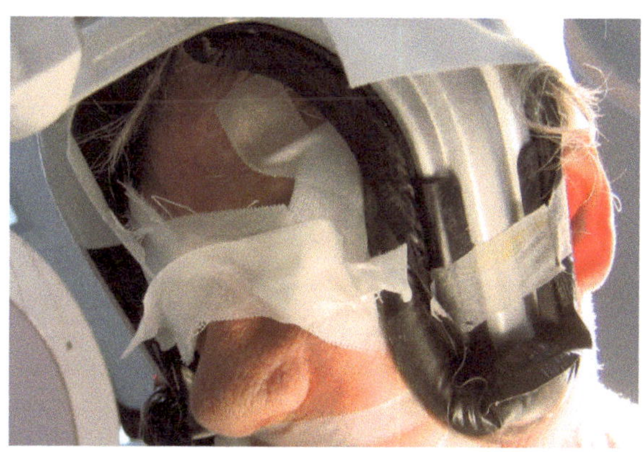

Fig. 6.2 The patient must be positioned avoiding direct pressure around the eyes

surgeon and the anesthesiologist [23]. Additionally, throughout the operation, patient position should be reassessed as often as feasible by the anesthesiologist to make sure that no change has occurred [24, 25]. External compression of the eyes may be an isolated mechanism of complete and definitive visual loss. This mechanism can be considered in patients with associated central retinal artery occlusion with local signs of compression, such as eyelid edema, ptosis, conjunctival hematoma, chemosis, periorbital numbness, or paresthesia [22, 24, 26–28].

External compression of the eye could increase intraocular pressure, decreasing perfusion pressure and causing retinal ischemia with central retinal artery occlusion. In the absence of obvious external compression of the eye, postoperative visual loss seems to be a multifactorial problem with no consistent underlying mechanism [22, 24, 26–28]. Causes of central retinal artery occlusion include spontaneous thrombosis of the central retinal artery, talc and starch emboli, frequently seen in association with drug abuse, collagen vascular disease, and cardiac disease. The mechanism of ischemic optic neuropathy is thought to be profound and sustained hypotension, resulting in infarction of the optic nerve from lowered perfusion pressure [21].

Even though loss of vision after spine surgery is rare, when it occurs is a devastating complication. The prognosis for visual recovery from ischemic neuropathy and retinal artery occlusion is very poor, resulting in definitive blindness in the majority of the patients [21]. Complete recovery of vision is very rare and is observed only when the postoperative visual loss is partial [29]. This is a devastating complication, which should be discussed with the patient preoperatively, particularly with the high-risk patient [30], clarifying that the risk for posterior ischemic optic neuropathy is approximately 1 in 3,000 [31].

The position of the head should be flexion of the head only and not of the neck with respect to the trunk [2]. Whenever possible, traction should be applied to the head to straighten the physiological lordosis of the cervical spine, and the head should be pulled slightly forward [2]. This positioning has several advantages. Superficially, the skin folds that cross under the occiput will be stretched out. The interspinal and interlaminal spaces between Cl and the occiput and Cl and C2 will be opened out, facilitating surgery in these areas once dissection reaches these deeper regions [8].

Great care should be taken to avoid the following:

- Rotation of the head on the neck. Incorrect positioning of the head and of the headrest produces an unfavorable position of the head and neck on the trunk. This can disadvantage the surgeon in carrying out his procedure because of the inappropriate positioning. This is of particular importance in the occipito-cervical region where it can produce significant difficulties.
- Lateral displacement of the neck on the trunk, which would produce problems during surgery in the lower cervical spine.

The operative table should be in the reverse-Trendelenburg position to decrease pressure and hence the risk of bleeding at the operative site. Having prepared for the skin incision, the surgeon must orientate himself by identifying specific landmarks that will help to outline the approach. The incision should be midline to avoid poor repair and scarring. From above, the external occipital protuberance, which can be felt through the skin, and the spinous processes of C2 and C7 (the most prominent) may be identified [32, 33]. A line is drawn connecting these landmarks, which have been marked preoperatively. Bleeding during the approach can be minimized using local anesthetic with epinephrine. Local anesthetic should be injected starting at the spinous processes and proceeding laterally into the paravertebral tissues [8].

6.3 Anterior Approach: Precautions and Recommendation

Many approaches can be used for the anterior cervical spine, depending on the pathological process (i.e. low and high presternocleidomastoid approaches, retrosternocleidomastoid approach, transoral, transmandibular, and submandibular approach) (Table 6.2).

The patient is placed supine; the head is taped to a headrest to hold it in a fixed position. There should be slight hyperextension, but not excessive traction, since the latter will only produce tension in the soft tissues of the neck, which will be detrimental to the exposure and the dissection [2] (Fig. 6.3). The combination of traction and excessive hyperextension of the head will compact tissue planes, making separation not only more difficult, but also more dangerous because structures will be difficult to identify, and therefore greater

Table 6.2 Complications of the supine position

Complications	How to avoid them: tips and tricks
Compression of the bony prominences	Use appropriate padded supports across all the bony prominences
Stretch injuries to the brachial plexus	Avoid excessive traction on the arm
Peripheral nerve damage	Pad all bony prominences in correspondence to the peripheral nerve and appropriately position the limbs The wrist band must produce sufficient traction to arm, but it must avoid excessive compression to the wrist, which may cause damage to the median nerve Use a soft pad in correspondence to the elbow to avoid damage to the ulnar nerve
Fall of the lower extremities from the operative table	Fix legs and thighs to the table by straps
Fall of the gluteal region during graft harvesting	Use a pillow to support the gluteal region in preparation for graft harvesting from the iliac crest
Movements of the head during surgery	Criss-cross tapes to position the head firmly in the headrest
Difficult approach	Avoid the combination of traction and excessive hyperextension of the head, which will compact tissue planes, making separation more difficult and dangerous because structures will be difficult to identify
Injuries to the cervical spine during surgery	Use a strong and rigid fixation and support of the neck to assure a good counterbalance to any surgical force applied

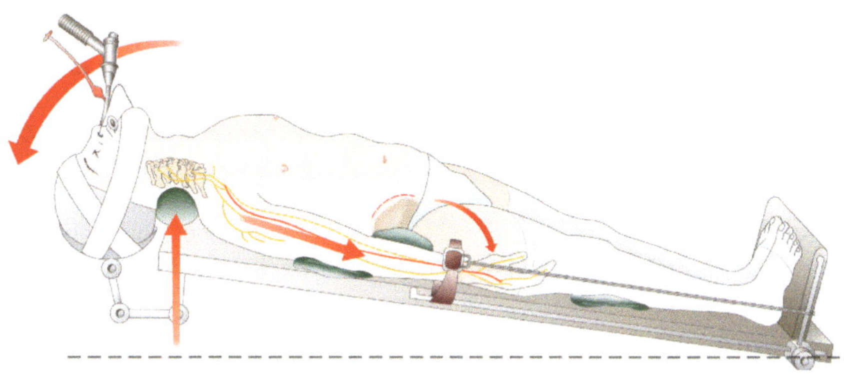

Fig. 6.3 The patient is placed in the anti-Trendelenburg position with a rigid support under the neck. The head is supported by a mobile and adjustable rest. Elastic bandages hold the head in position with slight hyperextension of the chin. The arm is subjected to traction to lower the shoulder

traction may be required. The laryngeal nerves may be at particular risk as a result of such positioning [8].

Rigid support is essential for the neck. The spinal processes should be well supported by a firm pillow. This will be particularly helpful in preventing complications when one is applying considerable force to the vertebral body (e.g. insertion of bony grafts and the use of Cloward's drill). In such cases, a strong and rigid fixation and support of the neck assures a good counterbalance to any surgical force applied [8].

We prefer a nasotracheal tube to an orotracheal tube, although both can be used [8]. It is imperative that a nasogastric tube be inserted to act as a marker for the pharynx and esophagus during dissection. The chin is taped to the bed and to the headrest, maintaining the slight hyperextension, which should be barely sufficient to stretch the skin of the neck. The arms should be extended with a wrist band that will produce sufficient traction to lower the shoulder, thereby permitting comfortable access to the patient [2, 8]. An excessive traction on the arm may cause excessive stretching of the roots of the brachial plexus, with postoperative stupor of the brachial plexus. The wrist band must produce sufficient traction to arm, but it must avoid excessive compression to the wrist, which may cause damage to the median nerve. In correspondence to the elbow, a soft pad is required to avoid damage to the ulnar nerve.

The gluteal region is supported by a pillow, towel, or sheet in preparation for graft harvesting from the iliac crest. The legs are well anchored to maintain stability on the surgical table. In fact, the patient should be in the reverse-Trendelenburg position. This position will not only produce lower pressure, but also favor venous drainage from the operative site in the neck [2, 8]. The patients must wear elastic stockings, as this position increases the venous pressure to the lower limbs.

Should the patient be in a halo jacket, the ring can be used to manipulate the head into the position of mild hyperextension; the head can then be anchored. Neuromonitoring is now the standard of care in all deformity surgery and when using spinal instrumentation. Monitoring should be initiated prior to start surgery, and continued until closure. With the patient awake, one applies the somatosensory evoked potential (SEP) electrodes preoperatively to obtain a baseline value, and a second baseline assessment is recorded once anesthesia has been induced. This is necessary because changes in the evoked potentials occur with induction of anesthesia. During the surgical maneuvers, it will be reassuring to have SEP monitoring, particularly when dealing with neural structures [2, 8].

6.4 Circumferential Approach: Precautions and Recommendation

Two types of circumferential approaches have been described. The combined approaches can be performed at the same surgical sitting, or can be performed at two stages (for example, the posterior approach can be performed first, and, after a variable length of time, the anterior approach is undertaken, or vice versa), depending on the type of lesion. In these instances, the surgical complications are the same to those reported for the single anterior and posterior approach. Great care should be taken when rolling the patient from the anterior to posterior position and vice versa, given the intrinsic instability of the lesion itself. Particular care has to be taken when positioning the patient in the lateral position (Fig. 6.4) (Table 6.3). The entire body lies on its side, completely on the table right up to the axilla. The shoulder and the arm should extend beyond the operating table. A wrist support holds the arm. An adjustable support holds the head in the lateral position (with or without halo traction) with the head adjusted to the same level as the shoulder. The upper arm is pulled toward the feet to lower the shoulder. The legs are well supported with a pillow between them. This position allows a simultaneous anterior presternocleiodomastoid approach and a posterior longitudinal approach along the spinal processes.

Potential complications of the lateral position may arise from compression of the axilla, excessive traction on the arm with stretching of the roots of the brachial plexus, compression of the median nerve at level of the wrist by the wrist band, and compression of the external popliteal branch of the sciatic nerve.

The simultaneous combined use of anterior and posterior approaches is undertaken in patients with tumors that require total or subtotal removal, and in patients with severe trauma, nonunion, or mal-union,

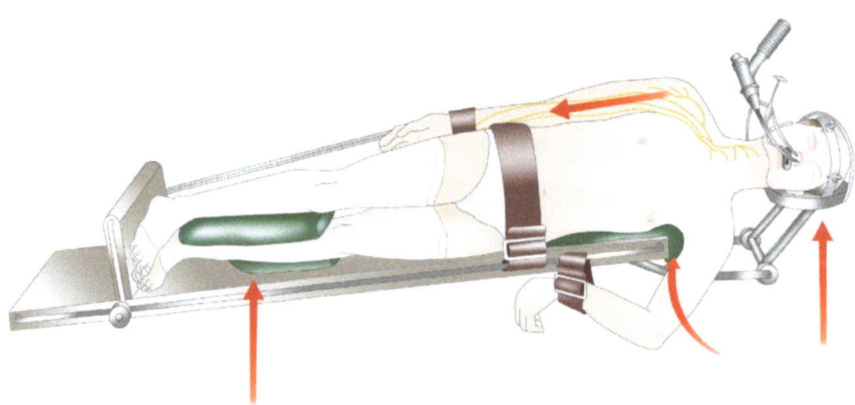

Fig. 6.4 Particular care has to be taken when positioning the patient in the lateral position. The entire body lies on its side, completely on the table right up to the axilla. The shoulder and the arm should extend beyond the operating table. A wrist support holds the arm. An adjustable support holds the head in the lateral position (with or without halo traction) with the head adjusted to the same level as the shoulder. The upper arm is pulled toward the feet to lower the shoulder. The legs are well supported with a pillow between them

Table 6.3 Complications of the lateral position

Complications	How to avoid them: Tips and tricks
Injuries to the brachial plexus	Use a soft pad to avoid compression to the axilla
Stretch injuries to the roots of the brachial plexus	Avoid excessive traction on the arm
Peripheral nerve damage	Pad all bony prominences in correspondence to the peripheral nerve and appropriately position the limbs The wrist band must produce sufficient traction to arm, but it must avoid excessive compression to the wrist, which may cause damage to the median nerve Use a soft pad in correspondence to the elbow to avoid damage to the ulnar nerve Use a soft pad in correspondence to the lateral aspect of the upper leg to avoid damage to the peroneal nerve
Compression of the bony prominences	Use appropriate padded supports across all the bony prominences
Fall of the lower extremities from the operative table	Fix legs and thighs to the table by straps

where both the anterior and posterior elements are involved. In patients with tumors, one can begin either from an anterior or a posterior approach. This initial approach is to begin the removal of the tumor and achieve stabilization [2, 8, 34]. Once this has been accomplished, the wound is completely closed. Conditions permitting, the patient is moved into the appropriate position for the second part of the combined approach. This second stage may also be deferred by several days if necessary [2, 8]. This strategy can be frequently applied in posttraumatic stenosis. In the presence of a recognized posterior lesion such as subluxation of the apophyseal joints, one may elect to begin from the back and surgically reduce the dislocation with fusion of the apophyseal joints [2, 8, 34].

There are no specific complications associated with the described methods using combined anterior and posterior approaches. Nevertheless, difficulties arise with patients in whom it becomes necessary to undertake a simultaneous anterior and posterior approach, to gain a simultaneous exposure of the anterior and posterior vertebral structures. A typical example of this is posttraumatic nonunion or mal-union, particularly in patients who have displaced vertebral bodies following a fracture subluxation, i.e. cases of subluxation of the apophyseal joints, especially neglected fracture subluxations, both of which have been consolidated in their position of displacement. Bony spurs and bony bridges will be formed, with calcification of the anterior longitudinal ligament [18, 35–37]. The bones are in a fixed position of malalignment of the apophyseal joints. Only after taking down the osseous buttresses and bridges of the anterior longitudinal ligament, the surgeon can reduce the fixed subluxation and restore the apophyseal joints to congruity. Obviously, neither the anterior nor the posterior approach alone will be sufficient to allow the surgeon to reduce such fixed dislocations. In these patients, the double approach must be used. The vertebral bodies must be freed and reduced with realignment of the walls of the bodies. This will restore the continuity and diameter of the vertebral canal. Obviously, this can be achieved only through a simultaneous combined approach [2, 8].

We prefer to perform this kind of surgery with the patient in the lateral position. In our experience, it is preferable to apply halo traction preoperatively. This provides postoperative immobilization and also helps in intraoperatively placing the head and neck [18, 35–37]. At all times, there must be fluoroscopic control. For monitoring cord function, to be warned if cord compression is produced by the maneuvering, we use SEP throughout the operation. During this procedure, the neck is entirely free and is basically held in suspension between the trunk and the head by the halo traction. Therefore, surgeons should be aware that they are maneuvering unsupported structures, and since they are devoid of any counterforce to the instrumentation. The use of chisels should be avoided and air drills should be used to remove osseous fragments and bone buttresses that obstruct reduction [18, 35–37].

As stated above, this approach has several difficulties, related to the difficult alignment of the cervical to be maintained, and the difficult position of the surgeon. For this reason, we prefer to perform circumferential approaches at two stages.

Core Messages

- Several complications have been reported as consequences of patient malpositioning during operative procedures to the cervical spine. Anterior, posterior, or combined approaches to the cervical spine determine different risks.
- In the anterior approach, rigid support is essential for the neck. The spinal processes should be well supported by a firm pillow. This will be particularly helpful in preventing complications when one is applying considerable force to the vertebral. A nasogastric tube can act as a marker for the pharynx and esophagus during dissection. The gluteal region must be supported by a pillow, towel, or sheet in preparation for graft harvesting from the iliac crest.
- The most common complications of the posterior approach are associated with positioning of the patient on the operating table, in addition to the surgical approach itself. The endotracheal anesthetic tube must be carefully anchored to the mouth to avoid loosening. The prone position commonly used in posterior spinal procedures may produce serious injury to the cornea and to the eye, including corneal abrasion (the most common ophthalmologic injury), and blindness as the result of posterior ischemic optic neuropathy, central retinal artery occlusion, or occipital cortical infarct or cortical blindness. Bleeding during the approach can be minimized using local anesthetic with epinephrine.
- Specific complications of the use of the Mayfield head clamp include breakage of Mayfield head rest, cranial fracture, epidural hematoma, and venous air embolism. The potential for venous air embolism exists any time the surgical wound is above the level of heart producing a subatmospheric pressure in the open veins. The head-fixating devices should be removed in the supine position to avoid venous air embolism and monitoring for venous air embolism should be performed throughout the entire intraoperative period until all potential sites for air entry into the circulation have been occluded.
- In the circumferential approach in lateral position, complications may arise from compression of the axilla, excessive traction on the arm with stretching of the roots of the brachial plexus, compression of the median nerve at level of the wrist by the wrist band, compression of the external popliteal branch of the sciatic nerve.

References

1. Callahan RA, Brown MD (1981) Positioning techniques in spinal surgery. Clin Orthop Relat Res 154:22–26
2. Denaro V, Denaro L, Gulino G et al (1998) Complicanze nella chirurgia cervicale. Giornale Italiano di Ortopedia e Traumatologia 24:681–688
3. Roy-Camille R, Judet TH, Saillant G, et al (1981) Tumeurs du rachis. Techniques chirugucales, Orthopedie. Encycl Med Chir Paris 44165:4.06.04
4. Alvine FG, Schurrer ME (1987) Postoperative ulnar-nerve palsy. Are there predisposing factors? J Bone Joint Surg Am 69:255–259
5. Kochilas X, Bibas A, Xenellis J et al (2008) Surgical anatomy of the external branch of the superior laryngeal nerve and its clinical significance in head and neck surgery. Clin Anat 21:99–105
6. Lange U, Bastian L, Muller CW et al (2007) How to prevent overlooking cervical spine injuries: pitfalls in spinal diagnostics. Arch Orthop Trauma Surg 127:953–958
7. Neal JM, Moore JM, Kopacz DJ et al (1998) Quantitative analysis of respiratory, motor, and sensory function after supraclavicular block. Anesth Analg 86:1239–1244
8. Denaro V (1991) Stenosis of the cervical spine. Springer, Berlin
9. Perez-Cruet MJ, Fessler RG, Perin NI (2002) Review: complications of minimally invasive spinal surgery. Neurosurgery 51:S26–S36
10. Bhardwaj A, Long DM, Ducker TB et al (2001) Neurologic deficits after cervical laminectomy in the prone position. J Neurosurg Anesthesiol 13:314–319
11. Aprile I, Caliandro P, Pazzaglia C et al (2004) Re: Yi HJ, Oh SH, Hong HJ, Lee KS. Common peroneal nerve palsy as a complication of anterior cervical operation: A case report. Surg Neurol 61:379–383. Surg Neurol 62:572; author reply 572–573
12. Taira T, Tanikawa T (1992) Breakage of Mayfield head rest. J Neurosurg 77:160–161
13. Baerts WD, de Lange JJ, Booij LH et al (1984) Complications of the Mayfield skull clamp. Anesthesiology 61:460–461
14. De Lange JJ, Baerts WD, Booij LH (1984) Air embolism due to the Mayfield skull clamp. Acta Anaesthesiol Belg 35:237–241

15. Grinberg F, Slaughter TF, McGrath BJ (1995) Probable venous air embolism associated with removal of the Mayfield skull clamp. Anesth Analg 80:1049–1050
16. Pang D (1982) Air embolism associated with wounds from a pin-type head-holder. Case report. J Neurosurg 57:710–713
17. Prabhakar H, Ali Z, Bhagat H (2008) Venous air embolism arising after removal of Mayfield skull clamp. J Neurosurg Anesthesiol 20:158–159
18. Boni M, Cherubino P, Denaro V (1983) The surgical treatment of fractures of the cervical spine. Ital J Orthop Traumatol 9(Suppl):107–126
19. Silvani V, Brambilla G, Rainoldi F et al (1987) Vertebral osteomyelitis with chronic cervical extradural abscess in a heroin addict. Neurochirurgia (Stuttg) 30:91–94
20. Myers MA, Hamilton SR, Bogosian AJ et al (1997) Visual loss as a complication of spine surgery. A review of 37 cases. Spine 22:1325–1329
21. Stambough JL, Dolan D, Werner R et al (2007) Ophthalmologic complications associated with prone positioning in spine surgery. J Am Acad Orthop Surg 15:156–165
22. Delattre O, Thoreux P, Liverneaux P et al (2007) Spinal surgery and ophthalmic complications: a French survey with review of 17 cases. J Spinal Disord Tech 20:302–307
23. American Society of Anesthesiologists (2006) Practice advisory for perioperative visual loss associated with spine surgery: a report by the American Society of Anesthesiologists Task Force on Perioperative Blindness. Anesthesiology 104:1319–1328
24. Manfredini M, Ferrante R, Gildone A et al (2000) Unilateral blindness as a complication of intraoperative positioning for cervical spinal surgery. J Spinal Disord 13:271–272
25. Yanagidate F, Dohi S (2003) Corneal abrasion after the wake-up test in spinal surgery. J Anesth 17:211–212
26. Hollenhorst RW, Svien HJ, Benoit CF (1954) Unilateral blindness occurring during anesthesia for neurosurgical operations. AMA Arch Ophthalmol 52:819–830
27. Kasodekar VB, Chen JL (2006) Monocular blindness: a complication of intraoperative positioning in posterior cervical spine surgery. Singapore Med J 47:631–633
28. Wolfe SW, Lospinuso MF, Burke SW (1992) Unilateral blindness as a complication of patient positioning for spinal surgery. A case report. Spine 17:600–605
29. Stevens WR, Glazer PA, Kelley SD et al (1997) Ophthalmic complications after spinal surgery. Spine 22:1319–1324
30. Chang SH, Miller NR (2005) The incidence of vision loss due to perioperative ischemic optic neuropathy associated with spine surgery: the Johns Hopkins hospital experience. Spine 30:1299–1302
31. Lee AG (1995) Ischemic optic neuropathy following lumbar spine surgery. Case report. J Neurosurg 83:348–349
32. D'Alpa F, Scandurra L, Savuto R et al (1989) Pre-, intra- and postoperative somatosensory evoked potentials in cervical vertebral and spinal cord injuries. Minerva Anestesiol 55:115–118
33. Mangiameli S, Denaro V, Cantarella G et al (1989) Moderated normovolemic hemodilution in surgery of the cervical rachis. Minerva Anestesiol 55:123–124
34. Denaro V, Gulino G, Papapietro N et al (1998) Treatment of metastases of the cervical spine. Chir Organi Mov 83: 127–137
35. Boni M, Denaro V (1982) The cervical stenosis syndrome with a review of 83 patients treated by operation. Int Orthop 6:185–195
36. Boni M, Denaro V (1982) Surgical treatment of cervical arthrosis. Follow-up review (2–13 years) of the 1st 100 cases operated on by anterior approach. Rev Chir Orthop Reparatrice Appar Mot 68:269–280
37. Boni M, Denaro V (1980) Surgical treatment of traumatic lesions of the middle and lower cervical spine (C3–C7). Ital J Orthop Traumatol 6:305–320

Section III

Complications of Surgical Approaches

Complications Related to Anterior Approaches

7

Luca Denaro, Domenico D'Avella, Umile Giuseppe Longo, and Vincenzo Denaro

Contents

L. Denaro (✉)
Department of Neuroscience, University of Padua, Via Giustiniani 5, 35128 Padua, Italy
e-mail: lucadenaro@hotmail.com

7.1 Transoral Approach

Transoral surgery is a procedure performed through the mouth to gain midline access from the sphenoid sinus rostrally to the third cervical vertebral body caudally [1], and it is particularly useful for lesions at the anterior aspect of the craniocervical junction [2, 3].

It has been used with varying degrees of success by numerous authors over the past century. The transoral approach, first described by Kanaval in 1919 [4] to remove a bullet locked between atlas and the base of the skull, was successively used by Scoville and Sherman in 1951 [5] for the removal of the odontoid process in basilar impression. Southwick and Robinson [6] and Mosberg and Lippman [7] described the transoral treatment of lesions of the second cervical vertebra.

Fang and Ong in 1962 [8] used the transoral approach in the management of six patients with traumatic Cl–C2 instability and tuberculosis of the upper cervical spine. They first emphasized the intra- and postoperative complications of this approach. Four of the six patients became infected and one of them died from infection following damage to the vertebral vessels. Modifications of the transoral approach were proposed by Greenberg in 1968 [9], Menezes 1980 [10], and Crockard in 1985 [2]. Because of the initial records of complications associated with this approach (infections, sepsis, unacceptable patient morbidity and mortality, cerebrospinal fluid leakage, limited exposure, and inappropriate instrumentation) [11–14], there was a flurry of interest in extra-pharyngeal approaches, which provided greater exposure and greater flexibility in the choice of surgery that could be performed [15, 16]. Despite the initial negative experiences, after the introduction of the operating microscope, of operative magnification and microinstrumentation [17], the improvement of preoperative

L. Denaro et al. (eds.), *Pitfalls in Cervical Spine Surgery*,
DOI: 10.1007/978-3-540-85019-9_7, © Springer-Verlag Berlin Heidelberg 2010

imaging with more definite localization of pathology [18], availability of antibiotics, and of new devices and techniques to manage dural tears, the transoral approach has gained its well-deserved place in the orthopedic armamentarium [19]. The operative microscope is perhaps the most necessary surgical tool, and the air drill, ultrasonic aspirator, and laser are useful adjuncts. Moreover, the introduction of lumboperitoneal shunting to reduce the incidence of a cerebrospinal fluid leak has been significant [20].

The transoral approach is the most direct midline approach to the anterior arch of the atlas, the base of the odontoid process, the body of the axis, the atlanto-axial articulation to the C2–C3 disk, and the more cranial portion of the body of C3 [21]. The posterior wall of the pharynx is the only structure present in front of the vertebral plane. It is composed of mucosa, a thin layer of constrictor muscles, and the buccal fascia, sits immediately in front of the anterior longitudinal ligament. Because of its softness and thinness, it allows easy access to the finger of the surgeon, which can easily palpate the arch of the atlas and its anterior tubercle (to which the long muscles of the neck are inserted), the body of the axis, and the C2–C3 intervertebral space (where the disk usually bulges anteriorly from the bodies) [22]. The surgical key to the ventral craniocervical junction is the tubercle and the arch of the atlas [1].

Today, the transoral approach is considered particularly useful to manage patients with midline pathologies of the craniovertebral junction, as malformations, tumors, and trauma [23]. The transoral approach has been described in the surgical management of a variety of extra- and intradural lesions [1, 2, 11, 15, 20, 24–34], including rheumatoid disease, glomus tumors, chordomas, meningiomas, schwannomas, platybasia, fractures, and metastasis [9, 20, 24, 33, 35–38].

The most important principle to avoid the reported complications with the transoral approach is patient selection. Moreover, modifications of the surgical technique make the approach simpler and avoid extended operating time [22]. Obviously, in patients with wider mouth opening and good neck extension, surgery will be easier than in patients with stiff neck and poor mouth opening [1]. The instruments cannot be placed in the mouth if the interdental distance is <25 mm [20].

The transoral approach has gained popularity with improved understanding of the biomechanics of the craniovertebral anatomy. However, because of the inherently deep and narrow surgical corridor, which is further restricted by the essential use of retractors, the extent of resection and medullary decompression may be difficult to visualize intraoperatively [18]. For this reason, intraoperative MR imaging systems have been used to monitor the extension of the resection in patients with lesions of the craniocervical junction [18], as well as navigated systems [39].

The most frequent complications encountered during the transoral approach are:

- Soft tissue injuries (lesion of tongue, soft palate, and pharynx)
- Neural injuries and cerebrospinal fluid leakage
- Injuries of the vertebral artery (especially when surgery is performed at level of the atlanto-axial joints)
- Injuries to the posterior wall of the pharynx (i.e., because of loosening of instrumentations, which can migrate anteriorly)
- Postsurgical infection (especially by bacteria of the mouth)
- Dental lesions

7.1.1 Surgical Technique

Prophylactic antibiotics are administered. In patients with a previous history of infections, or in patients susceptible to infections, a careful assessment of the bacterial flora of the pharynx is required to develop an appropriate preoperative antibiotic program [40]. Dental sepsis may be the site of postoperative septicemia. Hence, management of dental disorders should be performed preoperatively [20]. Moreover, many rheumatoid patients have poor dentition and hence a gum guard should be fashioned to fit the individual teeth to avoid damage by placement of the transoral retractor [20]. In patients with osteogenesis imperfecta, the oral cavity may present particular problems [20, 41, 42].

The patient is placed supine on the operating table. The head is in slight hyperextension and is held in position by an elastic band attached to the table. The neck is supported by a soft pad. If the patient is in a halo jacket, the ring can be used to manipulate the head into the position of mild hyperextension. The operating table is placed in the Trendelenburg position, to obtain better visibility of the operative site and better control of bleeding, as any drainage remains in the operative

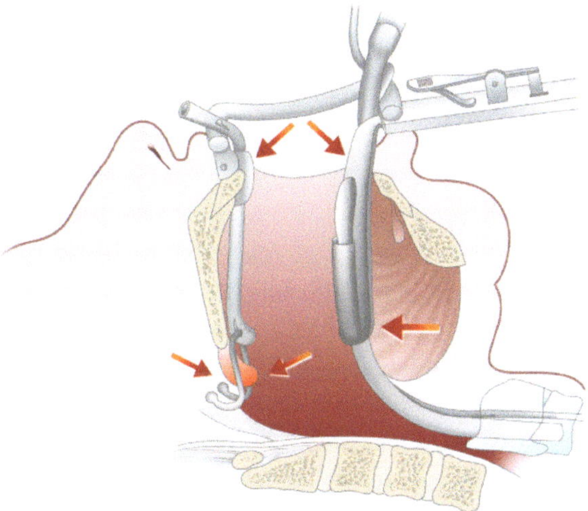

Fig. 7.1 The semi-rigid orotracheal tube for anesthesia is out of the operative field, and it is protected by the retractor itself. The instrument to raise the uvula is constructed with a double hook with blunted ends that latches onto and raises retracting the soft palate. An elastic band maintains the retraction on this specially designed hook and can be anchored onto the superior arm of the oral retractor. Arrows indicate the correct positioning of the retractor

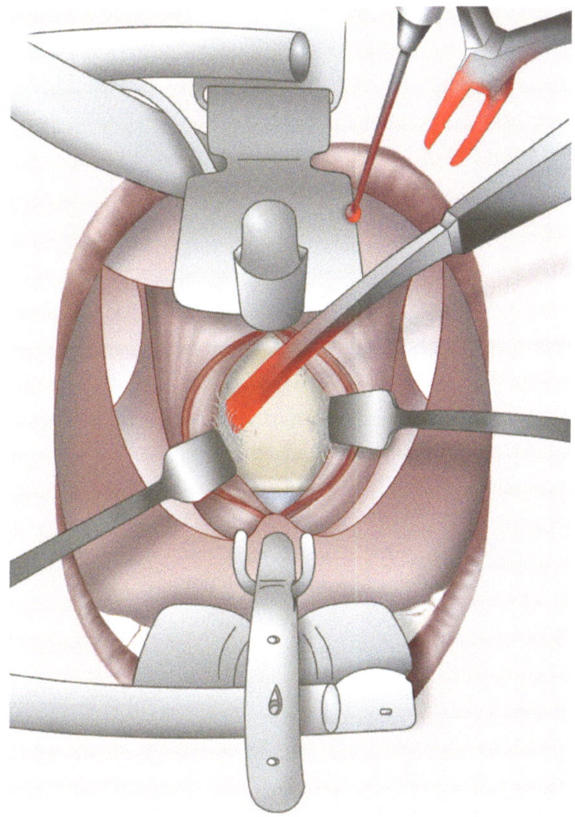

Fig 7.2 Any bleeding is controlled and gently packed with surgical

site and does not lie caudally [21]. Even though tracheostomy has been proposed by some authors [9, 10, 22, 43–45], nasotracheal intubation has been used for anesthesia in patients undergoing transoral approach. Crockard stated that tracheostomy is not required in the majority of patients [2], and a nasotracheal armored airway (Mallinckrodt) provides an adequate airway. It can be retracted out of the surgical field without compromise to its lumen [2].

The orally introduced tube does not hinder the surgeon [46], and respiratory disorders, caused by swelling of the pharyngeal soft tissue were not observed postoperatively. On the contrary, the risk of infection could be raised by the accumulation of secretion in tracheostomized patients [46].

We prefer to use transoral intubation, with the reinforced tube placed in the groove of the tongue retractor. This avoids the tube to cross the operative field and the necessity to repeatedly retract the tube when surgery is performed at level of the atlanto-axial joints.

To obtain adequate illumination of the operative site, it is mandatory to use a head lamp, which can shine directly into the pharynx and illuminate the depths of the operative site.

After preoperative cleansing, the upper teeth are protected and a tongue retractor with appropriate groove to hold the transoral intubation tube is secured over the mandible and tongue (Fig. 7.1) [47]. The base of the tongue, the pharynx, and soft palate can be displaced with packing. A special type of retractor is used to avoid the problems associated with self-retaining retractors (i.e., decreasing of the amount of light that reaches the depths of the operative site, and interference with access to the operative site through the mouth).

This retractor has a double hook with tapered tips, and as it is inserted below the soft palate, it retracts it posteriorly. The soft palate and the uvula commonly are not injured by the retractor, which is anchored externally with only sufficient tension to maintain it in the position desired by the surgeon. Occasionally, to obtain better exposure to the operative field, we have used suture retraction of the uvula and soft palate, and passed these sutures out through the nose and secure them externally. They must be used with great care since excessive traction will tear the tissues, leading to loss of retraction, of exposure, and to tissue damage. To reach the craniocervical junction and lower clivus without a soft palate split, a Jacques catheter passed nasally and sutured close to the uvula, allowing retraction of the soft palate into the nasopharynx, can be also used [48].

During a simple transoral procedure, retraction of the oropharyngeal structures allows access to the midline. Elevation of the soft palate will expose the arch of C1 and with some head extension the rim of the foramen magnum. Inferiorly, C2–C3 intervertebral space may be visualized [1].

To achieve extensive exposure to reach the base of the skull and the clivus, sometimes it is necessary to divide the soft palate and extend the exposure to the hard palate, which can be resected posteriorly to obtain unobstructed access to the clivus. When resection of the hard palate is performed, at the end of the procedure the portion of the hard palate removed is regrafted back into position. When it is necessary to operate on the clivus, transpalatal extension into the soft or the hard palate will provide good access to the lower third of the clivus [49]. To flush the operative site, a soft tube is placed on the lateral aspect of the operative field [29].

Once the area is prepared and retractors are in place, a midline incision is made in the posterior pharyngeal wall, cutting the full thickness of the mucosa right down to the anterior longitudinal ligament of the spine. Other authors prefer to use an H-shaped incision [50] or U-shaped incision [40].

Hemostasis must be carefully obtained immediately. Lateral widening of the incision is possible [47]. Any bleeding is controlled and gently packed with Surgicel (Johnson & Johnson Medical, Arlington, Texas) (Fig. 7.2). Self-retaining retractors tend to block access to the operative site, and for this reason we prefer to use silk sutures that evert the pharyngeal margins and which can be anchored to the lateral wall on the lateral pillars [29]. The anterior longitudinal ligament can be inspected and split longitudinally, obtaining access to the anterior surface of the vertebrae. At this point, surgery can be performed. At the end of the procedure, rarely drainage is necessary. We recommend the use of a drain when a large cavity has been produced, with incomplete debridment, or if there is possible oozing of blood despite overall adequate hemostasis [51]. In these patients, the drain is fixed through sutures that are passed to the outside via the nose and anchored externally.

Care must be taken to avoid that large grafts protrude beyond the limits of the host bone. If this is the case, the graft will make difficult the closure of soft tissues, with a tendency to produce dehiscence of tissue, and postoperative swallowing dysfunction. Closure of the pharyngeal wall should be full thickness with individual sutures, preferably made of reabsorbable material. When using this approach, there may be considerable difficulty in suturing an incision that reaches the C3 vertebral level or below. The pharyngeal wall is particularly thin in this lower part, and this can determine significant difficulties in obtaining adequate closure. If widely separated surgical margins are left in the pharyngeal wall, it may be necessary to release the lateral portions of the pharynx to permit approximation of the wound immediately. In clinical practice, if the underlying bony structure is intact, the surgeon can obtain adequate healing even if the surgical edges are not perfectly approximated and sutured. After the packing has been removed, a final rinse is performed to allow an accurate and complete inspection of the area for hemostasis. At this point, a nasogastric tube is introduced under direct vision and left in place for at least 24 h [51, 52] to prevent postoperative regurgitation of gastric contents, which might compromise the pharyngeal wound, and also cause pneumonia. Preoperative hyosine and postoperative antiemetics also reduce this possibility [2].

Alimentary abstinence after transoral surgery has been recommended for [44] 5–10 days [53]. According to other authors [46], we start oral nutrition with liquid food some days after the operation. A gastric tube inserted for a longer time will cause mucosal lesions by chronic pressure [46].

7.1.2 Complications

The transoral approach to upper cervical region is a direct and relatively safe route for high cervical and base of skull pathology [54]. It is avascular, with no intervening cranial nerves. For these reasons, the transoral approach is attractive and, with appropriate instruments (Crockard™ Transoral Instrument Set, Codman, Johnson and Johnson), the procedure is relatively straightforward, allowing an excellent view of the anterior cervical spine, from the clivus to the superior portion of the vertebral body of C3 [11, 25, 30–32, 55].

Table 7.1 Complications of the transoral approach

Complications	How to avoid them: Tips and tricks
Soft tissue injuries	Unskilled use of retractors or other instruments may injure soft tissues (from small contusions to very extensive lacerations) Avoid to catch the tongue between retractor and teeth
Neural injuries and cerebrospinal fluid leakage	Use appropriate micro-instrumentation and operating microscope to minimize neural injuries Cerebrospinalfluid leaks during transoral approach can have fatal consequences Insert a lumbar drainage (10–20 mL/h) preoperatively, and maintained for up to 5 days postoperatively to reduce the hydrostatic pressure on the wound and to remove blood and surgical debris In the presence of a large dural defect, covert the lumbar drainage to a lumbo-peritoneal shunt to maintain a low pressure for up to a month postoperatively
Injuries of the vertebral artery	Be cognizant, at every moment during surgery, of the position of the vertebral artery in relation to the planned bony resection
Dental lesions	Avoid unskilled use of retractors
Postsurgical infection (especially by bacteria of the mouth)	A careful assessment of the bacterial flora of the pharynx is required to develop an appropriate preoperative antibiotic program

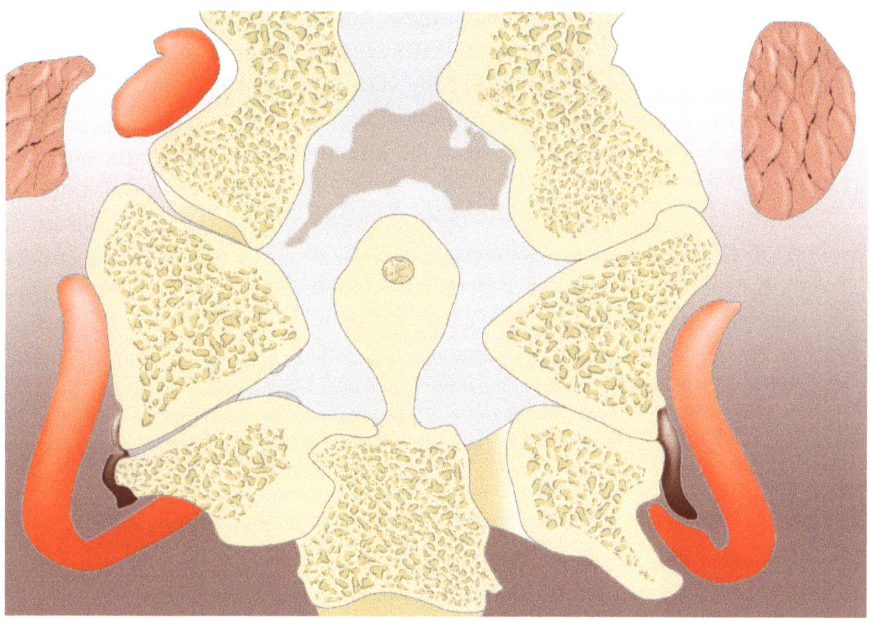

Fig 7.3 At level of the arch of the atlas, the vertebral artery is 24 mm from the midline; at level of the C2–C3 intervertebral space and of the anterior rim of the foramen magnum, it is 11 mm from the midline

Many of the initial described complications with this approach have resulted from the inappropriate selection of the patient. Most surgical procedures using transoral approach have high mortality, which reflects the severity of the underlying disease process [51, 52]. The main disadvantages are low visibility, complex retraction of the oropharyngeal structures, and the depth at which surgery is performed (10–15 cm from the dental margin) (Table 7.1).

7.1.2.1 Intraoperative Complications

Soft Tissue Injury

The risk of soft tissue injury is the most common complication of this route. The unskilled use of retractors or other instruments may injure the soft tissues including the tongue, the soft palate, and the lateral columns of the pharynx. These injuries range from small contusions to very extensive lacerations [51]. It is important to avoid to catch the tongue between retractor and teeth. The entire area can be coated liberally pre- and postoperatively in 1% hydrocortisone ointment [20].

Injuries to the vertebral artery are the most serious vascular complications, as the resulting hemorrhage is often massive and hard to control. At this level, the artery is inaccessible for suturing, and can be only clamped. The acute ischemia produced in the basilar circulation may be lethal. The surgeon must be cognizant of the position of the vertebral artery in relation to the planned bony resection [56]. The vertebral arteries are at least 11 mm away from the midline. At level of the arch of the atlas, the vertebral artery is 24 mm from the midline; at level of the C2–C3 intervertebral space and of the anterior rim of the foramen magnum, it is 11 mm from the midline (Fig. 7.3) [1]. Moreover, midline clival lesions distort neurovascular structures around their lateral boundaries [20]. A preoperative angio MRI is helpful to assess any anatomic variations of the vertebral artery. Care must be taken in particular when dissection is performed in correspondence to the atlanto-axial joints.

When vertebral artery is injured during surgery, packing off the bleeding with Gelfoam (Pharmacia & Upjohn, Kalamazoo, MI) and intraoperative or immediate postoperative angiography to evaluate the vessel with successive endovascular obliteration has been proposed [21, 56].

Neural Injury

Neural injuries may occur as a consequence of the deep surgical field and the difficulty in visualizing tissues, and obtaining complete hemostasis [47]. Lesions of the dura mater may produce cerebrospinal fluid fistulae, which must be sutured. The area should then be covered with a fibrin paste [28]. It is fortunate that the tentorial membrane and the posterior longitudinal ligament provide a fairly solid wall that protects the dura mater from inadvertent injury [51]. In patients with metastasis, involvement of this ligamentous barrier weakens it, making it particularly susceptible to penetration by instruments and leading to a greater risk of injury to the dura mater and spinal cord. For these reasons, the operating microscope is particularly useful [51].

Cerebrospinal fluid leaks during transoral approach have potentially fatal consequences [20]. A lumbar drainage (10–20 mL/h) is inserted preoperatively (it can be difficult to position it after CSF escapes) [20], and maintained for up to 5 days postoperatively to reduce the hydrostatic pressure on the wound and to remove blood and surgical debris [2, 48]. In the presence of a large dural defect, the lumbar drainage is converted to a lumboperitoneal shunt to maintain a low pressure for up to a month postoperatively. Meningitis, caused by oral bacteria invading the cerebrospinal fluid, and death have been reported with this complication [57].

Osseous Injury

Severe trauma or extensive tumor destruction can determine both instability and deformity. Through this approach, massive grafts cannot be adequately anchored and cannot be adequately incorporated. Internal fixation can be inadequately placed, insufficiently anchored, or protrude into the pharynx because of the technical difficulty of operating in such a deep and difficult field [21, 51, 52]. Crockard and Johnston [20] reported a low rate of fusion at the donor site and elevated morbidity at the donor site in 255 rheumatoid patients recruited in a prospective study. For this reason, they did not recommend bone graft in rheumatoid patients.

7.1.2.2 Postoperative Complications

Soft Tissues Injury

Postoperative edema and swelling may be severe enough to require tracheostomy. A hematoma in this area may become secondarily infected and lead to deeper infections that extend throughout the operative site and the spine and produce esophageal and tracheal fistulas. The infection may spread to the mediastinum. The consequent scarring and adhesions that occur in the pharyngeal wall may produce severe dysphagia. Among the vascular injuries, thrombosis of the medullary artery may produce paresis, while, if it involves the vertebral artery, it may produce cerebral damage [21, 51, 52].

Pharyngeal wound dehiscence and velopalatine incompetence have been also reported, the latter as a consequence occurred 3–6 months after the index surgery, where the palate had been split, secondary to fibrosis of the soft palate or in the pharyngeal wall [19, 22, 58].

Neural Injury

Injury to the neural tissues, particularly when resulting in thrombosis of the medullary artery, may produce paresis, while if it involves the vertebral artery, it may produce vertebral damage. Breakdown of the surgical site may lead to cerebrospinal fluid fistulas and eventually to life-threatening meningitis.

Osseous Injury

Postoperative instability should be always evaluated pre- and postoperatively [20]. If postoperative immobilization is insufficient, disruption of the operative site may lead to instability. If the surgical site becomes infected, this may lead to osteomyelitis with subsequent loosening and displacement of the graft.

Postoperative Infection

The incidence of infection has been high in some reported series using the transoral approach, but this can be reduced by gentle handling of the tissues and the use of an operating microscope and appropriate antibiotic cover [26]. To date, few studies have specifically addressed oropharyngeal morbidity using the transoral approach. The risk of infection was found higher in patients with tetraparesis, tracheostomy, and disorders of breathing and swallowing [46]. Inadequate care for preparation of surgical field has been indicated as an important point in sepsis after transoral surgery [20]. Crockard and Johnston [20] in one of the largest series available in literature attributed two deaths to recurrent wound abscesses and systemic sepsis. Merwing et al. [50] reported on 16 consecutive patients requiring exposure from clivus through C3 for pathology of the upper cervical spine. They found no deaths, wound breakdowns, infections, or persistent cerebrospinal fluid leakage. In no patient, they divided the mandible, tongue, soft palate, or uvula. Bonney and Williams [43] reported on 16 patients in whom transoral surgery was performed at the upper cervical spine for operative decompression and stabilization. Three patients had impaired posterior pharyngeal wall healing. Menezes and Van Gilder [22] reported on 72 patients who underwent a transoral approach to correct ventral irreducible compression of the cervicomedullary junction. In that series, there was one pharyngeal wound infection, requiring successive drainage. Louis [59] reported on a series of 80 patients who underwent transoral surgery for pathology of the upper cervical spine with a minimum follow-up of 2 years. Four pharyngeal wound infections were reported. Menezes et al. [10] reported on one patient with late sepsis and death after transoral odontoid resection and C1–C2 occiput fusion in a series of 17 patients. A higher rate of postoperative complications were found in patients who underwent a soft palate splint when compared with patients who did not undergo the soft palate splint [35, 40]. Crockard stated that splitting of the soft palate is not required for lesions below the foramen magnum [2]. When localization of pathology is higher, a Le Fort I down fracture or extend maxillotomy may be preferred [27, 49, 60]

7.2 Transmandibular Approach

The transmandibular approach is a direct, but rather disconcerting approach, which requires splitting of the lower lip, the mandible, the tongue, the floor of the mouth, the epiglottis, and the posterior pharynx down to, but not including, the hyoid bone. Transection of the hyoid bone can be added to achieve even greater exposure (transhyoid pharyngotomy).

7.2.1 Complications

This approach is quite aggressive and subject to significant postoperative difficulties, including:

1. Dental malocclusion, which may result from minimal asymmetry in the realignment of the transected mandible.
2. Possible loss of both motility and sensation in the tongue, partly because of scarring in the tongue

itself or through the frenulum. In addition, scarring may produce occlusion of the openings of the salivary glands, which may in turn produce cystic distension of ducts (in the manner of ranulae).

3. Scarring of the vestibular mucosa along the surface of the lip, which may produce deformity that will interfere with lip function.

In view of the above complications, this is not a popular approach. It is known to be a difficult approach that seldom provides any advantage over the direct transoral path or even the anterolateral retropharyngeal approaches, which are much more popular [28].

7.3 Submandibular Approach

Several extra-pharyngeal transvisceral approaches have been described. These follow the cutaneous and visceral planes in the submandibular region [23]. One of these is an approach above the hyoid bone, and another between the hyoid bone and the larynx. The suprahyoid approach reaches the spine anteriorly along a pathway that begins with a horizontal skin incision in the superficial cervical fascia and the hyoid muscles (mylohyoid and geniohyoid). After the skin incision, the superficial veins (anterior jugular) must be tied. The hypoglottis must be protected, while the tongue and the floor of the mouth are retracted upwards to allow access to the pharyngeal space. The posterior wall of the pharynx is opened longitudinally allowing the surgeon to reach the skeletal tissues. The subhyoid approach begins with a transverse cutaneous incision and crosses the subhyoid muscle and the interhyoid membrane. This exposes the pharynx, which is opened at first anteriorly and then posteriorly to obtain access to the bone [34].

7.3.1 Complications

The submandibular approach is mentioned for the sake of completion. It had serious complications and high potential for iatrogenic injury. The consequences include speech difficulties because of laryngeal injury, and difficulties in breathing and swallowing. In our experience, this approach has been totally supplanted by the extravisceral retropharyngeal approaches [47].

Core Messages. Take home messages

- The transoral approach provides direct access to the craniovertebral junction.
- The most frequent complications encountered during this approach include soft tissue injuries, neural injuries and cerebrospinal fluid leakage, injuries of the vertebral artery, injuries to the posterior wall of the pharynx, and postsurgical infection.
- If the patient has a history of previous infection, or is known to be susceptible to infections, undertake a careful assessment of the bacterial flora of the pharynx and to develop an appropriate preoperative antibiotic program.
- Use head lamp to shine directly into the pharynx and illuminate the depths of the operative site. Use retractor with a double hook with tapered tip to retract the soft palate to avoid the problems associated with self-retaining retractors, which may decrease the amount of light.
- To achieve sufficient exposure to reach the base of the skull and the clivus, the soft palate may be split longitudinally, and the hard palate may even be resected posteriorly to obtain unobstructed access to the clivus.
- The unskilled use of retractors or other instruments may injure the soft tissues including the tongue, the soft palate, and the lateral columns of the pharynx.
- Use a curette, spoon, or a clamp to remove distant fragment, which may cause injury to the vertebral artery. At this level, the artery is inaccessible for suturing, and can be only clamped.
- The resulting hemorrhage is often massive and hard to control. The acute ischemia produced in the basilar circulation may be lethal.
- Lesions of the dura mater may produce cerebrospinal fluid fistulae, which must be sutured. The area should then be covered with a fibrin paste.
- Avoid large grafts to protrude beyond the limits of the host bone.
- Massive grafts cannot be adequately anchored and cannot be adequately incorporated. Internal fixation can be inadequately placed, insufficiently anchored, or protrudes into the pharynx because of the technical difficulty of operating in such a deep and difficult field.

- Postoperative edema and swelling may be severe enough to require tracheostomy.
- A hematoma in this area may become secondarily infected and lead to deeper infections that extend throughout the operative site and the spine and produce esophageal and tracheal fistulas.
- Halo traction is essential to avoid motion and loosening of grafts or implants.
- The transmandibular approach is quite aggressive and can determine significant postoperative difficulties, including dental malocclusion, scarring of the vestibular mucosa along the surface of the lip, which may produce deformity that will interfere with lip function, and possible loss of both motility and sensation in the tongue. Scarring may produce occlusion of the openings of the salivary glands, which may in turn produce cystic distension of ducts (in the manner of ranulae).
- The submandibular approach has serious complications and high potential for iatrogenic injury, including laryngeal injury, and difficulties in breathing and swallowing.

References

1. Crockard HA (1995) Transoral surgery: some lessons learned. Br J Neurosurg 9:283–293
2. Crockard HA (1985) The transoral approach to the base of the brain and upper cervical cord. Ann R Coll Surg Engl 67:321–325
3. Crockard HA (1991) Ventral approaches to the upper cervical spine. Orthopade 20:140–146
4. Kanavel AB (1919) Bullet locked between atlas and the base of the skull: technique for removal through the mouth. Surg Clin 1:361–366
5. Scoville WB, Sherman IJ (1951) Platybasia, report of 10 cases with comments on familial tendency, a special diagnostic sign, and the end results of operation. Ann Surg 133:496–502
6. Southwick WO, Robinson RA (1957) Surgical approaches to the vertebral bodies in the cervical and lumbar regions. J Bone Joint Surg Am 39-A:631–644
7. Mosberg WH Jr, Lippman EM (1960) Anterior approach to the cervical vertebral bodies. Bull Sch Med Univ Md 45:10–17
8. Fang HSY, Ong GB (1962) Direct anterior approach to the upper cervical spine. J Bone joint Surg Am 44-A: 1588–1604
9. Greenberg AD, Scoville WB, Davey LM (1968) Transoral decompression of atlanto-axial dislocation due to odontoid hypoplasia. Report of two cases. J Neurosurg 28:266–269
10. Menezes AH, VanGilder JC, Graf CJ et al (1980) Craniocervical abnormalities. A comprehensive surgical approach. J Neurosurg 53:444–455
11. Crockard HA, Pozo JL, Ransford AO et al (1986) Transoral decompression and posterior fusion for rheumatoid atlanto-axial subluxation. J Bone Joint Surg Br 68:350–356
12. Di Lorenzo N, Fortuna A, Guidetti B (1982) Craniovertebral junction malformations. Clinicoradiological findings, long-term results, and surgical indications in 63 cases. J Neurosurg 57:603–608
13. Hayakawa T, Kamikawa K, Ohnishi T et al (1981) Prevention of postoperative complications after a transoral transclival approach to basilar aneurysms. Technical note. J Neurosurg 54:699–703
14. Tuite GF, Veres R, Crockard HA et al (1996) Pediatric transoral surgery: indications, complications, and long-term outcome. J Neurosurg 84:573–583
15. de Andrade JR, Macnab I (1969) Anterior occipito-cervical fusion using an extra-pharyngeal exposure. J Bone Joint Surg Am 51:1621–1626
16. Southwick WO, Robinson RA (1957) Surgical approaches to the vertebral bodies in the cervical and lumbar regions. J Bone Joint Surg Am 39:631–644
17. Hardy J (1969) Transphenoidal microsurgery of the normal and pathological pituitary. Clin Neurosurg 16:185–217
18. Kaibara T, Hurlbert RJ, Sutherland GR (2001) Intraoperative magnetic resonance imaging-augmented transoral resection of axial disease. Neurosurg Focus 10:E4
19. Menezes AH (2008) Surgical approaches: postoperative care and complications "transoral-transpalatopharyngeal approach to the craniocervical junction". Childs Nerv Syst 24(10): 1187–1193
20. Crockard HA, Johnston F (1993) Development of transoral approaches to lesions of the skull base and craniocervical junction. Neurosurg Q 3:61–82
21. Denaro V (1991) Stenosis of the cervical spine. Springer, Berlin
22. Menezes AH, VanGilder JC (1988) Transoral-transpharyngeal approach to the anterior craniocervical junction. Ten-year experience with 72 patients. J Neurosurg 69:895–903
23. Roy-Camille R, Judet TH, Saillant G et al (1981) Tumeurs du rachis. Techniques chirugucales, Orthopedie. Encycl Med Chir Paris 44165:4.06.04
24. Apuzzo ML, Weiss MH, Heiden JS (1978) Transoral exposure of the atlantoaxial region. Neurosurgery 3:201–207
25. Ashraf J, Crockard HA (1990) Transoral fusion for high cervical fractures. J Bone Joint Surg Br 72:76–79
26. Ashraf J, Crockard HA, Ransford AO et al (1991) Transoral decompression and posterior stabilisation in Morquio's disease. Arch Dis Child 66:1318–1321
27. Bhangoo RS, Crockard HA (1999) Transmaxillary anterior decompressions in patients with severe basilar impression. Clin Orthop Relat Res 359:115–125

28. Boni M, Denaro V (1982) The cervical stenosis syndrome with a review of 83 patients treated by operation. Int Orthop 6:185–195
29. Boni M, Denaro V (1982) Surgical treatment of cervical arthrosis. Follow-up review (2–13 years) of the 1st 100 cases operated on by anterior approach. Rev Chir Orthop Reparatrice Appar Mot 68:269–280
30. Crockard HA (1988) Anterior approaches to lesions of the upper cervical spine. Clin Neurosurg 34:389–416
31. Crockard HA (1995) Surgical management of cervical rheumatoid problems. Spine 20:2584–2590
32. Crockard HA, Essigman WK, Stevens JM et al (1985) Surgical treatment of cervical cord compression in rheumatoid arthritis. Ann Rheum Dis 44:809–816
33. Crockard HA, Sen CN (1991) The transoral approach for the management of intradural lesions at the craniovertebral junction: review of 7 cases. Neurosurgery 28:88–97; discussion 97–88
34. D'Alpa F, Scandurra L, Savuto R et al (1989) Pre-, intra- and postoperative somatosensory evoked potentials in cervical vertebral and spinal cord injuries. Minerva Anestesiol 55:115–118
35. Crockard HA, Bradford R (1985) Transoral transclival removal of a schwannoma anterior to the craniocervical junction. Case report. J Neurosurg 62:293–295
36. Delgado TE, Garrido E, Harwick RD (1981) Labiomandibular, transoral approach to chordomas in the clivus and upper cervical spine. Neurosurgery 8:675–679
37. Di Lorenzo N (1989) Transoral approach to extradural lesions of the lower clivus and upper cervical spine: an experience of 19 cases. Neurosurgery 24:37–42
38. Estridge MN, Smith RA (1967) Transoral fusion of odontoid fracture. Case report. J Neurosurg 27:462–465
39. Vougioukas VI, Hubbe U, Schipper J et al (2003) Navigated transoral approach to the cranial base and the craniocervical junction: technical note. Neurosurgery 52:247–250; discussion 251
40. Jones DC, Hayter JP, Vaughan ED et al (1998) Oropharyngeal morbidity following transoral approaches to the upper cervical spine. Int J Oral Maxillofac Surg 27:295–298
41. Harkey HL, Crockard HA, Stevens JM et al (1990) The operative management of basilar impression in osteogenesis imperfecta. Neurosurgery 27:782–786; discussion 786
42. Ibrahim AG, Crockard HA (2007) Basilar impression and osteogenesis imperfecta: a 21-year retrospective review of outcomes in 20 patients. J Neurosurg Spine 7: 594–600
43. Bonney G, Williams JP (1985) Trans-oral approach to the upper cervical spine. A report of 16 cases. J Bone Joint Surg Br 67:691–698
44. Lamas E, Estevez J, Castillo R et al (1977) Os odontoideum removed by a transoral approach. Surg Neurol 7:312–314
45. Pasztor E, Vajda J, Piffko P et al (1980) Transoral surgery for basilar impression. Surg Neurol 14:473–476
46. Gilsbach J, Eggert HR (1983) Transoral operations for craniospinal malformations. Neurosurg Rev 6:199–209
47. Boni M, Denaro V (1980) Surgical treatment of traumatic lesions of the middle and lower cervical spine (C3–C7). Ital J Orthop Traumatol 6:305–320
48. Spetzler RF, Selman WR, Nash CL Jr et al (1979) Transoral microsurgical odontoid resection and spinal cord monitoring. Spine 4:506–510
49. O'Reilly G, Crockard HA, Lightman S et al (1993) Excision of a clival and upper cervical pheochromocytoma by an extended maxillotomy approach: a case report. Skull Base Surg 3:87–90
50. Merwin GE, Post JC, Sypert GW (1991) Transoral approach to the upper cervical spine. Laryngoscope 101:780–784
51. Denaro V, Denaro L, Gulino G et al (1998) Complicanze nella chirurgia cervicale. Giornale Italiano di Ortopedia e Traumatologia 24:681–688
52. Denaro V, Gulino G, Papapietro N et al (1998) Treatment of metastases of the cervical spine. Chir Organi Mov 83: 127–137
53. Windle-Taylor PC (1977) Cervical chordoma: report of a case and the technique of transoral removal. Br J Surg 64: 438–441
54. Arvin B, Panchmatia JR, Casey AT (2008) Cervical C2 osteoma, unusual presentation and transoral approach for complete excision. Spine J 9(3):e9–e11
55. Crockard HA, Calder I, Ransford AO (1990) One-stage transoral decompression and posterior fixation in rheumatoid atlanto-axial subluxation. J Bone Joint Surg Br 72:682–685
56. Mummaneni PV, Haid RW (2005) Transoral odontoidectomy. Neurosurgery 56:1045–1050; discussion 1045–1050
57. Di Lorenzo N (1992) Craniocervical junction malformation treated by transoral approach. A survey of 25 cases with emphasis on postoperative instability and outcome. Acta Neurochir (Wien) 118:112–116
58. Cantarella G, Mazzola RF, Benincasa A (1998) A possible sequela of transoral approach to the upper cervical spine. Velopharyngeal incompetence. J Neurosurg Sci 42:51–55
59. Louis R (1992) Anterior surgery of the upper cervical spine. Chir Organi Mov 77:75–80
60. James D, Crockard HA (1991) Surgical access to the base of skull and upper cervical spine by extended maxillotomy. Neurosurgery 29:411–416

Complications Related to Anterolateral Approaches

8

Luca Denaro, Umile Giuseppe Longo, Rocco Papalia, and Vincenzo Denaro

Contents

L. Denaro (✉)
Department of Neuroscience, University of Padua,
Via Giustiniani, 5, 35128 Padua, Italy
e-mail: lucadenaro@hotmail.com

8.1 High and Low Presternocleidomastoid Approaches (Retropharyngeal and Precarotid)

The low and high retropharyngeal and precarotid presternocleidomastoid approaches to the cervical spine allow one to expose all the levels of the cervical spine, from the basis of the skull to the upper thoracic levels [1].

The low presternocleidomastoid approach is the most common direct approach to the middle and low cervical spine. It was first described to expose the proximal esophagus, and successively used in cervical spine surgery [2, 3].

The high presternocleidomastoid approach, on the other hand, allows one to easily expose the high cervical spine all the way up to clivus. It can be considered as a proximal extension of the classical presternocleidomastoid approach [3–5].

Absolute indications to the high presternocleidomastoid approach include:

- Surgery at the high cervical spine, particularly at level of the craniovertebral junction when asepsis is essential (see Chap. 7);
- The need to operate at different levels of the cervical spine. Indeed, this approach, when combined with the low presternocleidomastoid approach, allows one to expose the entire cervical spine from the base of the skull to the first thoracic vertebra.

8.1.1 Surgical Technique

8.1.1.1 Low Anterolateral Approach

In the low anterolateral approach, the skin incision can be either transverse or longitudinal, depending on the

L. Denaro et al. (eds.), *Pitfalls in Cervical Spine Surgery*,
DOI: 10.1007/978-3-540-85019-9_8, © Springer-Verlag Berlin Heidelberg 2010

extent of the required exposure. The transverse incision – cosmetically superior to the vertical one – can be performed when surgery has to be carried out at one or two levels of the cervical spine [2]. The longitudinal incision is preferred for wider multilevel exposure, and when it is essential to have an intraoperative visual control of the all neck. We modified the longitudinal incision. We do not follow the anterior border of the sternocleidomastoid muscle [6], but a half-way line between the mastoid process and the thyroid cartilage (Fig. 8.1). The incision extends downwards until the medial border of the sternocleidomastoid muscle at the level of the cricoid cartilage [7], and then proceeds in correspondence to the anterior border of the sternocleidomastoid muscle, down to the superior margin of the clavicle. This modification allows wider access to the anterior aspect of the vertebral bodies, which would not be possible with a more lateral incision [8]. The surgical dissection should be performed between the visceral structures of the neck and the neurovascular bundle [6].

Following the initial skin incision, bleeding vessels (usually branches of the external jugular vein) can be managed with bipolar electrocautery. When the external jugular vein is encountered, it can be swept aside or ligated [9]. The superficial tissues can be safely retracted with a self-retaining retractor. The platysma is split. In the plane deep to the platysma, the sternocleidomastoid muscle and the superficial cervical fascia can be easily identified [10]. The latter is split along the anterior margin of the sternocleidomastoid, and retracted with a hand-held retractor. Retraction of the sternocleidomastoid exposes the underlying neurovascular bundle, constituted by the vagus nerve, the common carotid artery, and the internal jugular vein [2]. The omohyoid muscle crosses the field embedded in the middle cervical fascia. It belongs to the group of infrahyoid muscles and consists of two bellies separated by an intermediate tendon. The middle cervical fascia is lifted at the proximal surface of the omohyoid muscle, and can be separated with blunt dissection from the underlying tissue all the way down to the distal end of the incision. Sutures are passed through the belly of the omohyoid muscle in its middle portion (Figs. 8.2 and 8.3). Muscle and fascia can be transected with diathermy (Fig. 8.4). The sutures can be used to raise the muscle and the middle cervical fascia [11]. This allows a wide visualization of the operative field, not obtainable with simple retraction. In such a way, the surgeon can easily control eventual complications. At the end of the surgical procedure, the omohyoid muscle is re-sutured.

At this point, one of the potential pitfalls is to damage the internal jugular vein at the distal end of the incision. This vein is usually quite superficial, but it is

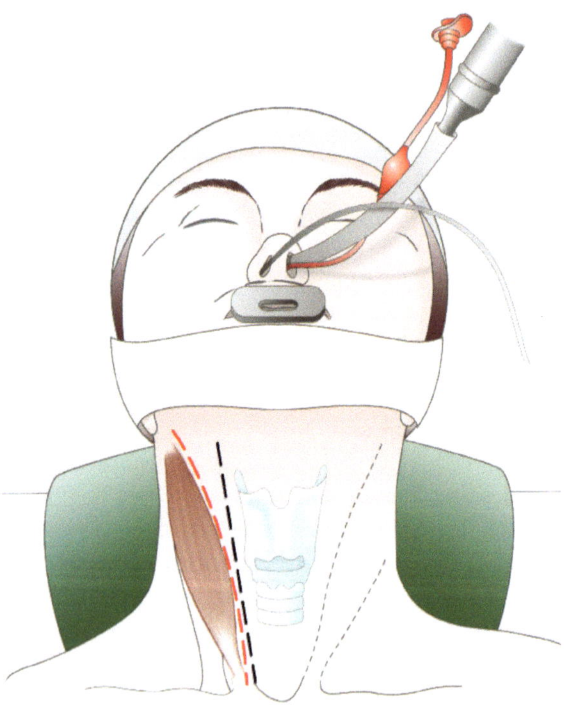

Fig. 8.1 We modified the longitudinal incision. We do not follow the anterior border of the sternocleidomastoid muscle, but a half-way line between the mastoid process and the thyroid cartilage

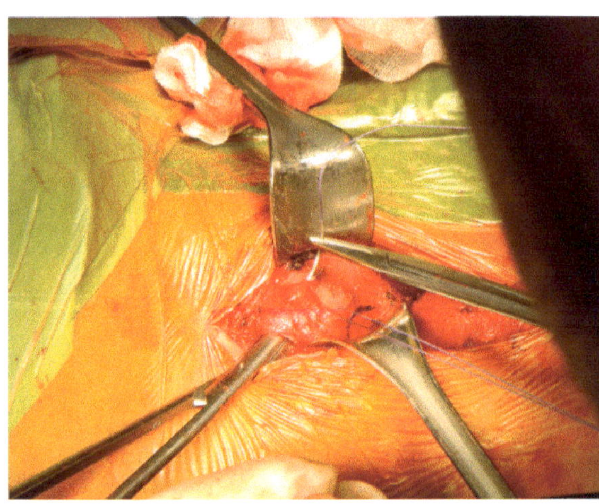

Fig. 8.2 Sutures are passed through the belly of the omohyoid muscle in its middle portion

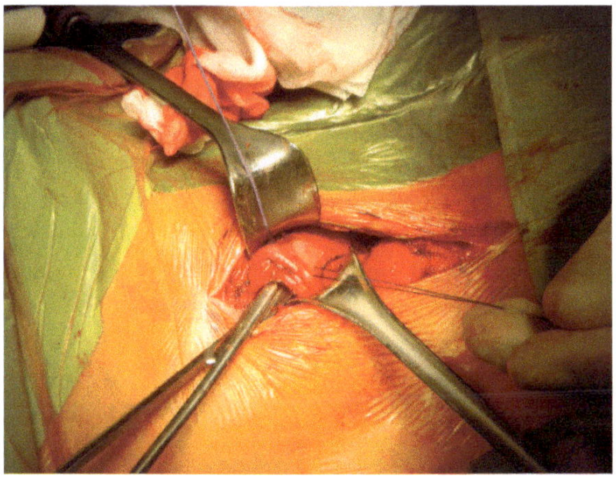

Fig. 8.3 The sutures passed through the belly of the omohyoid muscle in its middle portion can be used to raise the muscle

subject to great anatomical variation. Injuries to the vein are difficult to control because of the tension in the tissues that tends to retract the vessels out of the operative field making it more difficult to reach and to ligate [12].

The ends of the omohyoid muscle and the cervical fascia, once retracted, expose the neurovascular bundle in the carotid sheath. The artery is smaller and pulsating, the vein is wider and softer, and the vagus nerve, which lies posteriorly, is not directly visualized. The thyroid gland and the esophagus are covered by the sternohyoid and the sternothyroid muscles [8]. Blunt finger dissection will identify a plane of tissue separation between the neurovascular bundle laterally and the thyroid gland and muscles medially (Figs. 8.5 and 8.6). The middle thyroid vein, which variably may be

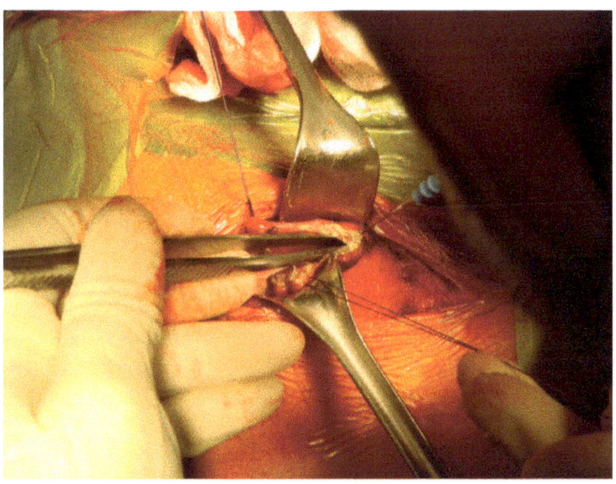

Fig. 8.4 Muscle and fascia can be transected with diathermy

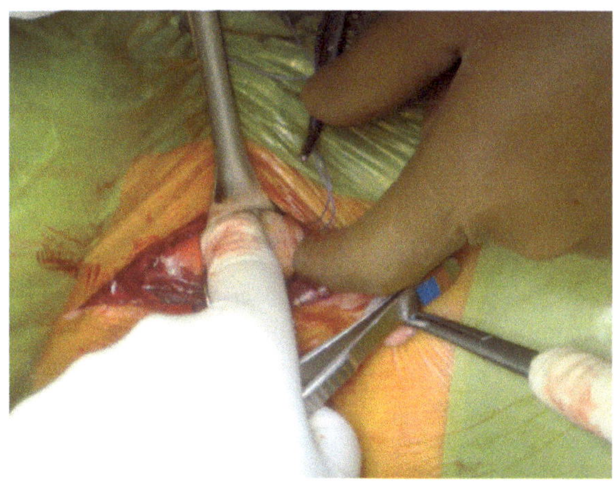

Fig. 8.5 Blunt finger dissection will identify a plane of tissue separation between the neurovascular bundle laterally and the thyroid gland and muscles medially

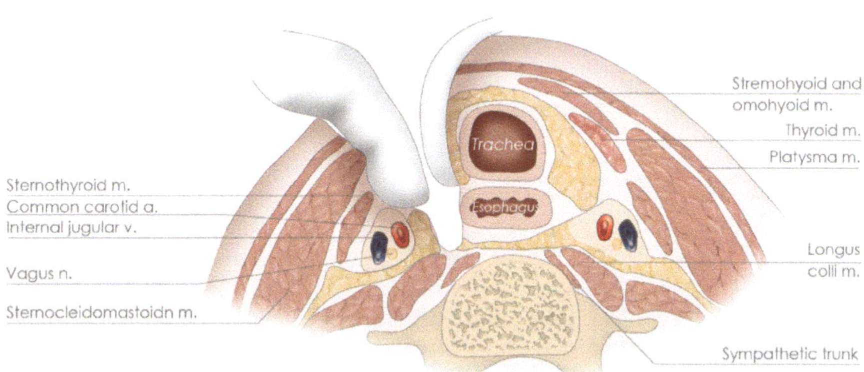

Fig. 8.6 Blunt finger dissection will identify a plane of tissue separation between the neurovascular bundle laterally and the thyroid gland and muscles medially

present, can be isolated and ligated. The retropharyngeal region has now been reached relatively easily with separation of the visceral structures of the neck that include pharynx, esophagus, trachea, and thyroid, which are retracted medially, and the neurovascular bundle, which can be retracted laterally together with the sternocleidomastoid muscle [11]. Once this blunt dissection has been completed, the deep cervical fascia (also known as alar fascia) is exposed [7]. At this point, the anterior longitudinal ligament and vertebral bodies are exposed. Once the deep cervical fascia and the anterior longitudinal ligament have been divided by diathermy, the periosteal surface of the vertebral bodies can be peeled off. The dissection can be performed laterally as required, but it is usually recommended to not dissect as far as the transverse processes, to avoid the cervical sympathetic chain [2]. Extensive bony bleeding (especially when the surgeon extends the dissection laterally) may be present once the anterior longitudinal ligament has been lifted from the vertebral body, often requiring sealing with Surgicel and bone wax to be controlled (Fig. 8.7) [6]. To avoid injuries to the soft tissues of the neck, the self-retaining retractor should be applied only to the anterior longitudinal ligament, when it is present, and its arms should not include or apply any pressure to nerves or other soft tissues of the neck. In the degenerative cervical spine, generally the anterior longitudinal ligament is disrupted and degenerated, and therefore it is difficult to apply a retractor. This is possible in young patients, or in some inflammatory conditions. At this point, it is necessary to check the cervical levels exposed by fluoroscopy [2].

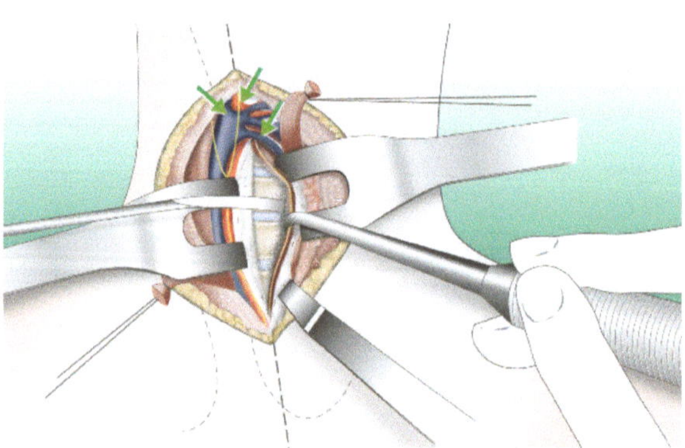

Fig. 8.7 Extensive bony bleeding (especially when the surgeon extends the dissection laterally) may be present once the anterior longitudinal ligament has been lifted from the vertebral body, often requiring sealing with Surgicel and bone wax to be controlled.

8.1.1.2 High Anterolateral Approach

In the high anterolateral approach [12], the skin incision starts in the submandibular region, one finger below the edge of the horizontal arm of the mandible [11]. The incision begins from the submental region and proceeds horizontally toward the mastoid, where it turns distally and medially along the anterior margin of the sternocleidomastoid muscle. In patients in whom greater exposure is required, it is possible to perform a T-shaped incision: the first horizontally, and the second (perpendicular to the first) in front of the sternocleidomastoid muscle [2].

The platysma is split and retracted. Once the platysma and superficial fascia are divided, a nerve stimulator can be used to find the mandibular branch of the facial nerve (seventh cranial nerve), which should be preserved [9]. The mandibular nerve is the first branch of the cervicofacial division of the facial nerve. It passes posteriorly to the angle of the mandible to supply the muscles of the corner of the mouth and lower lip [2, 10]. It is easy for this nerve to be injured by retractors, because it can get pinched between the retractor and the hard mandibular bone [9] [2].

The retromandibular vein is a landmark for its identification, as it generally courses above the retromandibular vein within the substance of the parotid gland in more than 90% of cases, while in the other 10%, it passes medially to the vein. The retromandibular vein is formed by the union of the superficial maxillary and temporal veins, descends in the substance of the parotid gland, superficial to the external carotid artery but beneath the facial nerve, and near the angle of the mandible divides into two branches, namely anterior and posterior. The anterior branch unites with the anterior facial vein to form the common facial vein. The posterior branch unites with the posterior auricular vein and becomes the external jugular vein [2].

The facial artery, a branch of the external carotid artery, crosses the parotid gland posteriorly, and passes over the mandible, always lying under the platysma. To expose the upper levels of the cervical spine, often it is necessary to ligate the retromandibular vein adjacent to its junction with the internal jugular vein, the thyrolinguofacial trunk, and the superior thyroid artery and vein. We have not encountered functional changes in the thyroid when thyroid vessels are ligated [2, 9].

Once the lingual and facial vessels have been ligated, the posterior belly of the digastric muscle can be identified. The digastric muscle lies below the body of the mandible, and extends, in a curved form, from the mastoid process to the symphysis menti. The hypoglossal nerve (12th cranial nerve) crosses the operative field from medial to lateral. It is more superior to the superior laryngeal nerve. Both should be protected by careful dissection and mobilization. The hypoglossal nerve can be retracted superiorly once it is dissected out from its exiting site at the skull base to its insertion near the tongue. The hypoglossal nerve follows a path that defines two suprahyoid anatomical zones. The first is Beclard's triangle, where the hypoglossal nerve lies superiorly, the stylohyoid muscle anteriorly, and the horn of the hyoid bone on the third side. The second is Pirogoff's triangle, which is defined superiorly by the hypoglossal nerve, anteriorly by the omohyoid muscle, and posteriorly by the tendon of the digastric muscle [2, 9].

It is rarely necessary to divide the tendons of the digastric and of the stylohyoid muscles to obtain better exposure. Retraction of the digastric muscle is sufficient to expose the prevertebral region. As a part of the final exposure to the actual operative site, it is sometimes necessary to remove the submandibular gland together with its vascular supply and salivary duct [2]. When the gland is resected to allow better exposure, the salivary duct must be ligated to prevent fistula formation.

8.1.2 *Intraoperative Complications*

Anterolateral approaches to the cervical spine are generally safe, even though many complications with serious life-threatening consequences have been reported [13]. Potential complications of this approach include:

- Vascular complications
- Neurological complications
- Soft tissue and visceral complications

A detailed overview of these complications of the anterolateral approaches to the cervical spine is reported (Table 8.1).

8.1.2.1 Vascular Injuries

Carotid Artery

The two common carotids are the principal arteries of supply to the head and neck. They ascend in the neck and divide into two branches: the external and the internal carotid. The right common carotid begins at the bifurcation of the innominate artery behind the sternoclavicular joint and is confined to the neck [14]. The left begins from the highest part of the arch of the aorta and consists of a thoracic and a cervical portion.

Injuries to the carotid artery during presternocleidomastoid approaches to the cervical spine are rare, because the artery, retracted laterally, is located within the carotid sheath and covered with connective tissue [15]. Difficult anatomy (i.e., in patients with advanced and widely disseminated tumors) and poor identification of the midline are risk factors for injuries of the carotid artery. Injuries to the artery can be either overt, with rapid blood flow from an injury, or insidious, with an occlusive stroke.

Direct injuries can result during dissection (when the artery is not adequately protected from sharp instruments such as drills and chisels), or because of the use of self-retaining retractors that apply direct pressure to the artery. Prolonged handle retraction may also be responsible for internal carotid artery thrombosis and hemispheric stroke [15]. This is the main reason why we recommend to intermittently release the retractors during surgery to restore adequate internal carotid artery flow. Embolic or occlusive strokes from the carotid artery are typically discovered postoperatively and are difficult to manage. Patient with injuries of the internal carotid artery may develop hemorrhagic infarction in the reperfused ischemic brain, or cerebrovascular morbidity such as cerebral edema and herniation.

The cross-sectional area of the internal carotid artery is reduced significantly following non-appropriate retraction. Pollard et al. [16] measured the carotid artery blood flow in 15 patients undergoing anterior cervical spine surgery to determine the effect of intraoperative retraction on carotid artery flow dynamics. Duplex ultrasonic measurements of common carotid artery flow velocity were taken. Measurements were recorded before surgery, intraoperatively after exposure was obtained and self-retaining retractors were placed, intraoperatively at the end of the procedure just before the release of retraction, after surgery in the recovery room, and on postoperative day 1. Using flow velocity data, the changes in cross-sectional area were calculated at each time interval and expressed as a percentage of change in area from baseline measurements. The authors found that vessel cross-sectional area decreased an average of 14% with the initial placement of self-retaining retractors, and decreased further to 70% of baseline by the end of the procedure.

Table 8.1 Complications of the anterolateral approach

Complications	How to avoid them: tips and tricks
Carotid artery	Adequately protect the artery from sharp instruments such as drills and chisels during dissection Do not apply direct pressure to the artery with self-retaining retractors Prolonged handle retraction may be responsible for internal carotid artery thrombosis and hemispheric stroke: intermittently release the retractors during surgery to restore adequate internal carotid artery flow When an injury occurs, minimize manipulation of the artery to avoid the risk of thrombus fragmentation and embolization Balance compression with the need to maintain flow in the artery Avoid to clamp the common or internal carotid artery unless the patient's condition is life-threatening because the interruption of theflow may cause embolism and cerebral ischemia
Vertebral artery	Avoid inappropriate use of retractors and surgical instruments Be careful in extensive dissection within the vertebral body, which may produce collapse of the lateral wall involving the vertebral artery, which can be caught in a sudden collapse of the surrounding bony structures Be careful in the following maneuvers: motorized dissection off midline, excessive lateral bone-disk removal, excessively lateral placement of instrumentation, removal of bone pathologically softened by tumor, infection, or irradiation Avoid the use of retractors with sharp or hooked end (e.g., Homann's retractor), to obtain exposure laterally to the vertebral body In cases of injury to the vertebral artery, direct surgical repair is mostly appropriate to prevent complications such as fistulas, late-onset hemorrhages, pseudoaneurysms, thrombosis, and emboli. Endovascular techniques are the first therapeutic option in injuries to the vertebral artery because of its location and surgical inaccessibility
Jugular vein	When damages occur, the resulting bleeding can be controlled by suturing the wall of the vein. The vessel must be totally accessible during the suture. This may require to open the carotid sheath to expose the vein and identify the artery and the vagus nerve to avoid to include these two additional structures in the sutures or ligatures
Thyroid vessels	Injury to the thyroid vessels are frequent when self-retaining retractors are used. Ligate the thyroid arteries when they cross the operative field
Esophagus and pharynx	Avoid excessive retraction to the esophagus during dissection Use a nasogastric tube, which can be palpated during dissection and can help to recognize the hypopharynx, preventing intraoperative injuries. Use sharp dissection rather than diathermy to expose the prevertebral fascia Protect the esophagus always by hand-held retractors to prevent thermal or direct injury If damages to esophagus and pharynx are identified intraoperatively and repaired immediately, maintain the nasogastric tube for 2–3 weeks postoperatively, with a compressive bandage on the neck.
Trachea	Avoid excessive retraction to the trachea during dissection Palpate the endotracheal anesthetic tube during dissection to help to recognize the trachea Use sharp dissection rather than diathermy during dissection Protect the trachea always by hand-held retractors to prevent thermal or direct injury
Thoracic duct	Always be aware of the considerable anatomic variations of the thoracic duct: the terminal arch of the thoracic duct in the neck may be situated inferior to, at, or as much as 5.5 cm superior to the clavicle The definitive management is ligation of the thoracic duct
Neurological injuries	Perform a careful identification and dissection Use soft, manually controlled retractors rather than self-retaining or hard retractors
Specific neurological injuries: laryngeal nerves	Be aware of the great number of anomalous paths of the inferior laryngeal nerve Laryngeal nerves can be injured whenever the retroesophageal prevertebral space is missed, and inadvertently the surgeon enters the space between the esophagus and trachea
Specific neurological injuries: cervical sympathetic chain	Remain subperiosteal in dissecting the lateral aspect of the vertebral body in the approach to the transverse apophyses

Extensive hemispheric infarct and lethal stroke have been reported after anterior cervical spine surgery because of thrombosis due to prolonged retraction both on an atherosclerotic common carotid artery [17], and on the normal common carotid artery [18].

Bleeding can be usually controlled by external compression [19]. During control by direct finger compression of the artery, manipulation must be minimized to avoid the risk of thrombus fragmentation and embolization. Also, compression needs to be balanced with the need to maintain flow in the artery. Sometimes, to control bleeding it can be necessary to clamp temporarily the common or internal carotid artery. This maneuver should be avoided unless the patient's condition is life-threatening because the interruption of the flow may cause embolization and cerebral ischemia. The risk of major stroke in these patients after carotid clamping is around 50%. Positioning of a shunt is the only therapeutic option to avoid a major stroke [19]. The procedure usually requires proximal and distal control, arteriotomy, and eventual extraction of the thrombus before to position the shunt. When the thrombus is extracted, a delicate technique is required to avoid fragmentation and dislodge as embolic masses [19]. The safest way to extract the thrombus is to use traction with forceps associated to suction. The result is satisfactory when the extraction is followed by brisk backflow. We do not recommend the use of thrombectomy catheters because of the risks fragmentation and dislodge into the circle of Willis [2, 6, 19].

The external carotid artery can be clamped almost always safely. When preparing for clamping, it is necessary to have performed a long incision to obtain proximal control of the common carotid on the left side and of the brachiocephalic trunk on the right. The facial vein and its confluence to the internal jugular vein must be identified. The internal jugular vein is a good landmark being located just above the carotid bifurcation. It can be safely clamped. Posterior retraction of the internal jugular vein exposes the common carotid and its bifurcation. At this stage, it is necessary to identify and protect the hypoglossal and vagus nerves [2, 6, 19].

Squeezing, trauma, and operative manipulation of the carotid arteries must be avoided because of the risk of embolization to the brain. The most cranial clamp is applied first to avoid embolization when the more proximal parts are clamped [19].

Many repair techniques are available, and include simple suture, patch, resection with end-to-end anastomosis, resection with an interposition graft, transposition of external to internal carotid artery, ligation, or balloon occlusion [19].

Generally, simple sutures are sufficient in patients with minor injuries. Patches can be used for minor wall defect. Resection with end-to-end anastomosis can be an option for limited injuries requiring minor resections, allowing an anastomosis without tension. Resection with an interposition graft (i.e., autologous vein graft harvested from the greater saphenous vein or prosthetic grafts) is required in patients with larger injuries to restore the continuity of the vessel. Transposition of external to internal carotid artery can be an option when vein grafts are not available. Ligation or balloon occlusion should be reserved for inaccessible injuries, which are impossible to repair. Ligation can be difficult in patients with very distal injuries to the internal carotid artery. In such instances, an occluding balloon catheter can then be positioned into the artery at the base of the skull and insufflated until bleeding stops. The balloon catheter can be left in place for 1–2 days or more and then be deflated and removed [19].

Postoperatively, to minimize the risks of bleeding and cerebral complications, it is necessary to monitor and correct blood pressure. The most common complications in the postoperative period include thrombosis and reperfusion problems [2, 6, 19]

Vertebral Artery

Serious vascular complications can arise from the injury to the vertebral artery [20]. In the high presternocleidomastoid approach, injuries to the vertebral arteries can easily occur when the surgeon operates at level of the cranio-cervical junction, laterally to the axis. At this level, the artery, out of the foramen transversarium, crosses anterolaterally, and forms the arterial circle of Willis at the base of the brain. In patients with massive osteolysis, damage to the vertebral artery in its extraskeletal portion can occur during the exposure of the lateral masses of C2 because of the inappropriate use of retractors and surgical instruments.

In the low presternocleidomastoid approach, the vertebral artery can be damaged when surgery is performed in the lateral portion of the vertebral body towards the transverse processes, and when osseous dissection involves the foramen transversarium, which contains the vertebral artery. Sometimes, extensive dissection within the vertebral body may produce a collapse of the lateral wall involving the vertebral artery, which can be caught in a sudden collapse of the surrounding bony structures. Fortunately, in the majority of patients, the artery is flexible enough to bend and adapt to the collapse of the surrounding bone. When injuries occur, the bleeding will be massive.

Vertebral artery laceration has been attributed to several factors: motorized dissection off midline, excessive lateral bone-disk removal, excessively lateral placement of instrumentation, bone pathologically softened by tumor, infection, or irradiation, and intraoperative loss of midline landmarks [21, 22]. The proximity of vertebral artery to the uncovertebral joint during foraminotomy or removal of the postero-lateral quadrant of the vertebral body is a predisposing factor to arterial laceration [23].

Injury to the vertebral artery may also occur as a result of specific technical maneuvers. The most common one is the use of retractors with sharp or hooked end (e.g., Homann's retractor), to obtain exposure laterally to the vertebral body. The exposure obtained by such retractors may appear to be advantageous, but the consequences can be catastrophic.

The rapid uncontrolled hemorrhage following damage of the vertebral artery can lead to exsanguination. The interruption of vertebral artery blood flow by ligation, attempted repair, or thrombus formation can cause numerous central nervous system complications. Wallenberg's syndrome, cerebellar infarction, isolated cranial nerve palsies, quadriparesis, and hemiplegia have been reported [22, 23]. In cases of injury to the vertebral artery, direct surgical repair is mostly appropriate to prevent complications such as fistulas, late-onset hemorrhages, pseudoaneurysms, thrombosis, and emboli. Endovascular techniques, clipping, or ligation of the artery can be considered [20].

The fragmentation occurring in the wall of the vertebral artery foramen may require the surgeon to ligate the artery at a lower level, often right down to C6.

When an injury to this artery occurs between atlas and axis, or more proximally (into the occipital foramen during dissection along the lateral wall of C1 and C2), the resulting hemorrhage can only be controlled by occluding the artery at the below intervertebral level. This emergency repair runs the risk of injury to the nerve root and, therefore, must be performed with great care.

Prevention of iatrogenic vertebral artery injury is the best management. Pre-operatively, the surgeon should study the position of the vertebral arteries on magnetic resonance imaging or CT scans to detect any ecstatic arteries or involvement in a tumor or infection. Preoperative magnetic resonance angiography or, as last instance, conventional angiography can be considered in patients in whom the artery is displaced, tortuous, or dilated [20].

Endovascular management is the first therapeutic option in injuries to the vertebral artery because of its location and surgical inaccessibility. Detachable balloons, coils, stents, and hemostatic agents are usually successful in managing bleeding. Immediate intervention with proximal and distal ligation is necessary in unstable patients with life-threatening bleeding [19].

Jugular Vein

The internal jugular vein collects the blood from the brain, from the superficial parts of the face, and from the neck. It is directly continuous with the transverse sinus, and begins in the posterior compartment of the jugular foramen, at the base of the skull [2, 6].

The jugular vein may be hidden behind the sternocleidomastoid muscle, and therefore difficult to visualize and identify during dissection. Its soft wall can be easily torn, particularly in older patients.

When damages occur, the resulting bleeding can be controlled by suturing the wall of the vein. The vessel must be totally accessible during the suture. This may require one to open the carotid sheath to expose the vein and identify the artery and the vagus nerve to avoid including these two additional structures in the sutures or ligatures [10].

In bilateral injuries to the internal jugular veins, however, reconstruction of one of the sides is necessary to avoid severe venous hypertension [19].

Thyroid Vessels

During dissection, the thyroid vessels may be injured. In the high presternocleidomastoid approach, the superior thyroid artery and vein can be ligated when it cannot be retracted from the operative field.

The middle thyroid vein, when present, should be ligated.

The inferior thyroid artery and vein must be carefully freed if they must be retracted. Injury to the inferior thyroid artery is a frequent event when self-retaining retractors are used, particularly in older patients in whom the vessels are hardened by arteriosclerosis, with loss of elasticity and calcification of the wall [10]. It is prudent to ligate the thyroid arteries when they cross the operative field.

8.1.2.2 Soft Tissue and Visceral Injury

Esophagus and Pharynx

Esophageal perforation is a recognized potentially fatal complication of anterior cervical spine surgery [24–33]. The incidence of esophageal injury is clearly higher in corpectomy, instrumented and traumatic surgery. Esophageal ischemic or direct injury usually is determined by excessive retraction during dissection. Injuries to the esophagus and pharynx require immediate surgical repair [6]. When the middle cervical fascia and the omohyoid muscle have been split, the esophagus and the pharynx are immediately exposed. The walls of these structures at these levels are thin and soft and, as a consequence, easily injured by aggressive dissection. Small tears to these structures can be missed intraoperatively.

The hypopharynx can be easily lacerated during dissection of the higher levels of the cervical spine, particularly if dissection is not performed with great care in patients with previous inflammatory diseases, or in patients with scarring and adhesions from previous surgery [6]. The latter cases are obviously associated with the loss of the natural planes of cleavage and of the normal tissue relationships. For this reason, the use of a nasogastric tube is recommended, which can be palpated during dissection and can help one to recognize the hypopharynx, preventing intraoperative injuries [10]. The use of diathermy rather than sharp dissection to expose the prevertebral fascia during the dissection of the longus colli muscle can lead to esophageal injury. The esophagus should always be protected by hand-held retractors to prevent thermal or direct injury.

If damages to the esophagus and pharynx are identified intraoperatively and repaired immediately, it is necessary to maintain the nasogastric tube for 2–3 weeks postoperatively, with a compressive bandage on the neck. Parenteral nutrition and feeding through the nasogastric tube will be sufficient, particularly when augmented by the use of atropine to decrease salivation. It is important to remember that if such intraoperative complications arise, the surgeon should avoid the use of massive osseous grafts or the application of foreign bodies such as metal devices. If the tear is not identified intraoperatively, then the surgeon must be on the alert for this possibility when drainage persists for several days postoperatively. An easy way to definitely confirm the presence of a tear is to give the patients 5–10 cc methylene blue to drink. After a few minutes, the dye will appear in the drainage from the wound. At this point, the surgical incision must be reopened and the tear must be repaired. Abscess cavities and sinuses can form deeply in the tissues of the neck. These can reach into the mediastinum, making management more difficult.

The morbidity and mortality of an esophageal injury, especially after delayed diagnosis, are high. With a complete perforation of the wall, oropharyngeal secretions with their micro-organisms are free to contaminate the visceral structures in the neck and mediastinum [34]. The occurrence of mediastinitis, pneumonia, pleuritis, pericarditis, and systemic sepsis is well documented in the literature [35–37]. Fistula formation is also a known late complication and in many instances leads to the diagnosis. Fistlulae can occur between esophagus and the respiratory tract. Esophageal–bronchial and esophageal–pleural fistula are both complicated therapeutic dilemmas [38]. The mortality of these conditions with conservative therapy has been reported up to 65%. With accurate early diagnosis and appropriate selection criteria, mortality rates of <7% are possible [39].

Salivary Duct

In the high presternocleidomastoid approach, the resection of the submandibular gland may be associated with the formation of a fistulous tract as a consequence of inappropriate ligature of the salivary duct. Usually, it results in the formation of an abscess and successively of a fistula because of retrograde passage of oral salivary contents into the stump of the resected duct, which can become obstructed and infected [2].

The Thyroid Gland

The thyroid gland is protected by the muscles of the neck and can only be injured by retractors or by sharp instruments used in dissection. Injuries are associated with hemorrhage, which can be controlled suturing the tear [2].

The Thoracic Duct

The thoracic duct is the main collecting vessel of the lymphatic system [40]. It drains three-quarters of the lymph in the body into the venous bloodstream [41]. Its length varies from 36 to 45 cm in adults. Its distal dilated origin is known as cisterna chyli, and it is usually located on the anterior surface of the first or second lumbar vertebra. The thoracic duct enters the thorax through the aortic hiatus to the right of midline and ascends through the posterior mediastinal cavity between the aorta and azygos vein [7, 8, 12]. Opposite to the fifth thoracic vertebra, it inclines toward the left side, enters the superior mediastinal cavity, and ascends posterior to the aortic arch [42]. It ascends forming an arch that rises approximately 3–4 cm above the clavicle to the level of the seventh cervical vertebra and crosses anterior to the subclavian artery, the vertebral artery and vein, and the thyrocervical trunk or its branches. It ends by opening into the angle of junction of the left subclavian vein with the left internal jugular vein. However, there may be considerable anatomic variations of the thoracic duct. The thoracic duct may terminate with single or multiple terminations in the left internal jugular vein, in the left subclavian vein, in the left external jugular vein, in the left innominate vein, in the vertebral vein [43], in the transverse cervical vein [44], and in the right internal jugular vein [43, 45, 46]. The terminal arch of the thoracic duct in the neck may be situated inferior to, at, or as much as 5.5 cm superior to the clavicle [46].

Thoracic duct injury is a rare but serious complication following cervical spine surgery [47]. It may lead to nutritional deficiencies, respiratory dysfunction, and immunosuppression with a mortality up to 50% [48, 49]. Despite the fragile nature of the lymphatic system and its proximity to the vertebral spine, chylorrhea is rarely encountered by spine surgeons, even though the real frequencies of the thoracic duct injuries may have been underestimated because some of them are considered as asymptomatic [50]. Since the anterior approach for cervical discectomy and fusion has been described in 1955 [3], only one case of thoracic duct injury occurring during cervical discectomy and fusion via an anterior approach has been described, as a consequence of the unusually cephalic location of the thoracic duct arch in the neck [51].

Nine cases of thoracic duct injury occurring during thoracic and/or lumbar spine have been reported [52–56]. In all these nine patients, thoracic duct injury manifested as an intraoperative chyle leak, postoperative chylothorax, chyloretroperitoneum, or a combination of these [52–56].

The variable anatomic course of the thoracic duct has been reported as the main reason for injuries during spinal surgery [2, 57]. Other factors include its small size, inconstant location, and proximity to the vertebral bodies.

Thoracic duct injury can present as cervical chylous fistula, chylothorax, or chylopericardium [58]. Chylous leakage in the thoracic cavity may complicate the primary disease and the management might be prolonged [11, 59].

When the thoracic duct is interrupted, chylothorax may occur from leakage due to reflux within substitution collateral pathways diverting the flow of chyle into the venoux confluents of the neck.

Conservative management consists of low-fat diet with medium chain triglycerides, total parenteral nutrition, correction of electrolyte imbalance, and adequate drainage by chest tube or neck drain [47, 60]. Somatostain 14 and Etilefrine have been reported to be effective [61]. However, it takes several weeks for the chylothorax to resolve with an overall failure rate up to 50%, requiring surgical intervention later [62].

The definitive management is ligation of the thoracic duct [63]. Despite excellent results, thoracotomy remains a procedure with high morbidity, pain, and associated risks. For this reason, early conservative therapy is recommended for 1–2 weeks at the beginning. Sufficient T-cell depletion, to place the patient at risk of septicemia, can occur within 8 days of chyle drainage despite optimal supportive care [48]. Any major surgery at this stage is logically associated with high morbidity and mortality [47].

Video-Assisted-Thoracic-Surgery has been used in the management of chyle leaks [62]. Many patients, after a period of failed conservative management receive clipping, ligation of the thoracic duct, and glue application to the site of the leak [62].

8.1.2.3 Neurological Injury

Damages of various nerves may occur during the anterolateral approach to the cervical spine, and severity is commonly defined using the Seddon's classification for nerve injury. This classification includes:

- Neurapraxia: temporary interruption of nerve conduction without loss of continuity of the axon.
- Axonotmesis: (Greek, axon + tmesis, cutting apart) interruption of the axon from nerve injury, with subsequent wallerian degeneration of the distal nerve segment and preservation of the connective tissue fragments, resulting in degeneration of the axon distal to the injury site.
- Neurotmesis: (Greek, neuron + tmesis, cutting apart) a peripheral nerve injury in which the nerve is completely disrupted by laceration or traction. It requires surgical approximation, with unpredictable recovery the neural tube is severed.

Facial Nerve (Seventh Cranial Nerve) and Hypoglossal Nerve (Twelfth Cranial Nerve)

The most common complications of the high presternocleidomastoid are neurological. In the submandibular and perimandibular region, the operative field will be crossed by the facial nerve (seventh cranial nerve), the hypoglossal nerve (twelfth cranial nerve), and the superior laryngeal nerve. The latter is the one most often injured. The occurrence of these neurological injuries is directly related to the degree of traction and retraction used. Excessive pull on these structures will certainly result in injury. The intention of the operation is to reach the vertebral bodies. To achieve this, there is a tendency to emphasize medial retraction. This can be prevented by accurate mobilization before any traction is applied, by careful identification and dissection, and by using soft, manually controlled retractors rather than self-retaining or hard retractors [2].

Damages to the mandibular branch of the facial nerve determine a very slight drooping of the corner of the mouth. The drooping may not be detectable when the mouth is closed, but only when it is in motion (i.e., smiling).

The orbicularis oris and the muscles innervated by buccal branches actually raise the commissure on the affected side. Injury to the anterior cervical branch produces minimal drooling that will disappear in 4–6 months.

Laryngeal Nerves

The superior laryngeal nerve can be injured during the high anterolateral approach. At this level, the nerve will be found to cross the field in its approach to the pharyngeal wall. The inferior laryngeal nerve is subject to a greater number of anomalous paths, arising from the vagus nerve anywhere from the middle to the inferior cervical region and often in association with the inferior thyroid vessels. These nerves are injured whenever the retroesophageal prevertebral space is missed, and inadvertently the surgeon enters the space between the esophagus and trachea [2].

The operating surgeon's dominant hand will determine the position that is more comfortable with reference to the patient. Usually, a right-handed surgeon will be more comfortable operating from the right side. All aspects of surgical operations on bone such as the use of chisels, knives, or curets favor a right-handed surgeon operating from the right side. In the past, there has been much debate in the literature if to prefer a right or left approach side, particularly with reference to complications arising from the recurrent laryngeal nerve [2]. Injury to this nerve produces vocal disturbance, which may be irreversible. Symptoms include hoarseness, vocal breathiness or fatigue, weak cough, dysphagia, or aspiration [64]. Although vocal cord paralysis may be permanent, in most cases symptoms last for weeks or months [65].

The course of the recurrent laryngeal nerves differs on the right and left sides. On the left side, it has a longer course, originating more distally in the vagus within the thorax, passing under the aortic arch, and then following the space between the esophagus and trachea in the neck. On the right side, the nerve follows a much shorter course. It arises quite proximally in the upper thorax, passes under the subclavian artery, and courses between the trachea and the esophagus. It is more superficial and, hence, more exposed. In addition, it may follow a number of differing anatomical pathways. It has been reported to arise as proximal as the inferior thyroid artery, which makes it particularly vulnerable to injury if this position is not immediately identified as a variant of normal. Injury may occur because of direct traction or retraction with excessive force if the nerve is stretched between two planes that are separated, and may lead to apraxia or axonotmesis. The surgeon should keep possible anatomical variations in mind [10].

Cervical Sympathetic Chain

The sympathetic trunk of the neck is in the prevertebral fascia between the carotid sheath in front and the longus colli and longus capitis muscles behind. It extends above into the skull as a plexus surrounding the internal carotid artery. It is continuous, downward, with the sympathetic trunk of the thorax. The cervical sympathetic chain is formed by the superior, middle, and inferior ganglia. Each gives gray rami communicantes to the cervical nerves, a cardiac nerve, and a plexus to an artery. The cervical sympathetic chain can be injured in its superior region near the stellate ganglion when the surgeon is dissecting (the long muscles of the neck) in the lateral cervical muscular plane. It is usually injured when the surgeon fails to remain subperiosteal in dissecting the lateral aspect of the vertebral body in the approach to the transverse apophyses. This injury leads to Horner's syndrome, characterized by homolateral anophthalmia, myosis, and palpebral ptosis.

Spinal Cord and to the Nerve Roots

Injury to the cord and to the nerve roots usually occurs as part of the specific surgical act being undertaken on these structures. Postoperative CSF leakage may occur at the dural suture line after intradural procedures or can be caused by inadvertent durotomy during discectomy.

Once occurred, surgical repair of dural tears via an anterior approach can be difficult or impossible because of the reduced space available during single level discectomy. When possible, tears should be sutured or a dural patch can be applied. Lyophilized dura or processed bovine pericardium are also materials that can be used in lesion repair. These latters can be directly sutured or sticked with fibrin glue: to be sure of the adhesion of the patch, the anesthesiologist should intraoperatively perform repeated Valsava maneuvers to increase CSF pressure. Fascial graft covered with gelfoam, fat graft, or fibrin glue can be used together with other sealant products (Duraseal Xact^{TM}) to obtain water-tight sealing of repaired dural tears [66].

A lumbar subarachnoid drainage must be always positioned both in case of failure and in doubtful cases of inadequate surgical repair [67]. The lumbar subarachnoid drainage decreases intradural pressure contributing to dural tear healing process. Drainage flow should be of 8–12 mL/h, with flow rate to be modified on the base of clinical response.

Spinal cord lesion can occur for direct or indirect injury. Direct lesion can be due to contusion at the level of surgery for inadvertent surgical maneuvers. In the immediate postoperative period, patients may have a worsening of preoperative neurological symptoms with areas of cord damage [68]. Indirect lesions occur following a vascular ischemic damage with subsequent postoperative neurological deficit. These lesions can occur for ipossia from eccessive distraction intraoperatively or postoperative edema or hematoma. Decompression of the already ischemic spinal cord in spinal stenosis can lead itself to a segmental paradoxical infarct the spinal cord, similar to that occurring in limb reimplantation surgery [69].

8.1.3 Postoperative Complications

The most frequent postoperative complications include:

- Pharyngeal or salivary fistula
- Infections (Chap. 13)
- Glottic edema, which results from tissue injury and which, in the most severe cases, may require tracheostomy.

Obstruction of the upper airway after surgery on the anterior aspect of the cervical spine is a rare but potentially lethal complication that occurs in the early postoperative period. It has been mentioned frequently as a possible complication but never actually quantified. Potential causes of airway obstruction include pharyngeal edema [70, 71] hematoma [72], cerebrospinal fluid leak [71], angioedema, and graft or plate dislodgment [73].

8.2 Presternocleidomastoid Approach (Retropharyngeal and Retrocarotid)

The retrocarotid retropharyngeal presternocleidomastoid approach has been originally used to obtain surgical access to the vertebral artery [74, 75], and successively adapted for the high cervical spine by Whiteside and Kelly [76].

It provides good exposure of both the intra- and extraosseous portion of the vertebral artery, the lateral side of the cervico-occipital region including the transverse apophyses, the intertransverse foramina, and the nerve roots of the first cervical vertebrae. When indicated, the incision may be extended distally to permit exposure of the lower cervical vertebrae.

8.2.1 Technique

The patient is placed supine. A hockey-stick incision is begun in the retromastoid region, 2 cm behind the apex of the mastoid, and is curved inferiorly. It is extended horizontally around the mastoid, and then down the anterior edge of the strenocleidomastoid muscle. The initial dissection should be directed to the identification of both the external jugular vein crossing in front of the sternocleidomastoid and the greater auricular nerve. The nerve must be freed and anchored superiorly to avoid injury, which would produce a retroauricular area of hypoesthesia. The sternocleidomastoid muscle is detached from the mastoid process, leaving only few fibers that will be useful in reinserting the muscle during closure. Removal of this muscle is necessary only if extensive exposure is required, and may not be necessary for limited surgical procedures such as biopsy, drainage of abscesses, or the removal of small lesions. It is necessary to identify the spinal accessory nerve, which can be located following the belly of the sternocleidomastoid muscle distally. The nerve lies approximately 3 cm from the insertion of the muscle, and may be partly embedded in the muscle itself. The nerve should be freed and retracted, either anteriorly or medially, together with the blood vessels that constitute the neurovascular bundle. If exposure is required below the level of C2 and even toward the distal end of the cervical spine, the nerve will remain in the way. To avoid sacrificing the spinal accessory nerve, it must be freed proximally up to its exit from the skull near the jugular vein, so that it can be retracted together with the strenocleidomastoid muscle. At this point, the transverse process of the atlas, which protrudes slightly laterally, is palpable half-way between the angle of the jaw and the mastoid process. The posterior belly of the digastric muscle must be identified and retracted either superiorly or medially to obtain adequate exposure.

This is the area through which the extraskeletal portion of the vertebral artery passes cephalad from the transverse process of C1. At this point, the transverse processes in the prevertebral plane are exposed behind the carotid sheath, which can be mobilized and retracted anteriorly. Further dissection will permit access to the retropharyngeal space separating the previsceral areolar tissues (Sharpey's fibers). The prevertebral muscular plane (longus colli muscle) is immediately visible. It covers the first cervical vertebra with fibers that extend as far as the anterior tubercle of the atlas on its medial side. To expose the anterior arch of the atlas, the body of the axis, or the base of the odontoid process, the surgeon must dissect this prevertebral muscular plane. The lateral joints between the masses of the atlas and the axis and the base of the odontoid process can be approached at the point in which they articulate with the atlas. The prevertebral muscular tissues can be dissected subperiosteally and retracted anteriorly, but care must be taken to not injure the cervical sympathetic chain. This dissection, however, will be essential if access to the transverse apophyses is required. To reach the vertebral body, the longus colli muscle must be separated from the central region of the vertebral body and retracted toward the transverse processes. Detachment of the muscles may be limited only to the area required by the specific procedure, and may require exposure of the entire vertebral surface or just of the lateral aspect including the transverse process.

8.2.2 Complications

8.2.2.1 Vascular Injury

In patients with trauma, inflammatory processes, or tumor, there is a risk of injury to the vertebral artery. This is often due to the anatomical changes brought about by the disease process. Rarely, and usually as a result of inexperience, lesions of the carotid artery and of the jugular vein have been reported. Usually, intracranial vascular injuries occur because of excessive retraction. In fact, the proximal end the carotid artery is anchored in the cranial foramen and excessive traction will be against this rigid and fixed position. The consequences of injury to the carotid artery will obviously be reflected in ischemic injury in its distribution [2].

8.2.2.2 Neurological Injury

Injuries can occur to a variety of nerves encountered in the surgical dissection, including the greater auricular nerve at the proximal edge of the sternocleidomastoid muscle, the spinal accessory nerve, the facial nerve, and the cervical sympathetic chain. The spinal accessory nerve can be injured either by careless dissection or unnecessary and excessive traction. The facial nerve may not only be overstretched by retraction, but may also be compressed between the retractors and the mandible. The cervical sympathetic chain can be injured in the dissection of muscle in the lateral cervical plane in the approach to the transverse apophyses [2].

8.2.2.3 Visceral Injury

Glottic edema is the most common postoperative complication because of the extensive tissue trauma induced by the surgical dissection. In our experience, preoperative tracheotomy is not always mandatory. We feel it essential only in patients with severe trauma or extensive tumor in which the dissection is expected to produce severe and extensive tissue injury. In all the other patients, we maintain postoperative intubation for at least 24 h and attempt to minimize or control edema with steroids [6].

8.2.3 Advantages

The retrocarotid approach avoids surgical dissection in areas where there are major vascular and neurological structures that must be identified, dissected, and retracted from the operative field. Once the neurovascular bundle of the neck has been identified and retracted anteriorly and medially, the surgeon has a clear pathway to the spine, devoid of any significant structure that must be dissected, retracted, or sacrificed. Second, this approach allows the exposure of the full length of the intertransverse region from Cl down to C7, with good access to the lateral aspect of the cervical spine. It is a very practical and useful approach in dealing with tumor compressing the spinal cord. When combined with the precarotid approach, it can provide a particularly extensive exposure that will permit spinal cord decompression and removal of extensive tumor masses [10]. This method, however, despite its great advantages throughout the cervical spine, does not give good access above C1. It cannot be used to expose the atlanto-occipital region. The carotid artery, the jugular vein, and the vagus and hypoglossal nerves have a fixed position as they exit the skull, and it is very difficult and dangerous to attempt to retract them. Serious problems include both neurological injury and vascular insufficiency involving the distribution of the internal carotid artery. A technical difficulty is that the dissection is angulated in such a way as to make good illumination of the operative site difficult, so that visualization of structures may be less than optimal [6].

8.3 Retrosternocleidomastoid Approach

The retrosternocleidomastoid approach allows access to the whole cervical spine, from C1 to C7, and it is used mostly to approach the cervical sympathetic chain, the anterior lateral surface of vertebral bodies, the transverse processes, the intertransverse spaces, and the vertebral artery [10].

Incision of skin starts from the upper portion of mastoid process and extends downwards, following the posterior edge of stenocleidomastoid muscle. After the subcutaneous tissue and platysma have been cut, the sternocleidomastoid muscle is exposed. The surgeon must be particularly careful to avoid injury to the superficial occipital vein and mastoid branches of the superficial cervical plexus. A good access to the underlying planes is obtained by cutting the superficial cervical fascia along the posterior edge of the sternocleidomastoid muscle, thus reaching the carotid artery [2]. The retrostyloid space is located in the upper part of incision. It is possible here to palpate the transverse process of the atlas 1 cm below the mastoid apex. Distally, it is easier to retract the sternocleidomastoid muscle, the neurovascular bundle, and the visceral structures of the neck. Prevertebral muscles are detached from the skeletal plane and then retracted. It is necessary first to locate the cervical sympathetic chain. After this has been done, it is easy to expose the anterolateral portion of the vertebral bodies, the transverse processes, the intertransverse spaces, and the vertebral artery [10].

Core Messages

- The low and high retropharyngeal and precarotid presternocleidomastoid approaches to the cervical spine allow one to expose all the levels of the cervical spine, from the basis of the skull to the upper thoracic levels.
- Potential complications of the anterolateral approaches to the cervical spine include: vascular, neurological, soft tissue, and visceral complications.
- Vascular Injuries include damages to the carotid artery, vertebral artery, jugular vein, and thyroid vessels.
- Injuries to the carotid artery during presternocleidomastoid approaches to the cervical spine are rare, because the artery, retracted laterally, is located within the carotid sheath and covered with connective tissue. Difficult anatomy and poor identification of the midline are risk factors for injuries of the carotid artery. Direct injuries can result during dissection, or because of the use of self-retaining retractors. Prolonged handle retraction may also be responsible for internal carotid artery thrombosis and hemispheric stroke. Intermittent release of retractors is recommended during surgery to restore adequate internal carotid artery flow. Bleeding can be usually controlled by external compression. Manipulation must be minimized to avoid the risk of thrombus fragmentation and embolization. Also, compression needs to be balanced with the need to maintain flow in the artery. Clamping of the common or internal carotid artery should be avoided unless the patient's condition is life-threatening because the interruption of the flow may cause embolization and cerebral ischemia. Repair techniques include simple suture, patch, resection with end-to-end anastomosis, resection with an interposition graft, transposition of external to internal carotid artery, ligation, or balloon occlusion. Ligation or balloon occlusion should be reserved for inaccessible injuries, which are impossible to repair.
- In the high presternocleidomastoid approach, injuries to the vertebral arteries can easily occur when the surgeon operates at the level of the cranio-cervical junction, laterally to the axis. In the low presternocleidomastoid approach, the vertebral artery can be damaged when surgery is performed in the lateral portion of the vertebral body toward the transverse processes, and when osseous dissection involves the foramen transversarium, which contains the vertebral artery. When injuries occur, the bleeding will be massive. Vertebral artery laceration has been attributed to several factors: motorized dissection off midline, excessive lateral bone-disk removal, excessively lateral placement of instrumentation, bone pathologically softened by tumor, infection, or irradiation, and intraoperative loss of midline landmarks. The proximity of vertebral artery to the uncovertebral joint during foraminotomy or removal of the postero-lateral quadrant of the vertebral body is a predisposing factor to arterial laceration. Prevention of iatrogenic vertebral artery injury is the best management. Endovascular management is the first therapeutic option in injuries to the vertebral artery because of its location and surgical inaccessibility. Detachable balloons, coils, stents, and hemostatic agents are usually successful to manage bleeding. Immediate intervention with proximal and distal ligation is necessary in unstable patients with life-threatening bleeding.
- When damages occur to the jugular vein, the resulting bleeding can be controlled by suturing the wall of the vein. The vessel must be totally accessible during the suture. This may require one to open the carotid sheath to expose the vein and identify the artery and the vagus nerve to avoid including these two additional structures in the sutures or ligatures.
- Esophageal perforation is a recognized potentially fatal complication of anterior cervical spine surgery. Esophageal ischemic or direct injury usually is determined by excessive retraction during dissection. If damages to

esophagus and pharynx are identified intraoperatively and repaired immediately, it is necessary to maintain the nasogastric tube for 2–3 weeks postoperatively, with a compressive bandage on the neck. Parenteral nutrition and feeding through the nasogastric tube will be sufficient, particularly when augmented by the use of atropine to decrease salivation. If the tear is not identified intraoperatively, then the surgeon must be on the alert for this possibility when drainage persists for several days postoperatively.

> Damages to the thoracic duct may lead to nutritional deficiencies, respiratory dysfunction, and immunosuppression with a mortality up to 50%. The variable anatomic course of the thoracic duct has been reported as the main reason for injuries during spinal surgery. Other factors include its small size, inconstant location, and proximity to the vertebral bodies. Thoracic duct injury can present as cervical chylous fistula, chylothorax, or chylopericardium. When the thoracic duct is interrupted, chylothorax may occur from leakage due to reflux within substitution collateral pathways diverting the flow of chyle into the venoux confluents of the neck. Conservative management consists of low-fat diet with medium chain triglycerides, total parenteral nutrition, correction of electrolyte imbalance, and adequate drainage by chest tube or neck drain. The definitive management is ligation of the thoracic duct.

> Damages of various nerves may occur during the anterolateral approach to the cervical spine, and severity is commonly defined as neurapraxia, axonotmesis, and neurotmesis. In the submandibular and perimandibular region, the operative field will be crossed by the facial nerve (seventh cranial nerve), the hypoglossal nerve (twelfth cranial nerve), and the superior laryngeal nerve.

> Damages to the mandibular branch of the facial nerve determine a very slight drooping of the corner of the mouth. The drooping may not be detectable when the mouth is closed, but only when it is in motion (i.e., smiling).

> The superior laryngeal nerve can be injured during the high anterolateral approach. And it is injured whenever the retroesophageal prevertebral space is missed, and inadvertently the surgeon enters the space between the esophagus and trachea. Injury to this nerve produces vocal disturbance, which may be irreversible. Symptoms include hoarseness, vocal breathiness or fatigue, weak cough, dysphagia, or aspiration. Although vocal cord paralysis may be permanent, in most cases symptoms last for weeks or months.

> The cervical sympathetic chain can be injured in its superior region near the stellate ganglion when the surgeon is dissecting (the long muscles of the neck) in the lateral cervical muscular plane. It is usually injured when the surgeon fails to remain subperiosteal in dissecting the lateral aspect of the vertebral body in the approach to the transverse apophyses. This injury leads to Horner's syndrome, characterized by homolateral anophthalmia, myosis, and palpebral ptosis.

References

1. Roy-Camille R, Judet TH, Saillant G et al (1981) Tumeurs du rachis. Techniques chirugucales, Orthopedie. Encycl Med Chir Paris 44165:4.06.04
2. Denaro V (1991) Stenosis of the cervical spine. Springer, Berlin
3. Robinson RA, Smith GW (1955) Anterolateral cervical disc removal and interbody fusion for cervical disc syndrome. Bull Johns Hopkins Hosp 96:223–224
4. de Andrade JR, Macnab I (1969) Anterior occipito-cervical fusion using an extra-pharyngeal exposure. J Bone Joint Surg Am 51:1621–1626
5. Riley LH Jr, Robinson RA, Johnson KA et al (1969) The results of anterior interbody fusion of the cervical spine. Review of ninety-three consecutive cases. J Neurosurg 30: 127–133
6. Denaro V, Denaro L, Gulino G et al (1998) Complicanze nella chirurgia cervicale. Giornale Italiano di Ortopedia e Traumatologia 24:681–688
7. Boni M, Denaro V (1982) Surgical treatment of cervical arthrosis. Follow-up review (2–13 years) of the 1st 100 cases operated on by anterior approach. Rev Chir Orthop Reparatrice Appar Mot 68:269–280

8. Boni M, Denaro V (1982) The cervical stenosis syndrome with a review of 83 patients treated by operation. Int Orthop 6:185–195
9. Eastlack RK, Currier BL (2008) Cervical Spine. In: Morrey BF, Morrey MC (eds) Master techniques in orthopaedic surgery: relevant surgical exposures, 1st edn. Lippincott Williams & Wilkins, Philadelphia, pp 268–297
10. Denaro V, Gulino G, Papapietro N et al (1998) Treatment of metastases of the cervical spine. Chir Organi Mov 83: 127–137
11. Boni M, Cherubino P, Denaro V (1983) The surgical treatment of fractures of the cervical spine. Ital J Orthop Traumatol 9(Suppl):367–369
12. Boni M, Denaro V (1980) Surgical treatment of traumatic lesions of the middle and lower cervical spine (C3–C7). Ital J Orthop Traumatol 6:305–320
13. Patel NP, Wolcott WP, Johnson JP et al (2008) Esophageal injury associated with anterior cervical spine surgery. Surg Neurol 69:20–24; discission 24
14. Alexander MJ, Smith TP, Tucci DL (2002) Treatment of an iatrogenic petrous carotid artery pseudoaneurysm with a symbiot covered stent: technical case report. Neurosurgery 50:658–662
15. Houkin K (2005) Iatrogenic carotid artery injury in neurosurgery. Neurosurg Rev 28:248
16. Pollard ME, Little PW (2002) Changes in carotid artery blood flow during anterior cervical spine surgery. Spine 27:152–155
17. Chozick BS, Watson P, Greenblatt SH (1994) Internal carotid artery thrombosis after cervical corpectomy. Spine 19:2230–2232
18. Yeh YC, Sun WZ, Lin CP et al (2004) Prolonged retraction on the normal common carotid artery induced lethal stroke after cervical spine surgery. Spine 29:E431–E434
19. Wahlberg E, Olofsson P, Goldstone J (2007) Vascular Injuries to the Neck. In: Wahlberg E, Olofsson P, Goldstone J (eds) Emergency vascular surgery – a practical guide. Springer, Berlin, pp 3–14
20. Daentzer D, Deinsberger W, Boker DK (2003) Vertebral artery complications in anterior approaches to the cervical spine: report of two cases and review of literature. Surg Neurol 59:300–309; discussion 309
21. Golfinos JG, Dickman CA, Zabramski JM et al (1994) Repair of vertebral artery injury during anterior cervical decompression. Spine 19:2552–2556
22. Smith MD, Emery SE, Dudley A et al (1993) Vertebral artery injury during anterior decompression of the cervical spine. A retrospective review of ten patients. J Bone Joint Surg Br 75:410–415
23. Curylo LJ, Mason HC, Bohlman HH et al (2000) Tortuous course of the vertebral artery and anterior cervical decompression: a cadaveric and clinical case study. Spine 25: 2860–2864
24. Eleraky MA, Llanos C, Sonntag VK (1999) Cervical corpectomy: report of 185 cases and review of the literature. J Neurosurg 90:35–41
25. Gaudinez RF, English GM, Gebhard JS et al (2000) Esophageal perforations after anterior cervical surgery. J Spinal Disord 13:77–84
26. Jamjoom ZA (1997) Pharyngo-cutaneous fistula following anterior cervical fusion. Br J Neurosurg 11:69–74
27. Jones WG II, Ginsberg RJ (1992) Esophageal perforation: a continuing challenge. Ann Thorac Surg 53:534–543
28. Kelly MF, Spiegel J, Rizzo KA et al (1991) Delayed pharyngoesophageal perforation: a complication of anterior spine surgery. Ann Otol Rhinol Laryngol 100:201–205
29. Morrison A (1960) Hyperextension injury of the cervical spine with rupture of the oesophagus. J Bone Joint Surg Br 42-B:356–357
30. Orlando ER, Caroli E, Ferrante L (2003) Management of the cervical esophagus and hypofarinx perforations complicating anterior cervical spine surgery. Spine 28:E290–E295
31. Sharma RR, Sethu AU, Lad SD et al (2001) Pharyngeal perforation and spontaneous extrusion of the cervical graft with its fixation device: a late complication of C2–C3 fusion via anterior approach. J Clin Neurosci 8:464–468
32. Smith MD, Bolesta MJ (1992) Esophageal perforation after anterior cervical plate fixation: a report of two cases. J Spinal Disord 5:357–362
33. Yee GK, Terry AF (1993) Esophageal penetration by an anterior cervical fixation device. A case report. Spine 18: 522–527
34. Witwer BP, Resnick DK (2003) Delayed esophageal injury without instrumentation failure: complication of anterior cervical instrumentation. J Spinal Disord Tech 16:519–523
35. Hankins JR, McLaughlin JS (1977) Pericarditis with effusion complicating esophageal perforation. J Thorac Cardiovasc Surg 73:225–230
36. Kiernan PD, Hernandez A, Byrne WD et al (1998) Descending cervical mediastinitis. Ann Thorac Surg 65: 1483–1488
37. Mayer JE Jr, Murray CA, Varco RL (1977) The treatment of esophageal perforation with delayed recognition and continuing sepsis. Ann Thorac Surg 23:568–573
38. Zenone EA, Trotman BW (1977) Boerhaave's syndrome. Spontaneous formation of an esophageal-bronchial fistula. JAMA 238:2048–2049
39. Sarr MG, Pemberton JH, Payne WS (1982) Management of instrumental perforations of the esophagus. J Thorac Cardiovasc Surg 84:211–218
40. Boffa DJ, Sands MJ, Rice TW et al (2008) A critical evaluation of a percutaneous diagnostic and treatment strategy for chylothorax after thoracic surgery. Eur J Cardiothorac Surg 33:435–439
41. Thompson KJ, Kernstine KH, Grannis FW Jr et al (2008) Treatment of chylothorax by robotic thoracic duct ligation. Ann Thorac Surg 85:334–336
42. Bourgeois P, Munck D, Sales F (2008) Anomalies of thoracic lymph duct drainage demonstrated by lymphoscintigraphy and review of the literature about these anomalies. Eur J Surg Oncol 34(5):553–555
43. Davis HK (1915) A statistical study of the thoracic duct in man. Am J Anat 17:211–244
44. Kinnaert P (1973) Anatomical variations of the cervical portion of the thoracic duct in man. J Anat 115:45–52
45. Greenfield J, Gottlieb MI (1956) Variations in the terminal portion of the human thoracic duct. Arch Surg 73:955–959
46. Van Pernis PA (1949) Variations of the thoracic duct. Surgery 26:806–809
47. Kumar S, Kumar A, Pawar DK (2004) Thoracoscopic management of thoracic duct injury: Is there a place for conservatism? J Postgrad Med 50:57–59

48. Bonavina L, Saino G, Bona D et al (2001) Thoracoscopic management of chylothorax complicating esophagectomy. J Laparoendosc Adv Surg Tech A 11:367–369
49. Crosthwaite GL, Joypaul BV, Cuschieri A (1995) Thoracoscopic management of thoracic duct injury. J R Coll Surg Edinb 40:303–304
50. Lubicky JP (1998) Chylous leakage after circumferential thoracolumbar fusion for correction of kyphosis resulting from fracture: report of three cases. Spine 23:1814–1815
51. Hart AK, Greinwald JH Jr, Shaffrey CI et al (1998) Thoracic duct injury during anterior cervical discectomy: a rare complication. Case report. J Neurosurg 88:151–154
52. Colletta AJ, Mayer PJ (1982) Chylothorax: an unusual complication of anterior thoracic interbody spinal fusion. Spine 7:46–49
53. Eisenstein S, O'Brien JP (1977) Chylothorax: a complication of Dwyer's anterior instrumentation. Br J Surg 64: 339–341
54. Nakai S, Zielke K (1986) Chylothorax–a rare complication after anterior and posterior spinal correction. Report on six cases. Spine 11:830–833
55. Propst-Proctor SL, Rinsky LA, Bleck EE (1983) The cisterna chyli in orthopaedic surgery. Spine 8:787–792
56. Shen YS, Cheung CY, Nilsen PT (1989) Chylous leakage after arthrodesis using the anterior approach to the spine. Report of two cases. J Bone Joint Surg Am 71:1250–1251
57. von Knoch M, Michiels I, Mueller S et al (2004) Chylous leakage after thoracolumbar fracture may cause paraplegia. Spine 29:E32–E34
58. Riquet M, Badia A (2004) Surgery for chylothorax. Rev Pneumol Clin 60:104–108
59. Boni M, Cherubino P, Denaro V et al (1984) Multiple subtotal somatectomy. Technique and evaluation of a series of 39 cases. Spine 9:358–362
60. Lapp GC, Brown DH, Gullane PJ et al (1998) Thoracoscopic management of chylous fistulae. Am J Otolaryngol 19:257–262
61. Collard JM, Laterre PF, Boemer F et al (2000) Conservative treatment of postsurgical lymphatic leaks with somatostatin-14. Chest 117:902–905
62. Inderbitzi RG, Krebs T, Stirneman T et al (1992) Treatment of postoperative chylothorax by fibrin glue application under thoracoscopic view with use of local anesthesia. J Thorac Cardiovasc Surg 104:209–210
63. Lampson RS (1948) Traumatic chylothorax; a review of the literature and report of a case treated by mediastinal ligation of the thoracic duct. J Thorac Surg 17:778–791
64. Netterville JL, Koriwchak MJ, Winkle M et al (1996) Vocal fold paralysis following the anterior approach to the cervical spine. Ann Otol Rhinol Laryngol 105:85–91
65. Apfelbaum RI, Kriskovich MD, Haller JR (2000) On the incidence, cause, and prevention of recurrent laryngeal nerve palsies during anterior cervical spine surgery. Spine 25:2906–2912
66. Riew KD, Cheng I, Pimenta L et al (2007) Posterior cervical spine surgery for radiculopathy. Neurosurgery 60:S57–S63
67. Kitchel SH, Eismont FJ, Green BA (1989) Closed subarachnoid drainage for management of cerebrospinal fluid leakage after an operation on the spine. J Bone Joint Surg Am 71:984–987
68. Bertalanffy H, Eggert HR (1989) Complications of anterior cervical discectomy without fusion in 450 consecutive patients. Acta Neurochir (Wien) 99:41–50
69. Wheeler DL, Enneking WF (2005) Allograft bone decreases in strength in vivo over time. Clin Orthop Relat Res 435:36–42
70. Emery SE, Smith MD, Bohlman HH (1991) Upper-airway obstruction after multilevel cervical corpectomy for myelopathy. J Bone Joint Surg Am 73:544–551
71. Penberthy A, Roberts N (1998) Recurrent acute upper airway obstruction after anterior cervical fusion. Anaesth Intensive Care 26:305–307
72. Boockvar JA, Philips MF, Telfeian AE et al (2001) Results and risk factors for anterior cervicothoracic junction surgery. J Neurosurg 94:12–17
73. Riew KD, Sethi NS, Devney J et al (1999) Complications of buttress plate stabilization of cervical corpectomy. Spine 24:2404–2410
74. Henry AK (1957) Extensile exposure. Churchill Livingstone, Edinburgh, pp 53–80
75. Henry GA (1957) Post irradiation damage to the pharynx; larynx and esophagus. Laryngoscope 67:709–712
76. Whitesides TE Jr, Kelly RP (1966) Lateral approach to the upper cervical spine for anterior fusion. South Med J 59:879–883

9 Complications Related to Posterior Approach

Luca Denaro, Domenico D'Avella, and Vincenzo Denaro

Contents

L. Denaro (✉)
Department of Neuroscience, University of Padua,
Via Giustiniani, 5, 35128 Padua, Italy
e-mail: lucadenaro@hotmail.com

9.1 Introduction

The posterior approach through a midline longitudinal incision provides the most direct access to the posterior elements of the cervical spine. Through this approach, the posterior elements of the cervical spine can be removed, and access to the posterior aspect of the spinal cord and nerve roots from the occiput to C7 can be obtained. The posterior approach to the cervical spine allows excellent exposure to perform several surgical techniques, with or without internal fixation. It can also be a useful rostral extension of a longer posterior thoracic spinal approach [1].

The posterior elements of the cervical spine play an important role in the stabilization of the cervical spine. Indeed, their removal in patients undergoing wide laminectomies (i.e., for the management of pathologies such as the spondylotic myelopathy, or extra- or intra-medullary tumors) may cause subluxation, or severe kyphotic angulation of the spine (i.e., swan neck), causing increased compression of the neural elements and worsening of neurological deficits [1].

In some patients, if necessary, with careful retraction and protection of the neural structures, it is possible to expose the anterior side of the spinal canal (actually the lateral side of the posterior wall of the vertebral body and the intervertebral disk space), the pedicles, and the posterior portion of the root canals. With this approach, however, the surgeon should not expect to be able to reach the central region of the posterior vertebral bodies [1]. This would involve particularly difficult (if not impossible) retraction or displacement of neural structures, which might produce severe neurological damage [2].

L. Denaro et al. (eds.), *Pitfalls in Cervical Spine Surgery*,
DOI: 10.1007/978-3-540-85019-9_9, © Springer-Verlag Berlin Heidelberg 2010

The choice of the side from which the surgery is performed depends on the side from which the surgeon is most comfortable, and therefore it is a personal choice of the surgeon [3]. Usually, a right-handed surgeon prefers the right side and vice versa.

The details of patient positioning on the operative table, the position of the head, and the protection of the eyes are described in Chap. 6. Briefly, when positioning the patient on the operative table, all the prominences must be well padded. Reverse-Trendelenberg position eases visualization of the occipito-cervical junction, and may reduce venous congestion and intraoperative bleeding. The hair of the patient is shaved from the neck to just above the external occipital protuberance to the ears laterally. The external occipital protuberance and the spinous processes of C2 and C7 (the most prominent) are specific landmarks, helping to outline the midline approach. A line uniting these landmarks can be drawn. Bleeding during the approach can be minimized by using pre-incision local anesthetic with a dilute 1:500,000 epinephrine solution. The infiltration with local anesthetic should begin at the spinous processes and proceed laterally from these into the paravertebral tissues [1]. It is important to perform a midline incision to avoid poor or unacceptable repair and scarring [4]. The length of the incision is determined by the level at which the surgery is to be performed. The incision usually begins 2–3 cm above the external occipital protuberance if the surgeon intends to reach the occipito-cervical region [4]. Following the initial skin incision, the subcutaneous fat layer is cut. A self-retaining retractor is used to open the wound and allow the achievement of hemostasis with diathermy [3]. Next, the midline should be identified to allow delineation of the lateral paravertebral regions. The superficial aponeurosis is then incised at the midline, the nucal ligament is identified. This is a membranous fibrous layer adherent on its anterior aspect to the spinous processes, and represents the medial insertion of the trapezius muscles of the neck. It is an important structure that plays a crucial role in the maintenance of stability in the cervical spine. It extends from the occiput to the posterior tubercles of the atlas and along the spinous processes from C2 to C7 [5]. Using diathermy and elevators, the posterior elements are exposed subperiosteally and self-retaining retractors are inserted. Dissection must remain outside the muscle bulk on either side, which now appears more superficial [6]. A considerable amount of muscle detachment from the posterior elements of the vertebrae is necessary. It is important to pay attention to the anatomic planes to avoid undesirable blood loss and neurological damage [7].

At the upper end, over the occipito-cervical junction, the incision is extended up to the occipital bone at the external occipital protuberance. The periosteum can be elevated from the occiput, using an appropriate periosteal elevator over the entire posterior surface of the occiput [8]. The periosteal elevation is not difficult. Beginning at the midline, it is extended for 15–20 mm laterally (Fig. 9.1).

It is important to preserve the greater occipital nerve of Arnold, which passes under the greater inferior oblique muscle of the head, and crosses the semispinal muscle of the head as well as the splenius and trapezius muscles. Superiorly, as it nears the occiput, it becomes more superficial, together with the terminal

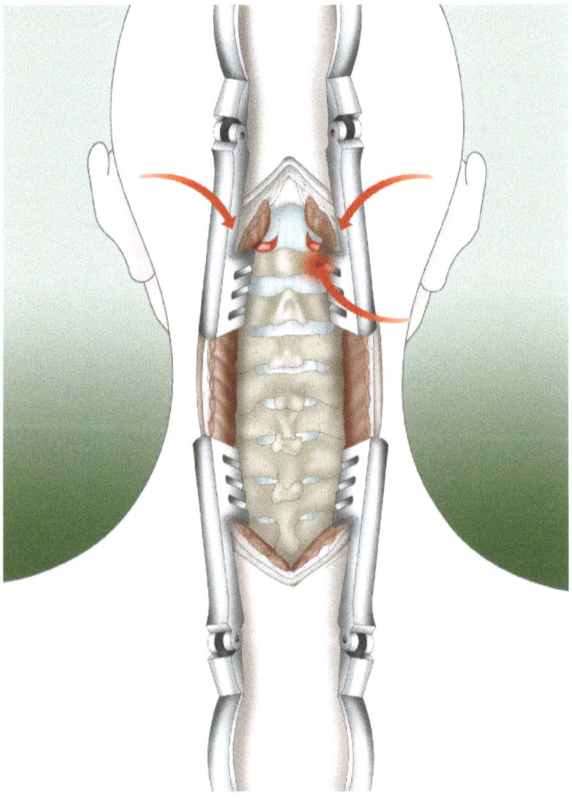

Fig. 9.1 At the upper cervical spine, it is important to avoid damages to the vertebral artery when self-retaining retractors are applied

branches of the occipital artery on either side of the occiput [7]. The greater occipital nerve is usually located 15 mm lateral to the midline, and is easily avoided if the surgeon scrupulously remains medially within the subperiosteal region during dissection [9, 10]. After exposure of the occipital surface and the external occipital protuberance, the surgeon must carefully identify the spinous process of C2. This will be a specific landmark in identifying the posterior arch of the atlas. After muscles detachment with diathermy from C2, the surgeon can identify the posterior arch of the atlas and its tubercle by palpation. The muscles are separated with a midline incision. Then, the elevation of the muscolo-ligamentous insertion from the tubercle of C1 is continued. The periosteum is stripped from the arch of the atlas laterally. The surgeon must be aware of the presence of the vertebral artery in this part of the dissection. This artery passes in the area by circumventing the lateral mass of the atlas at the same level as the posterior arch. As the surgeon follows the posterior arch of the atlas away from the central region (the tubercle), it is important that he remains meticulously in the subperiosteal plane. This elevation must be done carefully and need not extend beyond 15 mm from the midline. In dissection directed to the lower cervical spine, that is the more distal regions, the surgeon may use diathermy for stripping. Again, the surgeon must stay meticulously close to the periosteum of the spinous processes and the laminae of C2–C7. This will permit elevation of the lateral cervical muscles (these include the semispinal muscle of the head, the long muscles of the head and neck, and, situated in the deeper planes and higher, the oblique and rectus muscles along with the interspinal and transversospinal muscles) [5, 10].

The detachment and stripping of the paravertebral surface can be done easily with diathermy. Periosteal elevators are difficult to control and, in patients with tumors or with an element of instability, their use can determine neurological injuries. It is easier to use diathermy particularly to reach the more lateral portions of the dissection. Also, diathermy can always be fully controlled. Whenever periosteal elevators are used, the tip should be protected, making it suitable only for blunt dissection. At this point, muscle elevation and exposure of the apophyseal joints of the spine have been completed. The self-retaining retractors can now be positioned and the surgeon has full access to the entire posterior region of the neck [4].

9.2 Pitfalls

9.2.1 Bad Positioning

Complications related to the posterior approach are often associated with the positioning of the patient on the operating table (for a wider explanation, see Chap. 6). Briefly, it is absolutely essential to position the patient properly to reduce blood loss and improve intraoperative visualization. Bad positioning of the patient usually results from placing the patient directly onto the operating table in such a way that compression of the abdomen will interfere with diaphragmatic movements during respiration. The consequences are increased splenic venous pressure and greater intraoperative bleeding from the ensuing increased vascular pressure in the parameningeal vessels. Poor oxygenation of the patient can also occur. Incorrect positioning of the head and of the headrest results in an unfavorable position of the head and neck with respect to the trunk (see Chap. 6). This can disadvantage the surgeon during the surgical procedure, because of the inappropriate positioning of vertebrae. Ophthalmologic complications associated with prone positioning in spine surgery have been widely reported. They include corneal abrasion (the most common ophthalmologic injury), and blindness as the result of posterior ischemic optic neuropathy, central retinal artery occlusion, or occipital cortical infarct or cortical blindness. The patient must be positioned to avoid direct pressure over and around the eyes (Table 9.1).

Endotracheal tubes for anesthesia can be easily displaced, not only during positioning of the patient once anesthetized, but also during surgery (see Chap. 6). When this occurs, surgery must immediately stop, and the patient rolled on the operating table back to the supine position for re-intubation. This can be particularly dangerous in unstable spines (i.e., in patients with trauma or tumors), in which the removal of the supporting osteoligamentous structures performed in the early stages of surgery (before internal fixation is performed) makes the cervical spine even more unstable.

9.2.2 Neurological Injury

Neurological injuries include lesions to spinal cord, nerve roots, and dura mater. The more common

Table 9.1 Complications of the posterior approach

Complications	How to avoid them: tips and tricks
Injuries to the vertebral artery	Remains meticulously in the subperiosteal plane during dissection Limit the exposure of the posterior ring of the atlas to the medial aspect of the groove of the atlas, avoiding too laterally exposure (usually more than 15 mm from the tubercle) Be aware of the potential anomalous course of the VA at the atlas Because of its relatively inaccessible location, injuries to the vertebral artery are usually best managed by endovascular techniques
Neurological injuries	Carefully position the patient on the operative table Be aware of the potential damage to nerve roots when dissection is extended beyond the lateral limits of the apophyseal joints Be aware that ossification of the posterior longitudinal ligament is a risk factor for CSF fistula and pseudomeningocele High-speed drill should be used in the medial to lateral direction to avoid damages to the dura and the underlying spinal cord Protect the dura with a padded material against inadvertent penetration while bone is removed during surgery Close primarily dural tears when they are discovered before the end of surgery Use a surgical microscope to optimize lighting and magnification when closing a dural defect
Specific neurological injuries: damages to the greater occipital nerve of Arnold	Scrupulously remain medially within the subperiosteal region during dissection
Specific neurological injuries: postoperative C5 palsy	Avoid nerve root traction by posterior expansion and consequent displacement of the spinal cord during laminoplasty Perform a prophylactic foraminotomy, reducing the tension on the C5 nerve root Avoid aggressive opening of the lamina during laminoplasty to limit the posterior shift of the cord Avoid excessive reduction of the anterolisthetic C4 In patients with multilevel stenosis and spondylotic myelopathy, perform wide laminectomies, associated with fixation in lordosis of the operated segment: the laminectomy, with the removal of all the posterior elements of the canal, determines a widening of the spinal canal, the fixation in lordosis of the operated segment allows a back-shift of the spinal cord, so that the spinal cord lies away from the osteophytes

injuries are dural tears, which can lead to cerebrospinal fluid (CSF) fistulae. Indirect neurological injury may be the result of incorrect maneuvers of intubation or positioning of the patient on the operative table. On the other hand, direct neurological injuries are determined by surgery. The direct damage is a rare event, and it occurs more frequently in patients with tumors, trauma, inflammatory diseases, in whom the normal topographical anatomy is lost. Moreover, damages can occur more frequently when the surgeon is working near the dura mater in diseases that produce adherences on the dura (i.e., stenoses with hypertrophy of ligamentum flavum and loss of epidural fat).

At the upper level of the cervical spine, these complications are more frequent during the opening or widening of the foramen magnum, or in the detachment of atlanto-axial and atlanto-occipital tectorial membranes. When the dissection is extended beyond the lateral limits of the apophyseal joints, nerve roots may be injured.

The greater occipital nerve of Arnold arises from the jugular ganglion, and is joined after its origin by a filament from the petrous ganglion of the glossopharyngeal. It runs behind the internal jugular vein, and enters the mastoid canaliculus on the lateral wall of the jugular fossa. The nerve reaches the surface by passing through the tympanomastoid fissure between the mastoid process and the tympanic part of the temporal bone, and divides into two branches distributing to the skin of the back of the auricula and to the posterior part of the external acoustic meatus. Injuries may occur to the greater occipital nerve of Arnold during a too lateral dissection, which extends between the lateral occipital and lateral cervical muscle masses in the high regions of the neck.

9.2.3 Cerebrospinal Fluid Leaks

CSF leaks are one of the most common complications during posterior cervical spine surgery, with a prevalence of 0.5–13% [11–13], with the risk increasing to up to 18% with re-operations [14]. The surgical management of ossification of the posterior longitudinal ligament is associated with a high incidence of CSF fistula and pseudomeningocele (an extradural CSF collection arising from a dural defect) (4.5–32%) [14]. The rate of incidence is probably underreported because of the lack of associated morbidity with most dural tears. Although they are recognized as important complications, and they have been extensively reported in lumbar spine surgery [12, 15–17], dural tears have been poorly characterized in cervical spine [18]. The most feared complications associated with CSF leaks are life-threatening meningitis, spinocutaneous fistula, and pseudomeningocele [13, 19]. Their prevalence, ideal management, and long-term course remain debated [18]. Before operating on the cervical spine, the orthopedist should be familiar with the routine techniques used to open and close the dural sac and nerve root sheaths.

Strict adherence to basic surgical principles in the operating room may minimize the incidence of dural tears. Risk factors for dural tears include the use of a high-speed drill [20], which should be used in the medial to lateral direction to avoid damage to the dura and the underlying spinal cord in case of slippage. The dura should be covered with a padded material to protect against inadvertent penetration while bone is removed during surgery.

Careful preoperative planning and systematic surgical technique can help one to avoid damage to the scarred and often thin dura [20]. Dissection should begin where the tissue is normal and then proceed toward the area where the adherences are present.

The CSF may form a palpable mass, and can evolve in an external fistula [20]. The orthopedist must always suspect a CSF fistula in the presence of clear fluid emanating from a wound [20]. Common symptoms of patients with CSF fistula include headache, worsening when the patients stand. Magnetic resonance imaging remains the main imaging procedure to diagnose a CSF fistula, allowing to delineate the location, extent, and internal features of the lesion and eventual communication with the thecal sac.

When dural tears are discovered before the end of surgery, they should be closed primarily. When closing the dural defect, the use of a surgical microscope can optimize lighting and magnification, and allow the defect to be primarily sutured with 4-0, 5-0, or 6-0 nonabsorbable suture. When the dural defects are extensive and cannot be closed primarily, a patch graft of fascia lata, muscle tissue, or pericranium can be used. The use of cadaveric dura is discouraged because of the risk of Creuztfeldt–Jakob disease transmitted by cadaveric dura mater graft [21].

After the suture of the dura is performed, the surgeon must ask the anesthesiologist to increase intrathecal pressure (i.e., valsalva maneuver) to establish whether the closure is water-tight. If it is not water-tight, fibrin glue, another layer of fascia, and another layer of fibrin glue can be applied on top [20]. We prefer to apply fibrin glue to all dural repairs. Fibrin glue can be prepared from individual units of donor plasma, further reducing the risk of acquired infection [20].

In patients in whom the site of the CSF leak is inaccessible to repair or is discovered postoperatively, a lumbar subarachnoid drain should be placed, prophylactic antibiotics should be administered for a minimum of 72–96 h, and the patient should rest at bed. 200–300 mL CSF should be drained every 24 h. The drain is then clamped, and the patient allowed to ambulate. When a suspect of CSF leak persists, drainage can be continued for a maximum of 7 days. Then, drainage must be removed because of the risk of catheter-induced infection. Surgery should be performed in patients in whom lumbar catheter drainage fails.

9.2.4 Postoperative C5 Palsy

Posterior approach to the cervical spine has been associated with the risk of postoperative C5 palsy, which is the paralysis of the deltoid and/or biceps brachii muscles without any deterioration of myelopathy symptoms [22]. The incidence of postoperative C5 palsy in patients undergoing laminoplasty is around 4.6% (range, 0–30%) [23].

The pathogenesis of C5 palsy after posterior approaches to the cervical spine remains unknown. Many factors have been indicated, including nerve root traction by posterior expansion and consequent displacement of the spinal cord during laminoplasty [24–28], direct intraoperative nerve root injury [29], segmental damage to the spinal cord by mechanical insult [30], and ischemia from decreased radicular artery supply or reperfusion injuries [22, 31, 32]. Pre-existing foraminal stenosis can be a predictive factor [33], and prophylactic foraminotomy may help one to reduce its incidence [33, 34].

Postoperative C5 root palsy is common in patients undergoing cervical surgery for ossification of posterior longitudinal ligament [35], and for cervical compressive myelopathy with anterolisthesis of C4 [22]. In patients with multilevel cervical compressive myelopathy undergoing expansive laminectomy, in whom the instrumentation keeps the spine in lordosis, allowing the spinal cord to expand posteriorly after decompression, compression force for the vertebrae to create the lordotic alignment can also lead to the iatrogenic foraminal stenosis [22].

To decrease the risk of postoperative C5 palsy, it has been suggested to perform a prophylactic foraminotomy, reducing the tension on the C5 nerve root [33], to avoid aggressive opening of the lamina during laminoplasty to limit the posterior shift of the cord [22], and to avoid excessive reduction of the anterolisthetic C4 [22].

In our experience, we do not routinely perform laminoplasty in the management of patients with multilevel stenosis and spondylotic myelopathy. Indeed, we prefer to perform wide laminectomies, associated with fixation in lordosis of the operated segment. The laminectomy, with the removal of all the posterior elements of the canal, determines a widening of the spinal canal. The fixation in lordosis of the operated segment allows a back-shift of the spinal cord, so that the spinal cord lies away from the osteophytes. We have never observed postoperative C5 palsy in our experience since we perform this kind of surgery.

9.2.5 Vascular Injuries

Vascular complications may be associated with the deep cervical artery that passes along the posterior cervical region quite laterally near the apophyseal joints. Also, injuries to the posterior venous plexus can occur, but these do not determine severe consequences and can be easily controlled.

The vertebral artery (VA) is the most important vascular structure, which can be iatrogenic damaged during the posterior approach, with potential catastrophic consequences [36]. To avoid the injury of vertebral artery and to improve the accuracy of screw insertion during posterior spine surgery, many anatomic studies have been performed [37]. The VA can be divided into four portions (V1–V4) [38, 39]. The V1 portion extends from the subclavian artery, anterior to C7 transverse process, to the entry point of C6 foramen transversarium. V2 extends from the C6 foramen transversarium to C1 transverse foramina. V3 extends from the superior aspect of the arch of the atlas to the foramen magnum, coursing posteromedially in a horizontal groove on the upper surface of the posterior arch of the atlas. V4 extends intradurally from the foramen magnum to the contralateral VA to form the basilar artery [40]. The portions where the artery is most susceptible to injuries are anteriorly to C7, laterally at C3 to C7, and posteriorly to C1 and C2 [39, 41–46]. When posterior surgery to the atlanto-axial region is performed, the artery can be damaged especially during lateral extension of exposure or decompressive laminectomy of C1. Injuries to the artery may be avoided by limiting the exposure of the posterior ring of the atlas to the medial aspect of the groove of the atlas.

C1–C2 transarticular screw fixation has been associated with the majority of VA injury in posterior cervical spine surgery [43, 45–49].

To locate the VA and its venous plexus in the suboccipital region, two landmarks have been described [40]. The first one is the suboccipital triangle, constituted by the rectus capitis posterior major muscle, and obliquus capitis superior and inferior muscles [50], containing the horizontal part of the VA. The second one is the groove for the VA over the superior surface of the posterior arch of the atlas [51]. However, the course of VA is somewhat different. Yamaguchi et al. [40] used three-dimensional CT angiography images to quantify the protrusive course of the VA, and its diameter in 140 patients. They concluded that there may be significant variation in the location and branches of the VA that may place the vessel at risk during surgical intervention. The VA may run distant from the groove for the VA, making a posterolateral protrusion [52–54].

The VA may be injured when lateral exposure and instrumentation is performed at the atlanto-axial joint. The mean distance from the midline to the intersection of the VA and the inner cortex of the posterior arch of the atlas was about 15 mm [40]. The mean distance from the midline to the intersection of the VA and the outer cortex of the posterior arch was about 20 mm. The groove of the posterior arch of the atlas may not always be the exact location of the VA. Sometimes, a bony bridge over the VA groove of the atlas (namely atlantic ponticulus, posterior ponticulus, bony ponticles, or posterior bridging of the atlas) is found [40, 55–60].

Anomalous course of the VA at the atlas include the segmental course (in the case of vacancy of the ipsilateral transverse foramen of the atlas), duplication, or fenestration (in the case of occupancy of the transverse foramen of the atlas by another VA).

The artery may be injured by direct injury (i.e., during posterior decompression because of large tumor masses, during periosteal elevation and dissection of the posterior arch of the atlas) [61]. Injuries to the VA can also occur if the elevation is performed too laterally (usually more than 15 mm from the tubercle), and in an aggressive and poorly controlled manner. These events usually tend to occur more frequently with patients in whom the normal relationships have been changed, either by extensive trauma or by advanced tumor. Serious complications such as fistulas, pseudoaneurysm, massive bleeding, late-onset hemorrhage, thrombosis, embolism, cerebellar or brain stem infarction, and death have been reported after VA [45, 62–64].

Tears of the VA are difficult to repair. The region does not permit easy access, and is characterized by the presence of important neurological structures, such as the lower end of the medulla. Clips may be used to control hemorrhage only if the field is extended laterally.

Because of its relatively inaccessible location, injuries to the vertebral artery are usually best managed by endovascular techniques. Therapeutic options include intraluminal covered stents or endovascular embolization with coil. Bleeding, hematomas, pseudoaneurysms, and arteriovenous fistulas can occur after injuries to the vertebral artery, and they are successfully managed by transcatheter embolization. In unstable patients with life-threatening bleeding, immediate intervention with proximal and distal ligation is required [65].

Detachable balloons, coils, stents, or hemostatic agents are usually successful to manage bleeding, aneurysms, and fistulas. Antiplatelet and/or anticoagulation therapy should be administered postoperatively. A correlation between the incidence of stroke and mortality in carotid injuries has been showed, but not in injuries to the vertebral artery and the posterior circulation. Mortality directly related to vertebral artery injuries has been reported to be as low as 4% [65].

Core Messages

- During the posterior approach to the cervical spine, all the prominences must be well padded. Using diathermy and elevators, the posterior elements are exposed subperiosteally and insert self-retaining retractors. The detachment and stripping of the paravertebral surface can be done easily with diathermy.
- During the approach, it is important to preserve the greater occipital nerve of Arnold.
- Incorrect positioning of the head and of the headrest produces unfavorable position of the head and neck with respect to the trunk. This can disadvantage the surgeon during the surgical procedure, because of the inappropriate positioning of vertebral components.
- Injuries to the eyes (especially to the cornea) may result from incorrect positioning of the head.
- Endotracheal tubes for anesthesia may be easily displaced. When this happens, surgery must immediately stop, and the patient must be rotated on the operating table back into the intubation position. This can be particularly dangerous in an unstable spine, which may have been rendered even more unstable by the early stages of the surgical procedure before stabilization is performed.
- Neurological injuries include cord injury, of the root, of the dura mater. The more common are dural tears that can lead to CSF fistulae.
- The common reported complications associated with CSF leaks are life-threatening meningitis, spinocutaneous fistula, and pseudomeningocele. A CSF fistula should be always suspected in the presence of clear fluid emanating from a wound. When dural tears are discovered before the end of surgery, they should be closed primarily. If the CSF leak is

discovered postoperatively, CSF diversion by lumbar drainage may be the first management option. When the dural defects are extensive and cannot be closed primarily, a patch graft of fascia lata, muscle tissue, or pericranium can be used. The use of cadaveric dura is discouraged because of the risk of Creuztfeldt–Jakob disease transmitted by cadaveric dura mater graft. Fibrin glue can be applied after the suture has been performed.

› Posterior approach to the cervical spine has been associated with the risk of postoperative C5 palsy, which is the paralysis of the deltoid and/or biceps brachii muscles without any deterioration of myelopathy symptoms. To decrease the risk of postoperative C5 palsy, it has been suggested to perform a prophylactic foraminotomy, reducing the tension on the C5 nerve root, to avoid aggressive opening of the lamina during laminoplasty to limit the posterior shift of the cord, and to avoid excessive reduction of the anterolisthetic C4.

› The vertebral artery (VA) is the most important vascular structure, which can be iatrogenic damaged during the posterior approach. The artery may be injured during periosteal elevation and dissection of the posterior arch of the atlas. Injuries to the VA can also occur if the elevation is performed too laterally (usually more than 15 mm from the tubercle), and in an aggressive and poorly controlled manner. Serious complications such as fistulas, pseudoaneurysm, massive bleeding, late-onset hemorrhage, thrombosis, embolism, cerebellar or brain stem infarction, and death have been reported after VA.

References

1. Denaro V (1991) Stenosis of the cervical spine. Springer, Berlin
2. D'Alpa F, Scandurra L, Savuto R et al (1989) Pre-, intra- and postoperative somatosensory evoked potentials in cervical vertebral and spinal cord injuries. Minerva Anestesiol 55:115–118
3. Denaro V, Gulino G, Papapietro N et al (1998) Treatment of metastases of the cervical spine. Chir Organi Mov 83: 127–137
4. Denaro V, Denaro L, Gulino G et al (1998) Complicanze nella chirurgia cervicale. Giornale Italiano di Ortopedia e Traumatologia 24:681–688
5. Roy-Camille R, Judet TH, Saillant G et al (1981) Tumeurs du rachis. Techniques chirugucales, Orthopedie. Encycl Med Chir Paris 44165:4.06.04
6. Boni M, Cherubino P, Denaro V et al (1984) Multiple subtotal somatectomy. Technique and evaluation of a series of 39 cases. Spine 9:358–362
7. Boni M, Denaro V (1980) Surgical treatment of traumatic lesions of the middle and lower cervical spine (C3–C7). Ital J Orthop Traumatol 6:305–320
8. Boni M, Denaro V (1982) The cervical stenosis syndrome with a review of 83 patients treated by operation. Int Orthop 6:185–195
9. Boni M, Denaro V (1982) Surgical treatment of cervical arthrosis. Follow-up review (2–13 years) of the 1st 100 cases operated on by anterior approach. Rev Chir Orthop Reparatrice Appar Mot 68:269–280
10. Silvani V, Brambilla G, Rainoldi F et al (1987) Vertebral osteomyelitis with chronic cervical extradural abscess in a heroin addict. Neurochirurgia (Stuttg) 30:91–94
11. Bertalanffy H, Eggert HR (1989) Complications of anterior cervical discectomy without fusion in 450 consecutive patients. Acta Neurochir (Wien) 99:41–50
12. Cammisa FP Jr, Girardi FP, Sangani PK et al (2000) Incidental durotomy in spine surgery. Spine 25:2663–2667
13. Fountas KN, Kapsalaki EZ, Johnston KW (2005) Cerebrospinal fluid fistula secondary to dural tear in anterior cervical discectomy and fusion: case report. Spine 30: E277–E280
14. Clarck CR (2005) The cervical spine, 4th edn. Lippincott Williams &Wilkins, philadelphia
15. Eismont FJ, Wiesel SW, Rothman RH (1981) Treatment of dural tears associated with spinal surgery. J Bone Joint Surg Am 63:1132–1136
16. Hodges SD, Humphreys SC, Eck JC et al (1999) Management of incidental durotomy without mandatory bed rest. A retrospective review of 20 cases. Spine 24:2062–2064
17. Wang JC, Bohlman HH, Riew KD (1998) Dural tears secondary to operations on the lumbar spine. Management and results after a two-year-minimum follow-up of eighty-eight patients. J Bone Joint Surg Am 80:1728–1732
18. Hannallah D, Lee J, Khan M et al (2008) Cerebrospinal fluid leaks following cervical spine surgery. J Bone Joint Surg Am 90:1101–1105
19. Narotam PK, Jose S, Nathoo N et al (2004) Collagen matrix (DuraGen) in dural repair: analysis of a new modified technique. Spine 29:2861–2867; discussion 2868–2869
20. Graham JJ (1989) Complications of cervical spine surgery. A five-year report on a survey of the membership of the Cervical Spine Research Society by the morbidity and mortality committee. Spine 14:1046–1050
21. Yamada S, Aiba T, Endo Y et al (1994) Creutzfeldt-Jakob disease transmitted by a cadaveric dura mater graft. Neurosurgery 34:740–743; discussion 743–744
22. Takemitsu M, Cheung KM, Wong YW et al (2008) C5 nerve root palsy after cervical laminoplasty and posterior fusion with instrumentation. J Spinal Disord Tech 21:267–272
23. Sakaura H, Hosono N, Mukai Y et al (2003) C5 palsy after decompression surgery for cervical myelopathy: review of the literature. Spine 28:2447–2451

24. Epstein JA (1996) Extradural tethering effects as one mechanism of radiculopathy complicating posterior decompression of the cervical spinal cord. Spine 21:1839–1840
25. Hirabayashi K, Toyama Y, Chiba K (1999) Expansive laminoplasty for myelopathy in ossification of the longitudinal ligament. Clin Orthop Relat Res 359:35–48
26. Tsuzuki N, Abe R, Saiki K et al (1996) Extradural tethering effect as one mechanism of radiculopathy complicating posterior decompression of the cervical spinal cord. Spine 21:203–211
27. Uematsu Y, Tokuhashi Y, Matsuzaki H (1998) Radiculopathy after laminoplasty of the cervical spine. Spine 23: 2057–2062
28. Yonenobu K, Hosono N, Iwasaki M et al (1991) Neurologic complications of surgery for cervical compression myelopathy. Spine 16:1277–1282
29. Satomi K, Nishu Y, Kohno T et al (1994) Long-term follow-up studies of open-door expansive laminoplasty for cervical stenotic myelopathy. Spine 19:507–510
30. Shimizu T, Shimada H, Edakuni H (1996) Post-laminoplasty palsy of upper extremities, with special reference to the spinal cord factors. Bessatsu Seikeigeka 29:188–194
31. Chiba K, Toyama Y, Matsumoto M et al (2002) Segmental motor paralysis after expansive open-door laminoplasty. Spine 27:2108–2115
32. Komagata M, Nishiyama M, Endoh K (2002) Clinical study of the post operative C5 palsy after cervical laminoplasty; Efficacy of bilateral partial foraminotomy for prevention the C5 palsy. J Jpn Spine Res Soc 131:237
33. Sasai K, Saito T, Akagi S et al (2003) Preventing C5 palsy after laminoplasty. Spine 28:1972–1977
34. Minoda Y, Nakamura H, Konishi S et al (2003) Palsy of the C5 nerve root after midsagittal-splitting laminoplasty of the cervical spine. Spine 28:1123–1127
35. Chen Y, Chen D, Wang X et al (2007) C5 palsy after laminectomy and posterior cervical fixation for ossification of posterior longitudinal ligament. J Spinal Disord Tech 20: 533–535
36. Neo M, Fujibayashi S, Miyata M et al (2008) Vertebral artery injury during cervical spine surgery: a survey of more than 5600 operations. Spine 33:779–785
37. Zhao L, Xu R, Hu T et al (2008) Quantitative evaluation of the location of the vertebral artery in relation to the transverse foramen in the lower cervical spine. Spine 33:373–378
38. Lu J, Ebraheim NA, Georgiadis GM et al (1998) Anatomic considerations of the vertebral artery: implications for anterior decompression of the cervical spine. J Spinal Disord 11:233–236
39. Pateder DB, Carbone JJ (2006) Lateral mass screw fixation for cervical spine trauma: associated complications and efficacy in maintaining alignment. Spine J 6:40–43
40. Yamaguchi S, Eguchi K, Kiura Y et al (2008) Posterolateral protrusion of the vertebral artery over the posterior arch of the atlas: quantitative anatomical study using three-dimensional computed tomography angiography. J Neurosurg Spine 9:167–174
41. Abumi K, Shono Y, Ito M et al (2000) Complications of pedicle screw fixation in reconstructive surgery of the cervical spine. Spine 25:962–969
42. Deen HG, Birch BD, Wharen RE et al (2003) Lateral mass screw-rod fixation of the cervical spine: a prospective clinical series with 1-year follow-up. Spine J 3:489–495
43. Haid RW Jr, Subach BR, McLaughlin MR et al (2001) C1–C2 transarticular screw fixation for atlantoaxial instability: a 6-year experience. Neurosurgery 49:65–68; discussion 69–70
44. Heller JG, Silcox DH 3rd, Sutterlin CE 3rd (1995) Complications of posterior cervical plating. Spine 20: 2442–2448
45. Madawi AA, Casey AT, Solanki GA et al (1997) Radiological and anatomical evaluation of the atlantoaxial transarticular screw fixation technique. J Neurosurg 86:961–968
46. Wright NM, Lauryssen C (1998) Vertebral artery injury in C1–2 transarticular screw fixation: results of a survey of the AANS/CNS section on disorders of the spine and peripheral nerves. American Association of Neurological Surgeons/ Congress of Neurological Surgeons. J Neurosurg 88: 634–640
47. Gluf WM, Schmidt MH, Apfelbaum RI (2005) Atlantoaxial transarticular screw fixation: a review of surgical indications, fusion rate, complications, and lessons learned in 191 adult patients. J Neurosurg Spine 2:155–163
48. Mendez JC, Gonzalez-Llanos F (2005) Endovascular treatment of a vertebral artery pseudoaneurysm following posterior C1–C2 transarticular screw fixation. Cardiovasc Intervent Radiol 28:107–109
49. Prabhu VC, France JC, Voelker JL et al (2001) Vertebral artery pseudoaneurysm complicating posterior C1–2 transarticular screw fixation: case report. Surg Neurol 55:29–33; discussion 33–24
50. Arnautovic KI, al-Mefty O, Pait TG et al (1997) The suboccipital cavernous sinus. J Neurosurg 86:252–262
51. Ebraheim NA, Xu R, Ahmad M et al (1998) The quantitative anatomy of the vertebral artery groove of the atlas and its relation to the posterior atlantoaxial approach. Spine 23: 320–323
52. Abd el-Bary TH, Dujovny M, Ausman JI (1995) Microsurgical anatomy of the atlantal part of the vertebral artery. Surg Neurol 44:392–400; discussion 400–391
53. Cacciola F, Phalke U, Goel A (2004) Vertebral artery in relationship to C1–C2 vertebrae: an anatomical study. Neurol India 52:178–184
54. Rhoton AL Jr (2000) The far-lateral approach and its transcondylar, supracondylar, and paracondylar extensions. Neurosurgery 47:S195–S209
55. Buna M, Coghlan W, deGruchy M et al (1984) Ponticles of the atlas: a review and clinical perspective. J Manipulative Physiol Ther 7:261–266
56. Cushing KE, Ramesh V, Gardner-Medwin D et al (2001) Tethering of the vertebral artery in the congenital arcuate foramen of the atlas vertebra: a possible cause of vertebral artery dissection in children. Dev Med Child Neurol 43: 491–496
57. Hasan M, Shukla S, Siddiqui MS et al (2001) Posterolateral tunnels and ponticuli in human atlas vertebrae. J Anat 199:339–343
58. Le Minor JM, Trost O (2004) Bony ponticles of the atlas (C1) over the groove for the vertebral artery in humans and primates: polymorphism and evolutionary trends. Am J Phys Anthropol 125:16–29
59. Manjunath KY (2001) Posterior bridging of the atlas vertebra in south Indians. Indian J Med Sci 55:488–490
60. Senoglu M, Gumusalan Y, Yuksel KZ et al (2006) The effect of posterior bridging of C-1 on craniovertebral junction surgery. J Neurosurg Spine 5:50–52

61. Peng CW, Chou BT, Bendo JA et al (2009) Vertebral artery injury in cervical spine surgery-anatomical considerations, management, and preventive measures. Spine J 9(1):70–76
62. Coric D, Branch CL Jr, Wilson JA et al (1996) Arteriovenous fistula as a complication of C1–2 transarticular screw fixation. Case report and review of the literature. J Neurosurg 85:340–343
63. Smith MD, Emery SE, Dudley A et al (1993) Vertebral artery injury during anterior decompression of the cervical spine. A retrospective review of ten patients. J Bone Joint Surg Br 75:410–415
64. Weidner A, Wahler M, Chiu ST et al (2000) Modification of C1–C2 transarticular screw fixation by image-guided surgery. Spine 25:2668–2673; discussion 2674
65. Wahlberg E, Olofsson P, Goldstone J (2007) Vascular injuries to the neck. In: Wahlberg E, Olofsson P, Goldstone J (eds) Emergency vascular surgery – a practical guide. Springer, Berlin, pp 3–14

Section IV

Complications related to osteo-articular diseases

Degenerative Disk Disease

10

Vincenzo Denaro, Luca Denaro, Alberto Di Martino, Umile Giuseppe Longo, and Nicola Maffulli

Contents

V. Denaro (✉)
Department of Orthopaedic and Trauma Surgery, Campus Bio-medico University, Via Alvaro del Portillo 200, 00128 Rome, Italy
e-mail: denaro@unicampus.it

10.1 Introduction

When dealing with degenerative disease at the cervical spine, the target of any procedure must be the complete removal of the cause of the damage to the myeloradicular structures. When the pathological process causes an anterior compression, the anterior approach should be preferred. The release of the compressed neural structures via an anterior approach can be performed by several techniques, depending on the skill and experience of the surgeon in using a specific procedure (e.g., Cloward vs. Smith–Robinson vs. multilevel surgery).

In some patients, the stenosis is due to specific posterior abnormalities such as hypertrophy of the ligamentum flavum, anomalies of the laminae and pedicles, and degenerative changes at the facet joints. Moreover, the spinal canal can be narrowed in a uniform manner on a congenital basis, or be segmentally stenotic for an ossification of the posterior longitudinal ligament (OPLL) disease. All these diseases can benefit from a surgical decompression from the back.

Recent nonfusion technologies such as cervical spine arthroplasty (CSA) and minimally invasive decompressive procedures have elective indications in the treatment of the degenerative spine and aim at segmental motion preservation.

10.2 Anterior Surgical Techniques

10.2.1 Anterior Discectomy/Corpectomy and Fusion

Anterior cervical discectomy and fusion (ACDF) represents one of the most commonly performed spinal procedures and is related to a good clinical outcome in

L. Denaro et al. (eds.), *Pitfalls in Cervical Spine Surgery*,
DOI: 10.1007/978-3-540-85019-9_10, © Springer-Verlag Berlin Heidelberg 2010

the vast majority of patients. However, when complications occur, these can lead to severe consequences unless promptly recognized and managed [1]. In an analysis of complications in a population of 10416 patients operated of routine cervical discectomy [2], 6.7% (698/10,416) of patients developed one or more postoperative complications. These were noninfectious in 1.8% (189/10,416) of patients, and infectious in another 1.8% (189/10,416). Other medical complications occurred in 4.0% (413/10,416) of cases. Between the noninfectious complications, vascular injury or hemorrhage was reported in 134 out of 10,416 patients (1.3%). Urinary tract infection was reported in 1.1% (117/10,416) of patients. Pulmonary infections were reported in 36/10,416 (0.3%) patients and wound infections in 20/10,416 (0.2%). Myocardial infarction was reported in 0.02% (2/10,416) of patients, thromboembolic events in 0.09% (9/10,416), and cerebrovascular events in 0.13% (14/10,416). Statistical analysis demonstrated that congestive heart failure, alcohol or drug abuse, chronic obstructive pulmonary disease, previous spinal surgery, psychological disorders, together with chronic musculoskeletal disorders were independently associated with the risk of postoperative complications.

Current techniques of anterior cervical decompression and fusion are modifications of those originally described by Smith and Robinson [3], Cloward [4], Bailey and Badgley [5]. These are routinely performed for single or multilevel spinal fusion.

In the past, the main aim of these surgeries was to fuse the affected segment(s) without direct removal of the cause of patient disease. It was in fact believed that posterior osteophytes would resorb after time through the process of bone remodeling [6]. Nonetheless, bone remodeling and bony spurs reabsorption is a slow process, and consequent long-lasting neural compression can lead to neural compromise and/or permanent neurological deficits. Current techniques have been conversely developed with the aim to directly remove the etiology of neural compression (the disk–osteophyte complex) and fully decompress the neural structures. After accurate neural decompression, segmental fusion is usually performed.

The concept of spinal fusion after anterior decompression has not been widely accepted for a long time; in fact, even in recent years, some authors support that anterior discectomy without fusion is associated with acceptable results and "low" complication rates. These include worsening of the pre-existing myelopathy (3.3%), epidural hematoma, and instability of the cervical spine leading to postsurgical kyphosis (0.9%), nerve root lesion, and aseptic spondylodiscitis (0.4%). For these reasons, discectomy without interbody fusion has long been considered a reasonably safe procedure with acceptable operative morbidity [7]. In a recent review of literature on patients randomized to either discectomy alone or discectomy and fusion, patients treated with discectomy and fusion showed longer operative times and hospital stays, but a definite lower risk of kyphosis, when compared with patients treated with discectomy alone. Anyway, at present, fusion is routinely performed after anterior cervical discectomy, because segmental kyphosis can lead to neurological worsening and alterations in segmental loadings, with the risk of early degeneration of the adjacent disks.

An important advancement in surgical techniques for anterior cervical spine decompression and fusions has been the introduction of the procedure described by Cloward [4, 8]. It requires the use of a dedicated instrumentation and drill to perform the decompression.

We have extensively used a modified Cloward technique for the treatment of degenerative stenosis of the cervical spine [9, 10]. Once on the vertebral plane, the surgeon needs to remove the anterior osteophytes to obtain flat vertebral surfaces to make sure that the bodies are perfectly even and no eccentricity results (Fig. 10.1). This is particularly important because the Cloward drill has to be anchored anteriorly on the vertebral bodies: if anchoring surface is not even, then asymmetry may result and myeloradicular lesions could occur (Fig. 10.2). The guide is posed at the center of the vertebral bodies, and the lateral edges of the vertebral bodies to be drilled must be clearly visible to control orientation and centering during drilling. If drilling is eccentric or angled, serious complications may result, such as injuries to the vertebral artery and nerve roots at the infero-posterior end of the root canal, and spinal cord lesions. The sleeve of the Cloward drill guide has four tips to be tapped along the guide with a hammer until perfectly anchored in the vertebral bodies: if the sleeve is not perfectly anchored, the depth of drilling may be incorrectly measured and violation of the spinal canal with injury to the spinal cord occurs. With each drilling, the sleeve must be advanced with a tap of the hammer: this maneuver requires a rigid support for the patient's neck (Fig. 10.3). A soft support in fact allows some posterior displacement of the vertebral body at each attempt of penetration, thus pushing the bony edges

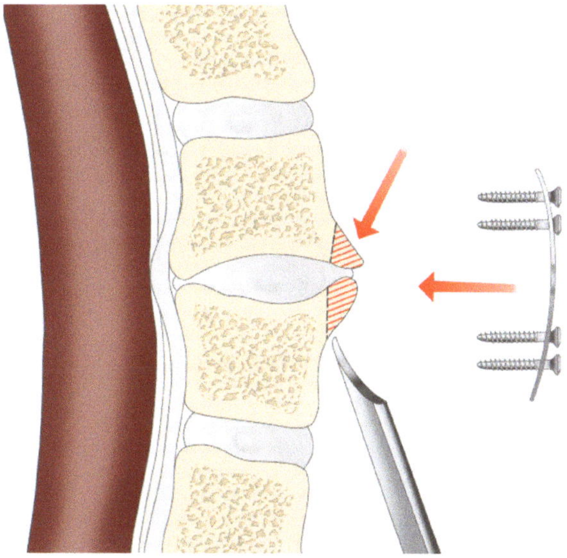

Fig. 10.1 The surgeon needs to remove the anterior osteophytes to obtain flat vertebral surfaces to make sure that the bodies are perfectly even and no eccentricity results. Moreover, a smooth surface will allow an easy application of instrumentation

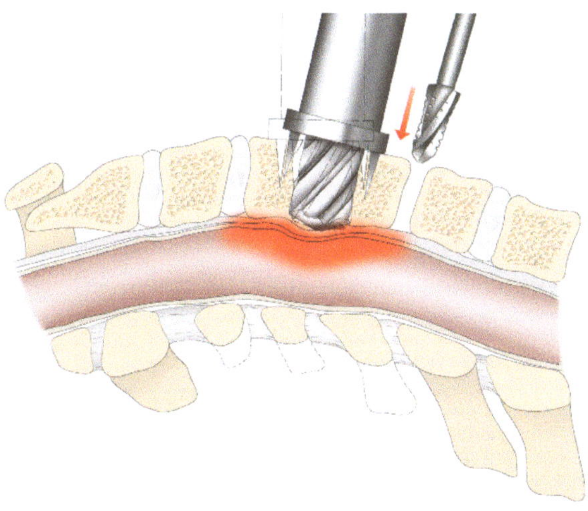

Fig. 10.2 The consequences of a malpositioned guide, which is not perpendicular to the vertebral bodies. As it is advanced, the drills follow an oblique path, reaching the posterior wall at one side, while, the other side of the drill is still within the vertebral body. Moreover, the position of the neck with the patient in reverse-Trendelemburg position can lead the inattentive surgeon to drill the endplate on a plane perpendicular to the surgical bed, with the risk to get too deep on one vertebral endplate and injure the meninges

toward the spinal cord and nerve roots with local injury. After drilling, the hole formed must be quickly examined while suctioning because of significant bleeding

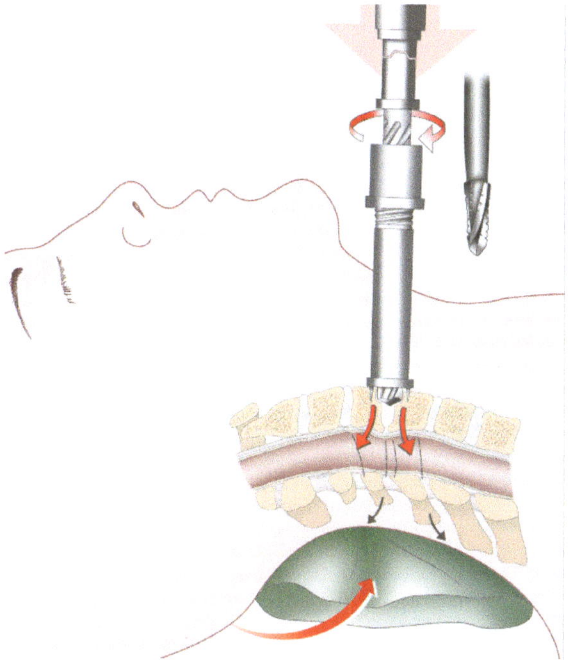

Fig. 10.3 A rigid support for the spinous processes avoids that the force of the drilling and the rotation cause posterior dislocation of the vertebral bodies, driving osteophytes and other fragments of the posterior wall of the vertebral body into the spinal cord, with potentially catastrophic consequences

originating from the posterior margin of the vertebral bodies where the nutrient vessels are located. Bleeding can be controlled by the use of bone wax pressed into the deep region and smeared along the walls of the cavity. Hemostasis is most important to visualize the operative site without any interference from excessive bleeding. Then, decompression is performed. Fusion requires iliac crest derived cylindrical bone that should be harvested with an instrument with a diameter of at least 3 mm greater than the hole drilled into the vertebra, obtaining a cylinder of bone including both cortices. Increased graft diameter is used to obtain a fusion in distraction and enlarge the root canal bilaterally. An important technical point is to ensure that the graft is pushed completely into the space left from decompression, with its anterior aspect even with the anterior surface of the adjacent vertebral bodies.

Some peculiar errors in surgery have been related to the use of Cloward instrumentation and drill [11, 12]. Between these, we already described the incorrect positioning of the guide and drill, which results in eccentric and angled direction of drilling (Fig. 10.2). Even when centered, incorrect use of the drill is the

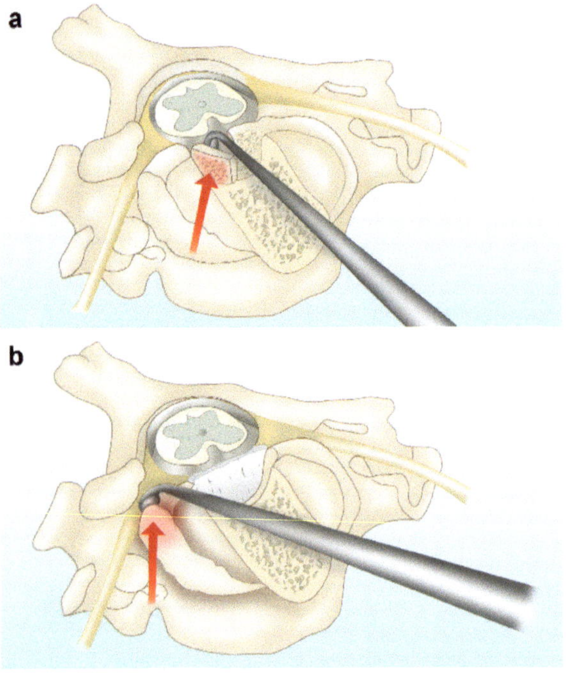

Fig. 10.4 The horizontal plan of dissection. (**a**) The curved curet scoops out the remnants of the posterior wall of the vertebral bodies, freeing them from the posterior longitudinal ligament. (**b**) The dissection is performed laterally with curets to remove any cause of compression or obstruction of the nerve root canal, which may be present in the posterolateral portion of the body

cause of the most severe complications observed in this procedure. Being cautious, advancing the drill slowly in predictable steps, and using curved curets to assess the depth reached by the drill, it is possible to identify the line of cleavage between the posterior cortex and the osteophyte; in fact, only at this point one should proceed for the removal of the osteophyte (Fig. 10.4). If the posterior wall is not accurately released, the neural tissue will not be free and the results will be poor. Graft collapse and loss of lordosis have also been frequently reported. To prevent this complication, anterior plate and screw instrumentation is routinely added after the Cloward procedure, particularly when performing multilevel procedures [13].

Despite many surgeons being comfortable with this technique, today other surgeons prefer to avoid using the Cloward's technique, because it requires to remove an excessive amount of vertebral bodies, it requires a cylindric graft, and the technique is complex and requires a long learning curve.

We prefer to reach the posterior osteophytes through the interbody approach, as initially described by Smith–Robinson, using air drills, which allow an easy removal of the posterior osteophytes and reduce the operative time. During these maneuvers, the intervertebral bodies are kept in distraction to allow an easier removal of the posterior aspect of the intervertebral disk and posterior osteophytes. A fundamental step of this technique is decompression of the disk space. Once decompression is performed, removal of more posterior disk fragments and posterior osteophytes in the foramen are commonly performed after application of a distractor, which allows for distraction of the vertebral bodies at the disk space increasing the light over the operatory field. The success of the procedure depends on the use of the distractor that separates the adjacent vertebral bodies in parallel. A distractor applied only anteriorly tends to open the anterior aspect of the intervertebral space and to close the posterior aspect (Fig. 10.5), with consequent possible difficult removal of the posterior osteophytes and cord damage. For this reason, in the past, we developed a dedicated distractor to help the surgery, where the distraction was held by four self-tapping screws (Fig. 10.6). More recently, Caspar or similar distractors can be used for this purpose. Caspar distractors have only two screws: the length of the screws that anchor the distractor to the vertebral bodies should not exceed 12 and 14 mm, to preserve the integrity of the posterior wall and protect the neural structures, because deeper screws may directly perforate the posterior wall and reach the anterior aspect of the spinal cord. Decompression is performed with the use of curets and kerrisons punches up to complete removal of posterior

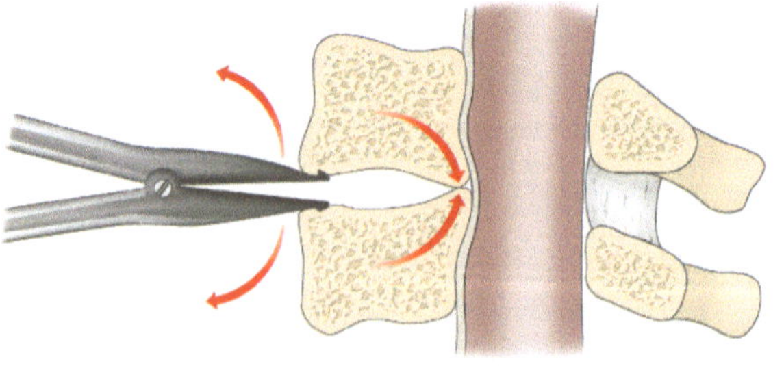

Fig. 10.5 The success of procedure depends on the use of distractor that separates the adjacent vertebral bodies in parallel. A distractor applied only anteriorly tends to open the anterior aspect of the intervertebral space and to close the posterior aspect, with consequent possible difficult removal of the posterior osteophytes and cord damage

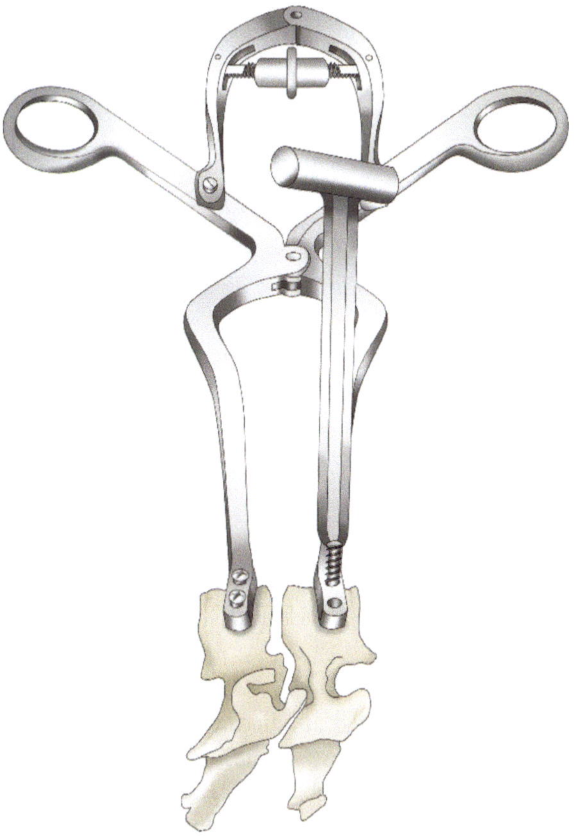

Fig. 10.6 In the past, we developed a dedicated distractor, where the distraction was held by four self-tapping screws, allowing a parallel distraction of the vertebral bodies, which facilitate the removal of the posterior osteophytes

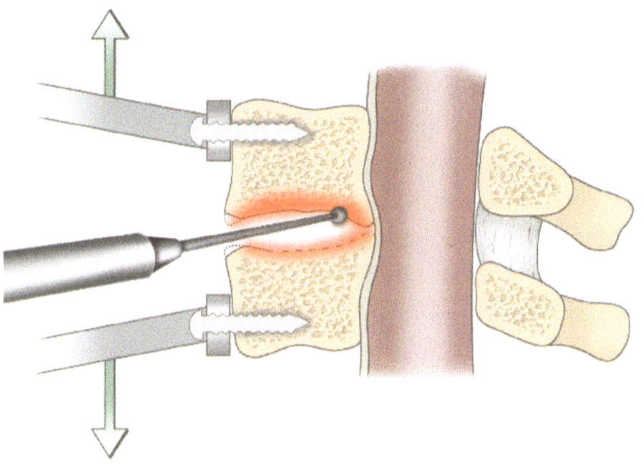

Fig. 10.7 Decompression is performed by using an air drill to remove the posterior osteophytes

osteophytes and the residual posterior part of the unci (Figs. 10.7 and 10.8).

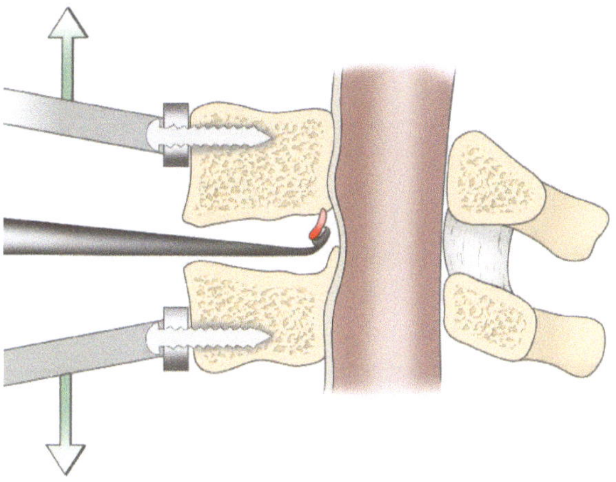

Fig. 10.8 Complete decompression of the posterior intervertebral disk space is performed using curet

After distraction is performed and disk and posterior osteophytes are removed, preparation of the vertebral endplate through drilling its central portion is required. Some authors suggest the use of chisels for this procedure, but the risk of shake lesions to the spinal cord during hammer use is elevated (Fig. 10.9), while air drills ensure a careful endplate preparation and obtaining a rectangular space with decreased risk of neural injury. Even in this case, drilling should be performed at the center of the vertebral endplate. It is mandatory to remove all the posterior aspects of the adjacent vertebral bodies, to completely visualize the freed posterior longitudinal ligament (Fig. 10.10). An incomplete cord decompression may cause poor outcome, with persistence of the clinical symptoms of the patient in the postoperative period. The position of the neck with the patient in reverse-Trendelemburg position can lead the inattentive surgeon to drill the endplate on a plane perpendicular to the surgical bed, with the risk to get too deep on one vertebral endplate and injure the meninges (Fig. 10.2).

As discussed in the chapter on complication of bone grafting (Chap. 17), stabilization requires the use of bone graft, bone graft alternatives, or cages. Autologous bone graft is to be preferred. It should be tricortical, solid, and rectangular in shape, and its dimensions superate in height the rectangular space in distraction; moreover, it should be taller in the front than the backside. This allows one to restore segmental stability and cervical lordosis at the same time, and to perform fusion in distraction. As already described for the Cloward

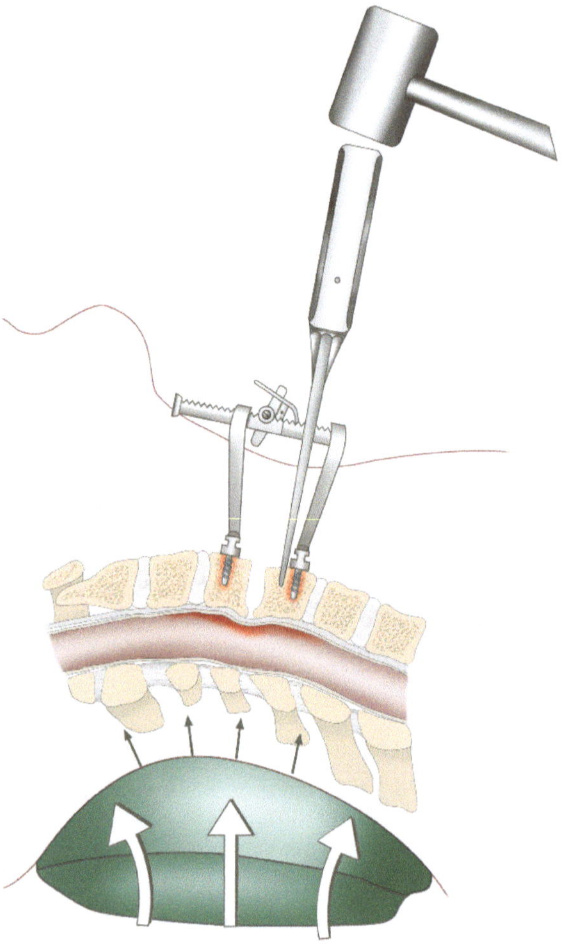

Fig. 10.9 The mechanism of the use of a hammer requires resistance, which is provided by rigid support of the spinous processes

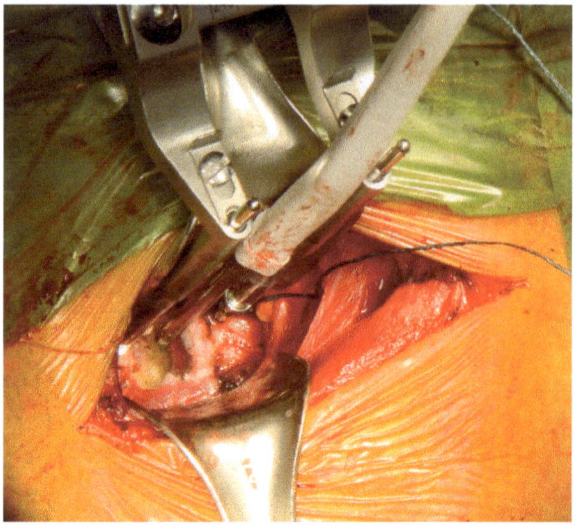

Fig. 10.10 Intraoperative picture, showing a wide anterior decompression with removal of the osteophytes and the posterior aspect of the vertebral bodies. The posterior longitudinal ligament is completely freed

procedure, when bone graft is introduced, the external cortex (wider than the posterior one) should correspond to the anterior surface of the adjacent vertebral bodies to prevent subsequent dislocation of the bone graft or graft collapse. The application of plate and screw fixation guarantees primary stability of the implant and gives the chance to leave the patient free from bracing in the postoperative period when screw anchoring is intraoperatively solid. The surgeon must be very careful when inserting the graft. A frequent error is to damage the spinal cord because of too deep insertion of the graft. To avoid this complication, we developed a custom-made instrument with lateral wings, which blocks a too deep penetration of the graft (Fig. 10.11).

The same procedure can be repeated at multiple levels. When spinal decompression and cord decompression is performed at adjacent levels, there is the risk to leave a too thin bony bridge between the two segments, unable to sustain bone graft or cages at the adjacent levels. To avoid this complication, the surgeon should obtain a thick bony bridge by removing more vertebral bone in the upper and lower part of the rostral and caudal vertebral bodies, respectively: this allows for an optimal posterior segmental decompression, and leaves enough bone to sustain the application of bone graft or cages. Alternatively, when discectomy is performed at two adjacent levels, the bony bridge between these can be removed to achieve a complete spinal cord decompression (corpectomy).

Complications occurring with anterior discectomy or corpectomy and fusion procedures range from vascular to myeloradicular; main complications and surgical recommendations are summarized in Table 10.1:

10.2.1.1 Vascular Lesions

Common Carotid Artery Lesions

Incidence reported in literature for direct lesion of the common carotid artery is 0.1% [14]. Also, thrombosis of the carotid artery secondary to prolonged retraction during anterior cervical surgery can lead to severe cerebral complications such as hemiplegia.

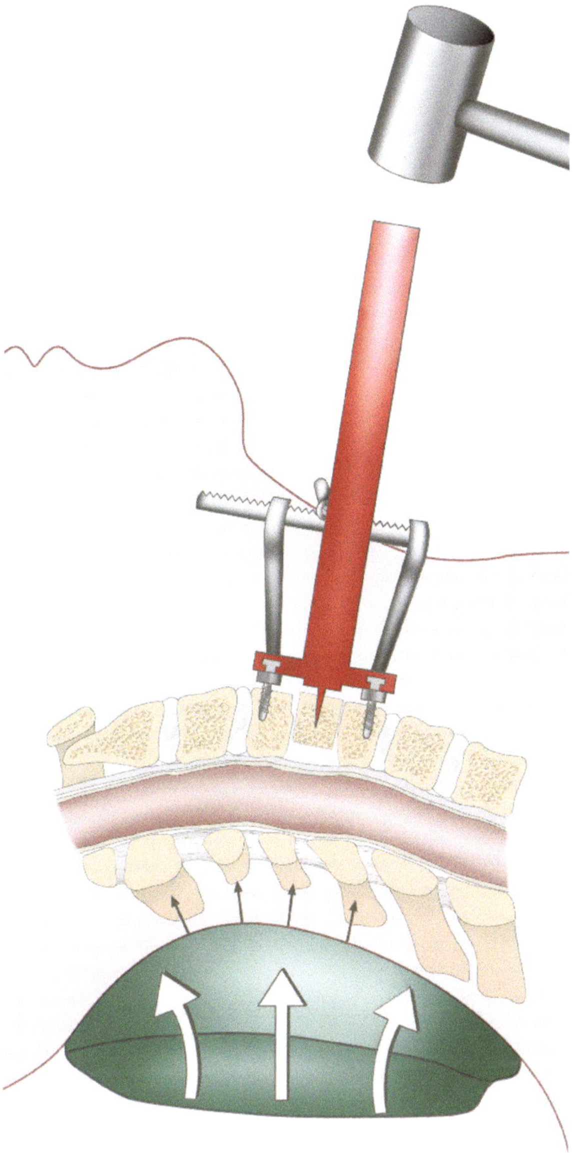

Fig. 10.11 A frequent error is to damage the spinal cord. To avoid a too deep insertion of the graft, we developed a custom-made instrument with lateral wings, which blocks the penetration of the graft. A rigid support for the spinous processes is required

The increased incidence of this complication is linked to several risk factors such as advanced age, prolonged surgical time, and diffuse vascular atherosclerotic disease (see Chap. 1) [15]. An adjunctive factor can be represented by the use of self-retractors which, differently from manual retraction, do not permit temporary release of vessel compression. Prevention is performed by the use of anticoagulants in the perioperative period, reduced surgical times, and the use of manual retraction.

Vertebral Artery Lesion

Lesions of the vertebral artery have been widely reported in anterior subaxial cervical spine procedures. Golfinos et al. [16] reported an incidence of 0.3% of cases after discectomy and corpectomy for myelopathy or radiculopathy. In this series of patients, lesions were secondary to retrograde drilling, soft tissue retraction, or screwing. Other authors [3] reported an incidence of lesions to the vertebral artery approximating 0.5% during discectomy or corpectomy surgery. In most cases, vessel injury was secondary to the inadvertent (too lateral) use of air drills, with subsequent neurological lesions (cerebellar infarction, root lesions due to direct trauma or secondary to artery ligation). Eleraky [17] and Daentzer [18] also described cases of intraoperative vertebral artery lesions, in some cases fatal.

In an analysis of vertebral artery injury during cervical spine surgery, five cases occurred out of more than 2,100 anterior cervical spine surgeries for degenerative diseases [19]. Tamponation of the injury site has been the treatment in four of five cases; in one patient, finding the site of vertebral artery lesion was impossible, and embolization was required to stop the bleeding. To stop the bleeding from the vertebral artery is necessary to isolate the superior and inferior segments of the lesion (performing a wide resection of the anterior portion of the transverse foramen) and to ligate the artery. When the artery is clamped caudally and rostrally without being isolated first, there is a high risk to damage the nerve roots, which are located close to the artery, with potential catastrophic consequences. In conditions of emergency, the safest way to clamp the artery is at the border of the transverse foramen of C6 caudally. Rostrally, after temporary ligation, vessel should be isolated inside the segmental transverse foramen after opening, avoiding involvement in ligation of the adjacent nerve root.

In posterior cervical spine surgery, when screws are placed into the articular apophyses or into the pedicles, bleeding may be controlled by bone wax and screw insertion [20].

One of the first tips to avoid intraoperative vertebral artery injury is to look for the midline during corpectomy

Table 10.1 Complications of anterior surgical techniques

Technique: ACDF(single/multilevel)/MSS	Consequences	Tips/tricks
Incomplete decompression	Persisting or worsening of neurological deficits	Direct visualization of the neuroforamen
Eccentric or too deep drilling	Lesions to vertebral artery, meninges,and spinal cord	Remove anterior osteophyte to obtain an even anterior spinal aspect
Kyphosis/Loss of lordosis	Adjacent disk degeneration Postsurgical deformity Persisting neurological compression	Graft in distraction
Vascular lesions	Vertebral artery: Hemorrhage, neurological deficits, need for ligation Carotid artery: Neurological sequelae Jugular vein: Hemorrhage (need for surgical revision)	Bony dissection not lateral to the unci Careful use of curets in the neuroforamen Protect the artery under the distractor Expose the vessel and separate vagus nerve and carotid artery before ligation Often injured while using sharp instruments
Soft tissue lesions related to surgical technique	Recurrent laryngeal nerve lesions Esophageal lesion with dysphagia	Use manual retraction when possible, in other cases decrease retraction temporarily during surgery Immediate repair required
Adjacent segment degeneration	New neurological symptoms Rare need for revision surgery	Perform fusion in distraction restoring physiological sagittal alignment

to avoid bone dissection going too lateral. Most authors suggest bony dissection not to reach the medial wall of the uncovertebral joint; moreover, the surgeon must be cautious in performing uncosectomy because inadvertent use of the instruments can injure the vertebral artery (Fig. 10.12), and the procedure should be limited to the posterior portion of the uncus only which contributes to the narrowing of the neuroforamen. Preoperative CT scan and angio-MRI to follow the vertebral artery in respect to the cervical spine can be helpful. Surgical technique can be modified in case of an aberrant loop of the vertebral artery penetrating the vertebral body [21].

Jugular Vein Lesion

If the jugular vein is not well visualized and identified during dissection, it may be out of the immediate visual field behind the sternocleidomastoid muscle. It is a very frequent lesion during decompression, occurring while using sharp instruments such as curets or air drill. The vessel wall is soft and can be easily torn, particularly in older patients. Bleeding is abundant, but can eventually be controlled by suture of the wall. The bleeding must be at first controlled by direct pressure; then the tear must be carefully assessed after adequate exposure of the vessel. This may require opening up the carotid sheath to expose the vein and to identify the artery and the vagus nerve, so that these two structures are not included in sutures or ligatures [11].

10.2.1.2 Soft Tissue Lesions

As already described for the complications related to vascular injury, lesions to the soft tissues can be encountered either during the surgical approach [22, 23] or during the surgical technique (retraction plus use of sharp instruments). Lesions related to the surgical approach and to the use of retractors are more extensively discussed in the complications of surgical approaches section (Chaps. 7–9).

Suggested risk factors are prolonged retraction of esophagus and trachea, multilevel cervical surgery, advanced age, postoperative edema or hematoma, use of bone graft or instrumentation in conflict with the esophagus, and revision surgery [6, 24–27].

Soft tissue lesions such as those to esophagus or trachea can usually be prevented by decreasing local pressure and ischemia, as for the self-retractors which, differently from manual retraction, may determine excessive compression [8, 28]. Once the lesions occur following direct trauma or necrosis of the esophageal wall, complications are often severe, leading eventually

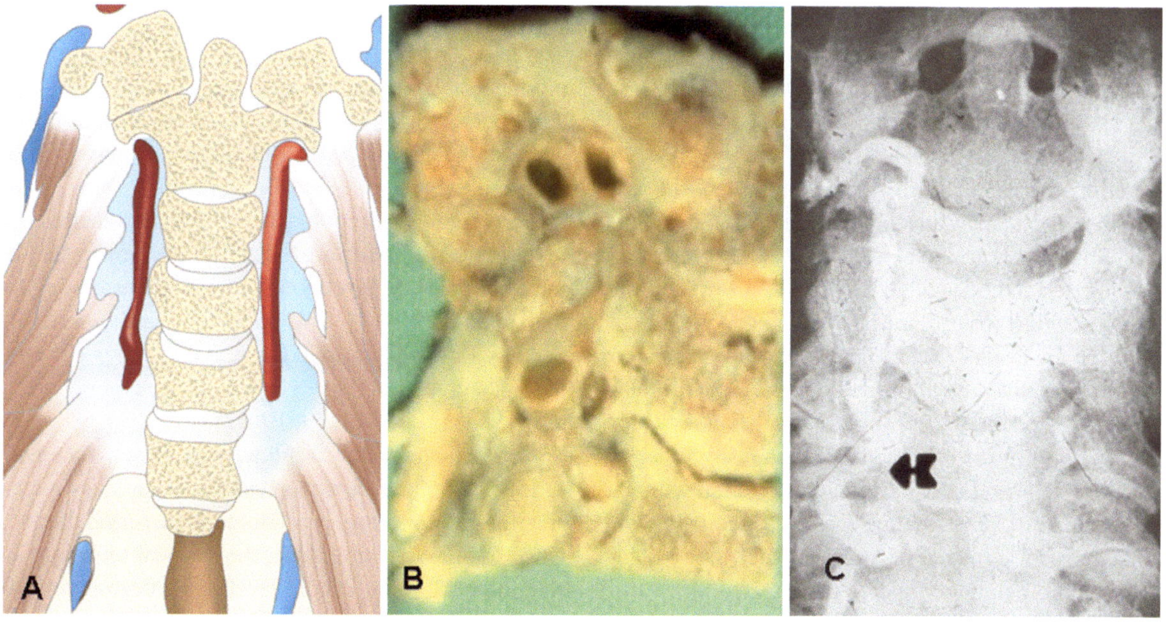

Fig. 10.12 (**a**) When operating, the surgeon should take into account the proximity of the vertebral artery to the vertebral bodies to prevent iatrogenic damage to the vessel. Frontal anatomic specimen (**b**), and angiographic study (**c**) of the same, before tissue processing, showing the proximity between the vertebral artery to the uncus. When the intersomatic decompression is performed too laterally, damages to the vertebral artery may occur

to esophageal drainage with mediastinitis, severe septicemia, and meningitis, and require revision surgery with direct visualization and repair of the defect and administration of wide spectrum antibiotics [22]. In a recent review on repaired esophageal perforations after anterior cervical spine surgery, the time to oral intake ranged from 7 days to 7 months. In the study, esophageal diversion and drainage, primary closure with or without omental free flap reinforcement, sternocleidomastoid flap repair, or a combination of multiple procedures have all been performed [29].

Postsurgical hematoma and prolonged retraction can also lead to postsurgical dysphagia. This can be self-resolving in similar cases, while others can show chronic deficits needing modification of the dietary regimen and swallow technique, and rarely also the implant of electrical stimulators [30, 31].

Dysphonia related to recurrent laryngeal nerve lesion during anterior cervical surgery has been reported in very low rate, approximating 1.27% (3/235). It has been suggested that possible causes for these complications are sharp dissection, pinching or stretching of the recurrent laryngeal nerve by retractors, postoperative edema, nerve involvement in suture, direct trauma to the cricoarytenoid joint by retractors, and reoperation at the same level. Authors suggest that careful endotracheal intubation and surgical technique, and safe retractor placement beneath the longus colli muscles are critical to preventing direct surgical trauma to the nerve and/or adjacent soft tissues [32].

10.2.1.3 Spinal and Dural Lesions

Spinal and dural lesions are among the most feared complications of cervical spine surgery. Many authors reported variable incidence of these severe complications in their studies [7].

In a recent revision on cerebrospinal fluid (CSF) leaks following cervical spine surgery, data from 1994 patients were reported [33]. Among the patients who had an anterior procedure, relative risk to develop an intraoperative dural tear was increased in cervical corpectomy and fusion procedures, revision anterior corpectomy and fusion surgeries, and OPLL. The authors reported an overall 1% (20/1994) rate of dural tears in the study population. Causes of injury were use of the rongeur or kerrison during an anterior discectomy and PLL removal.

An intraoperative trick is to perfom the decompress in distraction (Caspar), which put the PLL under tension, allowing a better definition of the surgical cleavage. It is important then to preoperatively plan such evidence and be ready to treat eventual dural tears when operating via an anterior approach. Another cause of inadvertent dural tear is the use of sharp surgical instruments and air drills.

Once occurred, surgical repair of dural tears via an anterior approach can be difficult or impossible because of the reduced space available during single-level discectomy. When possible, tears should be sutured or a dural patch can be applied. Lyophilized dura and processed bovine pericardium are also materials that can be used in lesion repair. The latter can be directly sutured or stuck with fibrin glue: to be sure of the adhesion of the patch, the anesthesiologist should intraoperatively perform repeated Valsava maneuvers to increase CSF pressure. Fascial graft covered with gelfoam, fat graft, or fibrin glue can be used together with other sealant products (Duraseal Xact^{TM}) to obtain water-tight sealing of repaired dural tears [34].

A lumbar subarachnoid drainage must be always positioned both in case of failure and in doubtful cases of inadequate surgical repair [35]. The lumbar subarachnoid drainage decreases intradural pressure contributing to dural tear healing process. Drainage flow should be of 8–12 mL/h, with flow rate to be modified on the basis of clinical response.

Spinal cord lesion can occur for direct or indirect injury. Direct lesion can be due to contusion at the level of surgery for inadvertent surgical maneuvers. In the immediate postoperative period, patients may have a worsening of preoperative neurological symptoms with areas of cord damage [7]. Indirect lesions occur following a vascular ischemic damage with subsequent postoperative neurological deficit. These lesions can occur for ipossia from excessive distraction intraoperatively or postoperative edema or hematoma. Decompression of the already ischemic spinal cord in spinal stenosis can lead itself to a segmental paradoxical infarct of the spinal cord, similar to that occurring in limb reimplantation surgery [36].

10.2.2 Anterior Decompression with Multiple Subtotal Corpectomies

When segmental stenosis with significant anterior spinal cord compression occurs at three or more levels, anterior spinal decompression via multiple subtotal corpectomies (MSC) can be performed. The technique is defined "multiple" because it is performed at multiple levels, "subtotal" because the lateral walls of the vertebral body are preserved, and "corpectomy" because the central part of the vertebral body is fully removed.

Performing a decompression with this technique, myeloradicular structures can be decompressed at multiple adjacent levels obtaining a real widening of the spinal canal [37]. This technique has been developed by Professor Boni in Pavia, Italy, who performed the first surgery in 1969. The results of surgeries were published successively [9, 10, 12].

Surgical approach is routinely performed via a pre-sternocleydomastoid route, and allows an easy exposure for multiple-level procedures at the cervical spine. Once on the vertebral plane, the surgical technique is started at the more caudal level to be decompressed, and then extended rostrally. The original technique, as described by Prof. Boni, required the use of a modified Cloward instrumentation. More recently, the diffusion of air drills allows an easier approach.

The technique is summarized as follows:

1. Incision of the anterior longitudinal ligament
2. Intervertebral disks removal
3. Drilling of the disk space with the drill to achieve holes of approximately 12 mm in diameter, then a bone trench is realized with the air drill
4. Widening of the holes at the multiple levels and deepening of the bony trench with removal of the posterior walls of the vertebral bodies (up to PLL) with removal of any element of conflict with the spinal cord

This procedure can be particularly dangerous in case of OPLL disease and in any case of massive posterior osteophytes protruding into the spinal canal compressing the spinal cord.

Careful cauterization and bleeding control at the surgical field is quintessential to obtain a better visualization of the spinal cord and nerve roots, because bleeding at that level is usually encountered while removing posterior osteophytes, adherent to the PLL, which should be removed without damage to the dura. Increased rate of lesions to the dura have been found in patients with ossification of the PLL. In these patients, we prefer to perform a wide laminectomy, stabilizing the cervical spine in lordosis to obtain the back-shift of the spinal cord.

During surgery, spongostan, simple or soaked with Tranexamic acid, together with bone wax for the bony walls, and multiple washes are effective for adequate hemostasis.

After decompression, the fusion bed for the bone graft is prepared. We routinely use autologous bone graft harvested from the iliac crest or allograft plus autologous bone marrow cells concentrate enriched with platelet-rich fibrin [38], because the convexity of the iliac crest reconstructs the physiological cervical lordosis. The graft should be 5 mm to 1 cm wider than the bone trench, and properly molded to follow and/or restore the physiological lordosis of the cervical spine. The graft is positioned in distraction to realize a contact between the vertebral body and the bone graft to facilitate the fusion.

Fibular grafts are constituted prevalently by cortical bone, with a little amount of cancellous bone. Therefore, the biological bony fusion is superior when using the tricortical graft from the iliac crest, which remains the gold standard. The reported complications with fibular grafts include nonunion and migration of the strut graft, fatigue fracture, or delayed graft fracture [39].

For the same reason, we prefer to avoid the use of titanium meshes filled with bone for the surgical management of cervical degenerative disease, because we observed bony fusion only at the cranial and caudal points of contact of the mesh, while the other bone remains not fused [36]. When using fibular strut graft in multilevel cervical reconstruction, a straight bone graft should be adapted to the cervical lordosis. Meticulous sculpting technique is one of the most important technical tips in this surgery. Docking sites with posterior lips should be created at the superior and inferior vertebrae. The fibular strut graft should be placed centrally in the vertebral bodies. More important, the ends of the strut should be molded in a dovetail fashion and inserted after careful distraction: release of the distraction provokes some mild compression on the graft to improve fit and give primary stability to the construct. When these technical points are respected, good clinical results have been demonstrated even in stabilization with strut graft without instrumentation [40].

The use of plate and screws when performing stabilization in distraction of the cervical spine allows to obtain an immediate stability of the cervical spine, and guarantees a fast biological bony fusion and the possibility to use more simplex postoperative orthoses. In the past, Halo or Minerva cast (not always well tolerated by the patients) were required for at least 3 months to guarantee the stability of tricortical bone graft, and its fusion.

10.2.2.1 Complications

Complications encountered during MSC technique are similar to general and local complications already described for anterior cervical discectomy/corpectomy and fusion procedures (vascular, neurological, and deep structures of the neck). Obviously, the percentage is higher because the surgical approach is wider.

Peculiar complications of a more extensive approach include:

- Dural tears

Dural tears occur mainly in cases of OPLL disease. As known, ossification of the PLL is responsible for spinal stenosis in approximately 2–3% of patients, and less frequently in Caucasians [11]. Surgery aimed at myeloradicular decompression exposes the patient to a high risk for dural tears because of the strict relationship between the PLL and the dural plane [33]. In the type most commonly encountered in the Caucasian population (segmental type), the risk of dural tear increases because in multilevel procedures, it is easier for the surgeon to find a cleavage proximally or caudally and try to dissect the calcified LLP from the dural plane.

The removal of posterior osteophytes and the adherent PLL may determine the formation of microtears, which are not immediately evident, but can lead to the formation of a fistula few days postoperatively (Fig. 10.13).

To prevent this complication, as already reported in revision lumbar spine surgery, it is possible to improve and ease surgical dissection by delivering locally a mucolytic agent (MESNA) [41]. When it is impossible to find a safe cleavage, it is suggested to decrease the width of the calcification with a diamond-coated burr and leave the remnant on site: the widening of the segmental stenosis leaves enough space for the spinal cord that is not more compressed. In case of dural tears, as already reported, anterior repair could not be suitable for suture, and coverage with gelfoam, fat graft, fibrin glue, or other sealants can be used [34]; in case of failure, use of a lumbar subarachnoid drainage is suggested [35].

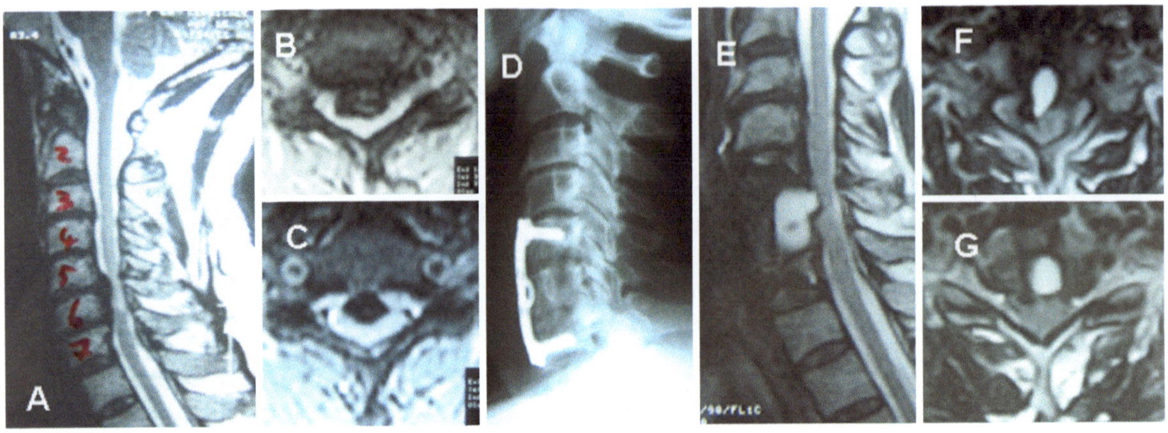

Fig. 10.13 Patient with C5–C7 severe stenosis. (**a**) Sagittal, (**b, c**) Transversal MRI section showing the osteophytes compressing and deforming the spinal cord. The patient underwent somatectomy and wide decompression with removal of the posterior longitudinal ligament. Intraoperatively, no dural tears were detected. (**d**) Postoperative lateral radiograph of the cervical spine. Three days postoperatively, the patient started to complain of headache. Liquorrhea drained from the surgical wound. (**e**) Sagittal, (**f, g**) Transversal MRI showing the liquoral fistula. The patient was successfully managed by lumbar drainage

- Violation of the lateral walls

As described above for the ACDF procedures, the risk of iatrogenic lesion of the vertebral artery is increased when eccentric drilling is performed toward the lateral wall of the vertebral body. Vessel injury is increased in multilevel procedures [12, 19]. In case of severe tears, artery ligation is required [42].

- Inadequate decompression

Inadequate decompression of the nerve roots at the neuroforamen is usually related to persistence of the posterior osteophytes or poor distraction. Complete removal of the posterior wall of the vertebral body is mandatory to achieve proper decompression of the neural structures, and requires extension toward the lateral margins of the PLL. Widening of the neuroforamens is to be performed at all the affected levels, and should be checked intraoperatively by direct visualization and fluoroscopic examination.

- Postoperative kyphosis or inversion of cervical lordosis

This complication is of great concern in MSC when compared with single-level surgery, because the operated segment is wide, and therefore postoperative kyphosis may be worst. This complication occurs for implant of bone graft or cages positioned not in distraction. Restoring of spinal lordosis allows for the back-shift of the spinal cord. When cervical sagittal alignment remains in kyphosis, spinal cord lies adjacent to the posterior wall of the vertebral bodies, and persisting spinal cord or nerve roots compression occurs. This sagittal imbalance with fusion in incorrect position is also responsible for adjacent disk degeneration [9].

- Anterior or posterior graft migration or graft collapse

Anterior or posterior graft migration or graft collapse can occur if the bone graft size is smaller than the bony trench: in this case, the graft can easily dislodge posteriorly leading to a direct compression to the spinal cord, even in case of anterior instrumentation. Anterior dislodgement of the graft is often encountered in noninstrumented fusions, and leads to chronic dysphagia requiring surgical revision. To avoid these complications, the bone graft should be applied in distraction, with its extremities contoured in dovetail fashion to lock the graft and prevent further migrations. The use of stabilization with plate and screws drastically reduced the incidence of these complications [9].

Late Postoperative Complication: Adjacent Segment Degeneration

It is logical to think that intervertebral disk degeneration adjacent to a previous fusion is the direct consequence of the fusion surgery. In particular, abolition of segmental movement after fusion would shift the loads at the adjacent motion segment and determine early disk degeneration.

On average, adjacent segment motion remains unchanged after 2 years from a previous fusion [43–45]. In the experimental study of Fuller on cervical spine from cadavers, the author demonstrated how single-level fusion leads to a uniform increase of motion in all the remaining mobile units, harmonically distributing motion degrees to all the cervical spine [46].

On the contrary, it has been demonstrated that fusion leads to a significant increase in intradiscal pressure of the adjacent disks during physiological range of motion, potentially leading to early intervertebral disk degeneration [43]. In this controversial context, several clinical studies have been designed to clarify the natural history of the intervertebral disk degeneration adjacent to a fusion.

Goffin, on his study on 180 anterior cervical fusions, observed a radiological evidence of adjacent disk degeneration in 92% (166/180) operated patients, and performed revision surgery at the adjacent level in 6,11% (11/180) of cases of symptomatic disease [47]. An important criticism to the paper of Goffin is the inclusion of trauma patients in his study, because post-mortem studies on accidental injuries demonstrated occult spinal lesions even in patients without radiological evidence of cervical spine injury [48].

In the report on the first 100 cases of single or multilevel cervical disk herniation treated by discectomy and fusion with the Cloward's technique, we found radiological evidence of adjacent disk degeneration in 32% of patients [49]. In contrast to the findings of Goffin, all the patients were asymptomatic. We observed that 2/3 of the cases of degeneration of the adjacent disk degeneration occurred at the intervertebral disk below the arthrodesis, and 1/3 at the intervertebral disk above the arthrodesis. This is probably a consequence of the greater mobility of the lower segments of the cervical spine.

This result is consistent with the findings of Hilibrand [50], who reported on 409 procedures of anterior cervical interbody fusions for degenerative disk disease. Despite this, in this study population symptomatic adjacent disk degeneration had a prevalence of 14.2% (58/409), only 29 out 409 (7%) required surgery. Hilibrand concluded that adjacent level degeneration is the physiological progression disk degeneration, and independent from fusion; these data are similar to reports of other authors [51].

In a study on adjacent segment degeneration after cervical fusion on a sample of 55 patients treated for single or multilevel fusion via an anterior, posterior, or combined approach and followed for 3–18 years [52], results showed that in young patients, whose disks are not yet involved in the degenerative process, even in the long term follow-up signs of adjacent disk degeneration are not found; conversely, in the adult patients, whose disks are already affected by arthritic changes, an evolution of disk degeneration adjacent to a fusion can be observed.

One of the major determinants of adjacent segment disease after fusion surgery is most probably the post-operative segmental alignment after fusion [53–56]. Degenerative changes adjacent to a previous fusion are, in fact, more frequent in patients with kyphosis and sigmoidal curves, and less observed in patients in postoperative physiological lordosis [57], similarly to what occurs in patients with Klippel–Feil syndrome.

The functional overload to the adjacent intervertebral disks is more important when arthrodeses are performed at levels C5–C6 and C6–C7, which are considered the more mobile points of the cervical spine. The risk of adjacent intervertebral disk disease is lower when fusion is performed at level C2–C3 or C4–C5 (Fig. 10.14).

When MSC is performed, adjacent segment degeneration is more common when compared with interventions with fusion of one or two levels. In our series of patients undergoing MSC, we followed 16 patients for 5–13 years. We studied the radiographic evolution of the disk spaces above and below the involved levels. In seven patients, we observed radiographic changes indicating lesions of the intervertebral disk above and below the fused level. In three patients, we observed a progressive hypermobility of the spaces above the arthrodesis developed. In four patients, a static overload with degenerative changes in the inferior disk was noted. All the patients were asymptomatic, not requiring any management (Fig. 10.15).

10.2.3 Anterior Instrumentation

Anterior instrumentation for the cervical spine has been subjected to a technical evolution in the recent years. Before the 1970s, there was no instrumentation dedicated to the stabilization of the cervical spine

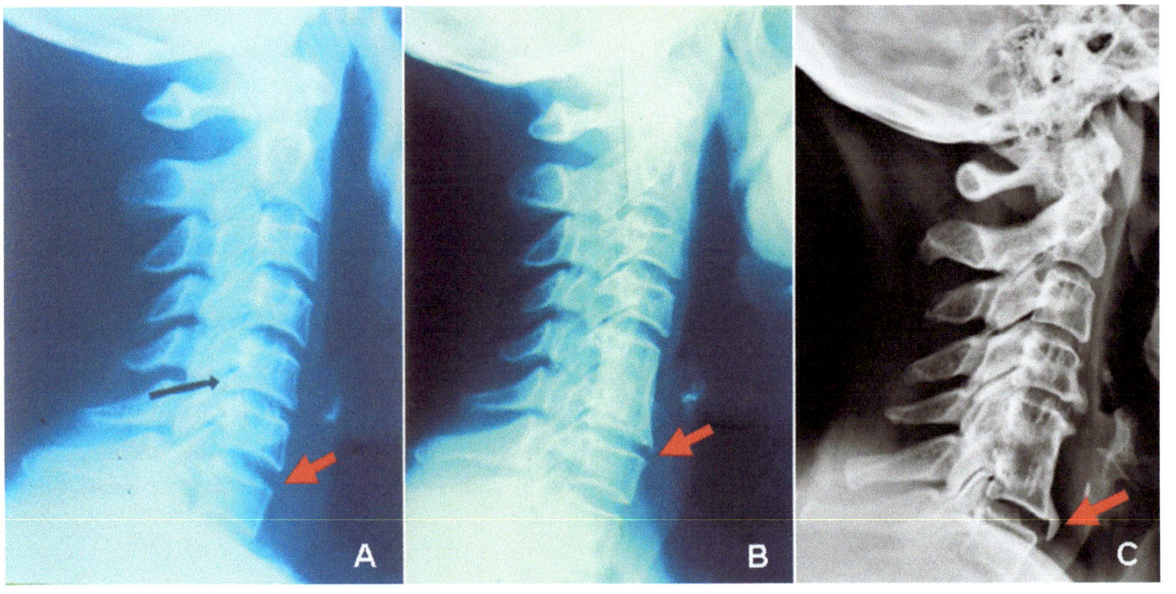

Fig. 10.14 (**a**) Lateral radiograph of a patient managed with a Cloward procedure. (**b**) 3-year postoperative lateral radiograph. The *red arrow* indicates the adjacent intervertebral disk, which does not show evident signs of adjacent level degeneration. (**c**) 11-year postoperative lateral radiograph. The intervertebral disk is conserved and an asymptomatic ossification of the anterior longitudinal ligament is present

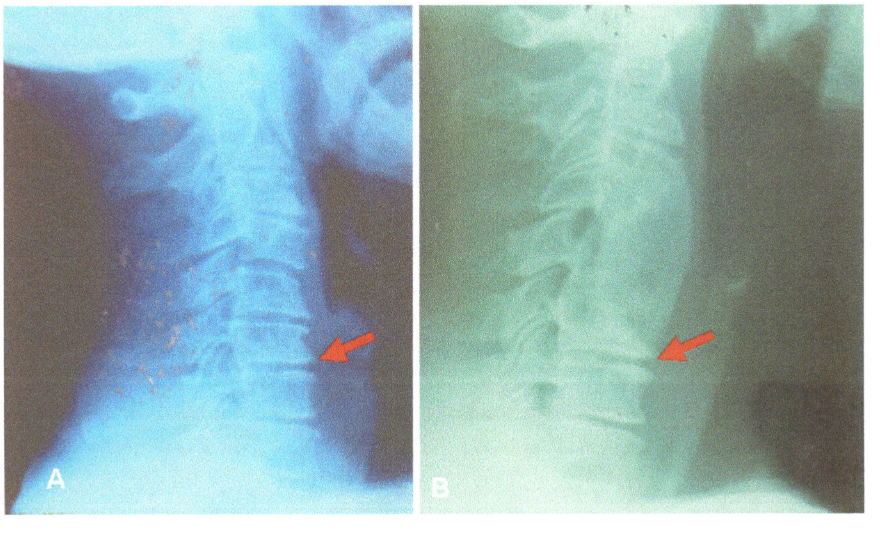

Fig. 10.15 (**a**) Lateral radiograph of a patient with spondylotic cervical myelopathy. The patient was managed by multiple subtotal somatectomy in 1969. (**b**) 4-year postoperative lateral radiograph. The *red arrow* indicates the adjacent intervertebral disk, which does not show particular signs of worsening of the adjacent level

when required to treat post-traumatic or neoplastic instability. When needed, fixation was performed with plates and screws studied for the stabilization of other segments such as the forearm or the long bones (Fig. 10.16). Since then, plate and screw systems dedicated to the anterior spine were developed, and instrumentation was first used in patients operated for multilevel degenerative disk disease [58].

In degenerative disk disease, in fact, reported fusion rates for noninstrumented single-level ADCF exceeds 90%, while decreases to 70% in two-level surgery [49, 58]. In the study by Wright and Eisenstein [58], single-level uninstrumented cervical fusion resulted in 6 out of 54 (11%) patients that required adjunctive posterior fixation, and refusion in four out of six. In the double-level surgeries, 12/54 patients (22%) underwent nonunion,

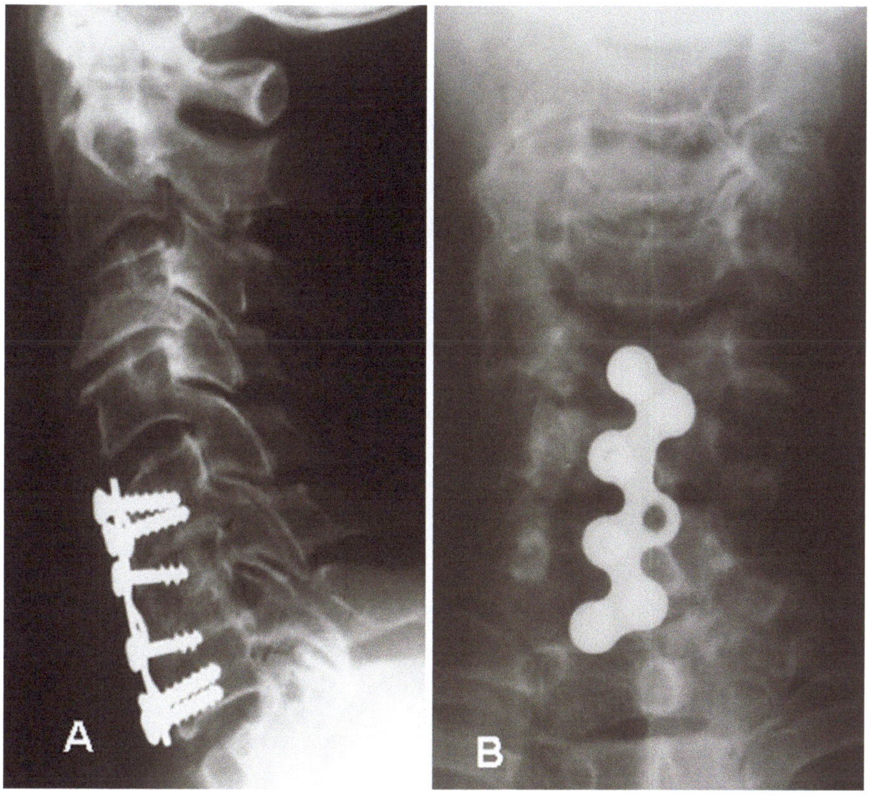

Fig. 10.16 Fixation of the cervical spine by means of a bone long plate used in the 1970s, when no instrumentation dedicated to the stabilization of the cervical spine was available

and 5 out of 12 required resurgery via a posterior route. Authors concluded that plating could not add benefit in single-level ACDF, but support the routine plating fixation in double-level surgery. Nonetheless, at present, plate fixation is routinely performed even in single-level anterior fusion procedures with bone grafting [59].

Anterior cervical plates can be grossly divided into "Rigid" and "Dynamic" implants, remembering that evolution of the implants is often a commercial requirement.

In the rigid constructs, there is a fixed relationship between plates and screws, which can be inserted at variable angles [60]. The use of these implants is associated with the nonunion of the bone graft and subsidence of approximately 1–1.5 mm per operated level. Dynamic plates instead allow for movement at the plate–screw interface [61]. This allows for subsidence and codivision of loadings between the construct and the graft, and theoretically for an increased rate of fusion, but decrease the stability of the graft itself [62, 63].

In the study by DuBois comparing static vs. dynamic anterior cervical plates, clinical outcome was found to be similar between the static and dynamic plate groups, with good clinical results in 84% of patients [64]. Nonetheless, the author observed a significantly higher rate of nonunion in patients treated with dynamic plates than with a static plate (16 vs. 5%), maybe due to increased motion at the bone–plate interface in comparison with more rigid static plates. One of the concerns regarding the use of dynamic plates is progressive plate migration toward the adjacent unfused disk secondary to graft collapse and sliding of screws, potentially leading to adjacent segment degeneration [65–68]. For this reason, plates should be placed 3–5 mm away from the adjacent disk spaces to decrease the likelihood of moderate to severe adjacent level degeneration [64, 67]. At present, no evidence is available to support the superiority of dynamic plates when compared with static plates, and further evaluation is still needed; nonetheless, adherence to careful surgical techniques can decrease the incidence of surgery-related complications in the use of dynamic plate implants. In a study over 116 patients operated of ACDF with iliac crest strut autograft with dynamic plate fixation, Epstein reported that 11 patients developed postoperative complications within the first 2 years of the study, while via intraoperative surgical tips the author has been able to decrease the complication rate in the following 4 years [69]. In the first 2 years, three patients did not fuse for plate/graft extrusion at 3 weeks ($n=1$), and nonunions at 6 months ($n=2$). The three patients required a posterior adjunctive fixation and in the extrusion case also anterior revision surgery. Symptomatic adjacent level degeneration occurred in one patient who required surgery; in other five patients some kind of adjacent degeneration occurred, but remained asymptomatic and did not require surgery. Seven patients developed delayed strut fractures, four of which required revision surgery. The author suggested that the following tips in surgical techniques eliminated these complications in the latter phases of the study: more extensive endplate removal exposing cancellous bone, avoidance of fibula allograft, and better placement of the screws in the cephalad 1/3 or caudad 1/3 of the contiguous vertebral bodies. Moreover, inadequate initial bracing was suspected to contribute to delayed strut graft fractures, and routine use of a cervicothoracic orthosis for 6 weeks postoperatively was started. Complications related to the use of instrumentation in the degenerative cervical spine can be divided in those related to plate and screws systems and those associated with the use of cages (Table 10.2).

10.2.3.1 Plates and Screws

Implant positioning and dimension selection depend on the instrumentation system used. The plate is posed over the interface between bone graft and vertebral body, allowing for rostral and caudal screw insertion. Plate should be posed at the midline of the vertebral body to avoid local complications: an easy way to find the midline is bilateral visualization of the unci. Severely malpositioned implants can be associated with direct injury to neurovascular structures such as the sympathetic trunk, vertebral artery, or spinal nerve roots, and there are several clinical case series describing implant-associated complications [70]. Nonetheless, radiological studies have shown a relatively wide variation among patients in implant position with respect to both lateralization and rotation, with greater rotation variability observed in association with single-level as opposed to multiple-level fusions, but long-term results on clinical impact of these variations are not available.

Another fundamental surgical point is the plate to bone graft reciprocal contouring, aimed at maximization of interface surface contact. Intuitively, plate molding could modify the reciprocal direction of the screws

Table 10.2 Complications associated with the use of anterior instrumentation

Implant	Complication	Consequences	Tips/tricks
Plates	Migration toward the adjacent disk	Early adjacent disk degeneration Graft collapse	Leave at least 3 mm from adjacent disk space
	Malpositioning (lateralization/rotation)	Possible neural and vascular lesions	Find the midline by visualizing the unci Fluoroscopic check for rotation
	Rupture	Plate migration Need for revision surgery	Risk increased in long implants
Screws	Excessive length	Subdural hematoma Dural tears Spinal cord lesions	Preoperative vertebral body measure by CT scan Monocortical fixation
	Breakage	Implant failure Need for revision surgery	Use 4 mm diameter screws
	Violation of the endplate or diskspace	Disk degeneration Segmental instability Repositioning required	Check fluoroscopically the position of the screw and eventually reposition
	Loosening and pull-out	Implant mobilization	Use high-profile thread screws with 4 mm diameter
Cages	Weakening of vertebral endplate	Subsidence	Use in degenerative disease only Notin patients with osteoporosis
	Dislocation/migration	Damage to neurovascular structures Soft tissue damage	Adequate postoperative immobilization
	Pseudoarthrosis	Cage migration	Adequate endplate preparation to promote device osteointegration

in respect to the vertebral body. For this reason, the surgeon should remove anterior osteophytes before decompression begins (Fig. 10.1). This procedure not only eases the identification of the disk space, but allows for a perfect adhesion of the plate to the anterior aspect of the vertebral bodies.

Screws can be self-tapped or require tapping before insertion. It is useful to estimate the width of the vertebral body with preoperative radiological examination to calculate screw length. Despite this, some systems require a bicortical fixation; in most cases monocortical fixation provides adequate segmental stability, with low risk to enter the spinal canal. Proximal and distal screws should be inserted diagonally opposite to achieve symmetrical stability, and then the other screws are inserted. In case of somatectomies of 2–3 segments, when a long graft is implanted, it is useful to stabilize the implant with plates and screws. Some implants allow to also insert screws into the graft, connecting the graft to the plate.

Before closure, the esophagous should be inspected to put in evidence eventual lesions of the muscular wall that occurred during plate insertion. Complications associated with the use of anterior plate and screws systems can be divided into those specific to the soft tissues, and those strictly dependent on the use of the implants. Injury to soft tissue can be observed either during the insertion process of the screws or when implant migration occurs postoperatively [71–77].

Other feared complications associated with the use of instrumentation are implant failure, screw mobilization, plate rupture, and plate or graft mobilization [71, 72, 74, 78, 79]. Screw or implant mobilization can occur after bony fusion occurrs, or being secondary to traumas. Screw or implant mobilization can lead to severe esophageal lesions and consequent local infection, spondylodiscitis or mediastinitis, acute airways obstruction, and even death. Once an esophageal lesion is suspected, revision of the surgical wound after administration of methylene blue helps the surgeon in finding the lesion and ease repair [80].

In vitro testing of cervical plating systems has shown loosening of the screw–bone interface over time with repetitive loading [81]. Other factors that could possibly stimulate screw loosening are cancellous bone osteoporosis, motion at the screw–bone interface occurring in the bone itself and degree of constraint provided by the design of the implant that could apply stress at the screw–bone interface that can play a role in relative loosening [82]. This latter is more often encountered in multilevel constructs and is associated with serious life-threatening complications such as acute airways obstruction and even death.

In a retrospective study, complications that occurred in a mixed population of 2,233 consecutive patients affected by subaxial cervical disorders (trauma, $n=553$; spondylosis, $n=1{,}267$; OPLL, $n=198$; vertebral body tumors, $n=158$; infections, $n=46$; cervical kyphosis, $n=11$) treated with single or multilevel surgeries with the use of an anterior cervical plate were pooled [83]. Overall complication rate was 10.7% (239/2233) patients. Authors divided plate-related complications in implant malpositions, biomechanical complications, and tracheoesophageal or neurovascular structural injuries. Oblique plating (plate axis more than 15° from the midline) was observed in 56/2,233 (2.5%) patients. Two out of the 56 (3.6%) patients complained of radiculopathy and neck pain after surgery: one underwent revision and plate repositioning in 2 weeks and a screw was retrieved in the soft tissue and impinging the nerve root; the other patient underwent plate removal after fusion. Screw pullout was observed in 37/2,233 (1.7%) patients. Five screws pulled out more than 5 mm, and three esophageal perforations occurred; in the other two patients, the loosened screw was removed before occurrence of esophageal perforation. Plate loosening occurred in 72/2,233 (3.2%) cases; between them, 45/72 (62.5%) nonunions were found, which were managed by anterior revision surgery using iliac bone autograft and a new plate. Screw breakage was found in four cases and broken plate in two (occurring in nonunion patients). Conflict between the adjacent disk space and the plate leading to adjacent degeneration occurred in 14 patients (0.6%), mainly with semi-constrained plates (13/14), and all patients required revisions. In four patients out of 2233 (0.2%), screw penetration into the disk space occurred; patients developed plate loosening 1–2 months post operation, and plate revision was required. Screw violation of the endplate with the tip into the disk space occurred in 42/2,233 (1.9%) patients, but none required revision surgery. In 42 cases, 76 screws penetrated the endplates and 11/42 (26.2%) developed triangular fracture at the bottom endplate. The same complication was reported in other eight patients with screws close to the endplate without violation. Conservative treatment was performed in all the patients.

In one patient from our university, the inferior screw was positioned penetrating into the intervertebral space.

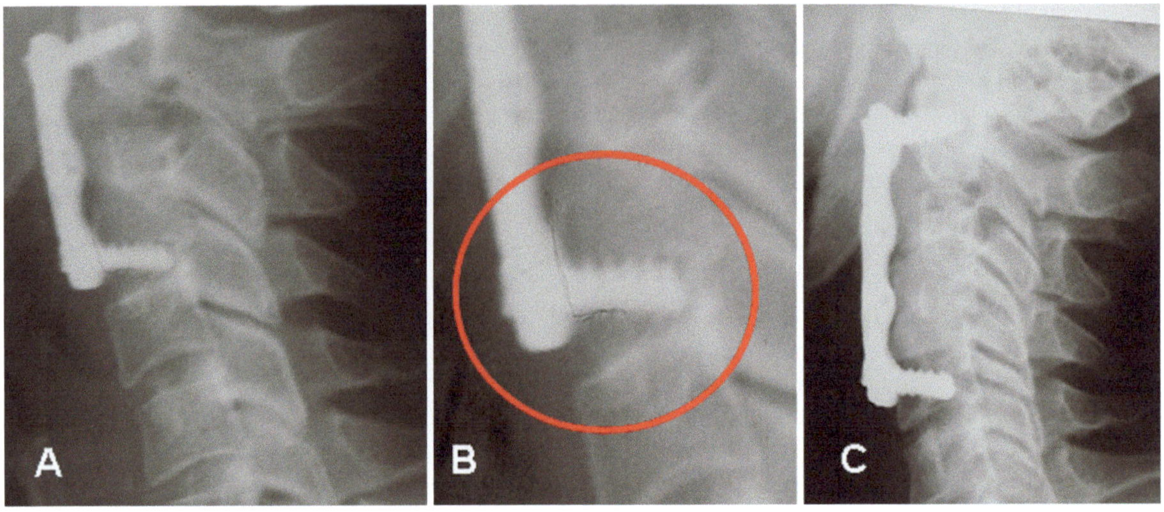

Fig. 10.17 (**a**, **b**) Lateral radiograph of a patient in whom the inferior screw was positioned penetrating into the intervertebral space. Circle shows a magnification of the malpositioned screw. Intraoperatively, the plate was stable, because it was fixed to the anterior aspect of the vertebral body, but invaded the intervertebral disk. (**c**) Six months after the index procedure, a revision surgery was required because of persistent neck pain. Symptoms resolved after revision surgery

Intraoperatively, the plate was stable, because it was fixed to the anterior aspect of the vertebral body, but invaded the intervertebral disk. Six months after the index procedure, a revision surgery was required because of persistent neck pain. Symptoms resolved after revision surgery (Fig. 10.17).

The rate of instrumentation failure increases in multilevel constructs [84]. In the study of Papadopulos [85] on 46 patients operated by three-level ACDF with plate fixation, five instrumentation-related complications occurred, namely two plate impingement on the cephalad unfused disk associated with early adjacent degeneration, one broken distal screw, and one violation of the inferior endplate by the distal screws. Moreover, one patient developed a horizontal fracture of the vertebral body at the level of the distal screws, which required adjunctive bracing to achieve fusion. It is then suitable in multilevel fusion patients (when compatible to patient disease) to use an instrumented posterior approach, or hybrids of corpectomy plus discectomy at the bottom level, which are biomechanically more stable [86, 87].

10.2.3.2 Anterior Cervical Cages

Cages were developed at the beginning to avoid morbidity related to bone graft harvesting from the iliac crest during anterior cervical spine surgery, and in most cases, when implanted in distraction, do not require associated implantation of plate and screws [62].

It is possible to divide cages into two categories, cylindrical and cubical. Moreover, these can be of different materials such as poly-ether-ether-ketone (PEEK), titanium alloys, carbon fibers, tantallium. Finally, cages can be full or hollow to allow for bone graft filling with either bone graft or graft extenders to stimulate implant integration. Cage implant requires a dedicated instrumentation. Cubical cages are implanted as an allograft or autograft spacer in Smith–Robinson-like procedures. Cylindrical cages require instead the use of Cloward-type reaming tools to obtain a proper space for cage positioning. The bone removed during corpectomy or reaming, is added when hollow cages are used to fill the void [88]; alternatively, bone allograft or PMMA have also been described to fill the cage. Some authors suggested the use of osteoinductive factors such as rh-BMP-2 to improve fusion. When rh-BMP-2 was used in conjunction of PEEK cages and an anterior cervical plate, high rates of fusion were observed (100% of rhBMP-2 cases). Nonetheless, endplate erosion and marked prevertebral soft tissue swelling with dysphagia is observed more frequently with respect to patients operated of ACDF with standard allograft, together with a significant increase in costs of the procedure [89].

Current studies demonstrated the efficacy of anterior cervical cages in surgical treatment of radiculopathy secondary to single and bi-level degenerative disk disease, and in the reconstruction after multilevel corpectomies [88, 90]. In a recent review on the results of prospective clinical trials comparing cervical fusion with iliac crest bone graft vs. interbody cage and autogenous bone graft, some evidence was found that cages could result in higher fusion rates in single-level surgeries, but lower fusion rates in the two-level surgeries. Conversely, clinical scores and patient satisfaction tended to be higher in patients treated without cage implant.

Potential complications associated with the use of these devices are nonunion, implant dislocation, endplate collapse with implant subsidence, vascular and neurological lesions secondary to implant migration or malpositioning [27]. Structural failure and subsidence occur mainly when one or both vertebral endplates are fully removed during discectomy and the cage is positioned into the cancellous bone, which may easily collapse in cases of osteoporosis. Moreover, implant of a hollow cage without bone graft inside avoids integration, favors mechanical failure, implants mobilization of the subchondral trabecular bone and leads to subsidence, and should not be performed [91].

Many factors can affect the subsidence behavior of cages. It is commonly thought that the incidence is higher in older patients and in women, especially after menopause, because the bone quality of the vertebrae and the thickness of the endplates decrease in these patients (Fig. 10.18) [92].

Reconstruction after multilevel corpectomy is one of the main risk factors for cage subsidence [93, 94]. In a study on multilevel implant using cubical cages, it has been suggested that cage subsidence determined kyphotic deformity in up to 16% of patients, leading to instrumentation failure, and subsequent neurological deterioration; these complications often required revision surgery [95].

Other authors support that use of cylindrical cages is associated with a lower incidence of postoperative complications [88]. In a study on 488 patients, the implant-related complications of a BAK/C cage (with or without hydroxyapatite (HA) coating) were lower with respect to the use of noninstrumented ACDF with auto or allograft (3.4% for the BAK/C and 1.2% for the HA-coated BAK/C, compared with 7.7% for the ACDF procedures). The device-related complications included six cases of nonunion (four of which required a second surgery), one fractured vertebrae, and one stenosis secondary to excessive bone formation around the implant. Nonunion was associated with the use of the BAK-C cage, with lower rates when hydroxyapatite-coated cage was used.

In other studies, PEEK cages compared favorably against autograft in the treatment of cervical spine degenerative disk disease [96, 97]. In a study where over 180 consecutive patients participated in multilevel cervical surgery [96], patients were randomized into one of three study groups. Sixty patients underwent anterior discectomy and PEEK cage fusion, 50 patients underwent ACDF with autologous bone graft and plate fixation, and 70 patients underwent ACDF with autologous bone graft only. The analysis of complications showed a significant increase of complications in patients with ACDF with autologous bone graft alone

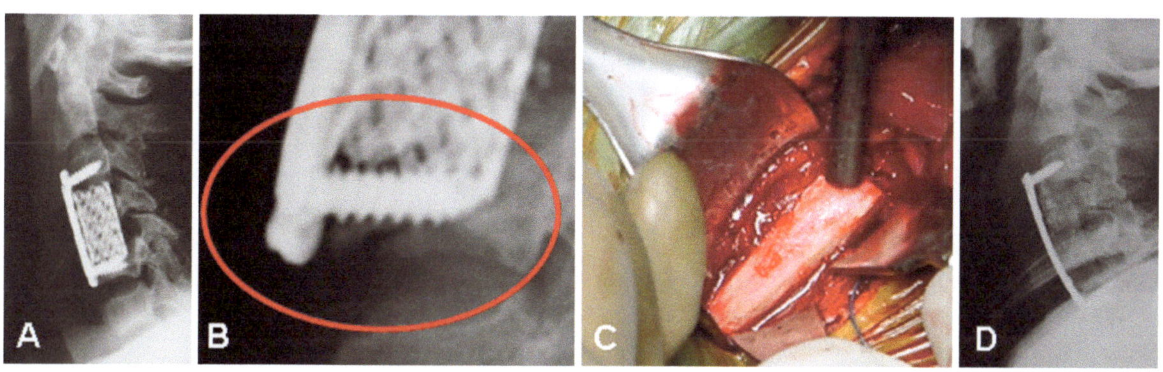

Fig. 10.18 (**a, b**) Lateral radiograph of a dialyzed patient with spondylotic cervical myelopathy, showing subsidence of a titanium mesh cage. The circle shows the distal screw was wrongly implanted in an osteoporotic vertebral body, with little quantity of bone. (**c**) Revision surgery. The mesh cage was removed, and an arthrodesis performed with iliac bone autograft and anchorage to the adjacent healthy vertebral bodies. (**d**) Postoperative radiograph

that reached 54.3%, compared with PEEK (3.3%) and plate group (16%), but only 13 patients with graft complications showed clear symptoms (severe neck pain, radicular pain, or neurologic deficits) and required treatment.

Recently, bioabsorbable cages have been used in surgery for cervical degenerative spine. In a pilot study on the use of bioabsorbable cages, eight patients underwent ACDF in which a bioabsorbable (poly L-lactide-co-D,L-lactide) anterior cervical interbody spacer was filled with demineralized bone matrix or rh-BMP-2 (one patient); segment fixation was performed with an anterior metallic cervical plate [98]. At an early available follow-up (average 7 months), 17/18 (94%) grafted levels appeared to be solidly fused. One patient experienced a perisurgical complication consisting of a symptomatic hematoma, which was successfully drained. Inflammatory responses to the components of the bioabsorbable spacers appeared not to be a problem in the study population.

Prevention: It is fundamental to respect correct indications. The use of these implants should be avoided in patients affected by metabolic bone diseases (osteoporosis), posttraumatic instability, infective, inflammatory, and neoplastic cervical spine disease. Moreover, it is useful to remember that implants should be inserted under fluoroscopic view to prevent posterior or lateral dislocation, vertebral artery lesions, as well as spinal cord or nerve root compressions. Preservation of the vertebral endplate is mandatory to avoid structural collapse and implant subsidence.

10.3 Posterior Surgical Techniques

10.3.1 Laminectomy and Fusion

For several years, the complete removal of the posterior structures of the spinal canal consisting in bony laminae, ligamentum flavum, and the spinous processes has been the only procedure performed to treat stenosis at cervical spine. Surgery in those patients classically affected by multilevel spinal stenosis is the so-called "wide laminectomy," which still today represents the treatment of choice for patients affected by multilevel stenosis of the spinal canal sustained mainly by posterior structures (hypertrophy of the pedicles, hypertrophy of the ligamentum flavum, deformity of the laminae), and in patients with circumferential spinal stenosis on a congenital base. It is moreover the treatment of choice for patient affected by multilevel OPLL disease.

Laminectomy can be considered when decompression is required at more than three levels, particularly in elderly patients. All levels with radiological evidence of stenosis should be fully decompressed. Concerns about postlaminectomy kyphosis and segmental instability (swan neck, kyphosis) stimulated the implementation of adequate solid fusion and then to the use of posterior instrumentation.

Although surgical techniques can vary, few intraoperative tricks can help the surgeon in avoiding complications.

Great care must be taken when positioning the surgical instruments (kerrison, rongeurs) under lamina where major spinal cord compression should be avoided because of the risk of spinal cord lesion, dural tears, and worsening neurological picture.

Laminectomy is performed on the basis of the surgeon's experience. The first stage of the laminectomy consists in the removal of the interspinal ligament. Then, using Luer forceps, the tow of spinous processes are cut at the base at the point of confluences of the two laminae at each level. At the upper cervical spine, when the arch of the atlas is removed, the surgeon must be aware that too laterally dissection may cause damages to the vertebral artery (Fig. 10.19).

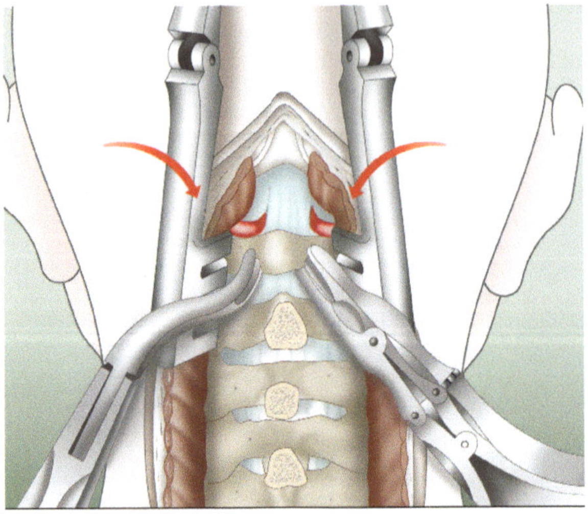

Fig. 10.19 At the upper cervical spine, when the arch of the atlas is removed, the surgeon must be aware that too laterally dissection may cause damages to the vertebral artery

Once the spinous processes have been removed, bone wax is used to stem the bleeding from the cancellous bone, which is now exposed. At each operative level and using curved curets, the ligament flavum is elevated, but must remain intact and in place, since it will act as a buffer between the instrument and the subjacent nerve structures. As the laminectomy proceeds, the surgeon can contemporaneously begin to remove the ligamentum flavum. Once this has been done, the peridural fat appears indicating that the dura mater has been reached.

Alternatively, when the surgeon wants to perform an en bloc removal of the posterior wall of the canal, including the laminae and the ligamentum flavum, air drill can be used to outline the limits of the lamina at the interface with the articular mass. The cut across the lamina is gradually deepened to reach the internal cortex bilaterally. The ligamentum flavum is detached at its most proximal and distal parts with curved curets. The anterior cortex of the lamina can then be removed with very fine Kerrison forceps (which have a cutting edge), curets, or a very fine drill with a pointed bit. Great care must be taken to protect the underlying neural structures with a spatula. Afterwards, en bloc asportation of the resected segments by the spinous processes and transection of remaining adherences is performed, paying special attention to avoid tilting of the lamina, which would create tears to the dura mater [99].

Laminectomy without instrumentation at present should be restricted to patients with preserved cervical lordosis and stiff neck. Conversely, when a flexible cervical kyphosis is evident, laminectomy and instrumented fusion should be performed. In all the other cases, especially in patients with segmental kyphosis, instrumentation after laminectomy is mandatory. The latter is performed modeling the hardware in lordosis, to restore cervical lordosis and maximize back-shift of the spinal cord [100].

In addition to the complications already described when positioning the patient on the operating table (Chap. 6) when performing a posterior surgical access, there are several complications strictly related to the laminectomy and fusion procedure itself (Table 10.3):

Dural tears and neural lesions
Bleeding from venous plexus
Lateral masses violation
General complications

Table 10.3 Complications of posterior cervical spine surgery in the degenerative cervical spine

	Consequences	Tips/tricks
Laminectomy and fusion		
Dural tears	CSF fluid leakage needing suture or repair	Leave in situ the ligamentum flavum during flavectomy Reverse-Trendelemburg position during surgical repair
Bleeding from venous plexus	Postsurgical hematoma Decreased visual control during surgery	Use surgicel and spongostan soaked with-tranexamic acid
Facet joints violation	Postsurgical instability and kyphosis	Use instrumentation Revision surgery often required
Laminoplasty		
Wrong patient selection	Increased risk of postoperative instability and kyphosis	*Avoid patients with:* Neutral or kyphotic spine Myelopathy Segmental instability
Closure of the lamina ("door") in the follow-up period, fusion of the laminae	Potential loss of decompression	Need for decompressive revision surgery
Fracture or dislocation of the hinge	Migration of the bony fragment with potential injury to spinal cord and nerve roots	Intraoperatively evaluate hinge stability Eventual reinforce with a minifragment plate Conversion to laminectomy and fusion procedure
Selective paralysis of C5 root	Weakness atdeltoid and biceps brachii muscle	Affects the "hinge side" root Self-resolving within 1–2 y

10.3.1.1 Dural Tears and Neural Lesions

Dural tears are mainly secondary to surgical instruments used for spinal decompression (curettes, Kerrison, air drill). A technical tip is to leave in situ the ligamentum flavum during laminectomy as a protection for the delicate dural tissue. Removal of the ligamentum flavum after laminectomy can also lead to dural tears for the strict adherences between the two tissues: this maneuver can be performed in an easier fashion by the intraoperative use of MESNA (Uromixetan) (Sodium 2-mercaptoethane sulfonate) released locally (Fig. 10.20) [41]. In fact, in patients with severe deformity of the cervical spine and severe congenital stenosis, the spinal cord is surrounded by scant peridural adipose tissue suitable for dural protection during surgical dissection, and in these patients the ligamentum flavum and the laminae leave a footprint over the dural sac, expression of the strict relation between them. Adherences to the dura are between the main responsible for occurrence of dural tears during surgical dissection.

The use of diamond-coated burrs decreases the risk for direct lesion to the neural structures and surrounding soft tissues during surgical decompression. As already described, surgical repair of dural tears during spine surgery via a posterior approach are usually easier to repair with respect to those that occurred during anterior surgery. Positioning the patient in reverse Trendelemburg position decreases hydrostatic pressure of CSF and can ease surgical repair. It is fundamental when suturing dural tears in the cervical spine to avoid a decrease in the transverse diameter of the dural sac due to sutures, because of the high risk to develop an iatrogenic stenosis, so when possible using patches of liodura can be used; conversely adding Duraseal™ tear suture is not always needed. If not well repaired, even small lesions inevitably lead to the occurrence of liquoral fistulas in the postoperative setting with a high risk of meningitis. After repair of the dural tear, keeping the patient in supine position is preferred. In case of postural headache, the patient should take bed rest. If this continues, the patient should be sent for MRI examination and eventual surgical wound revision, or should be considered for application of a lumbar subarachnoid drainage. As we already stated, patients with lumbar drainage should undergo continuous monitoring, and start spectrum antibiotic therapy to avoid superinfection. Drainage flow should be of 8–12 mL/h, with flow rate modified on the basis of the clinical response to the headache. Bed rest is suggested for 24 h after drainage removal.

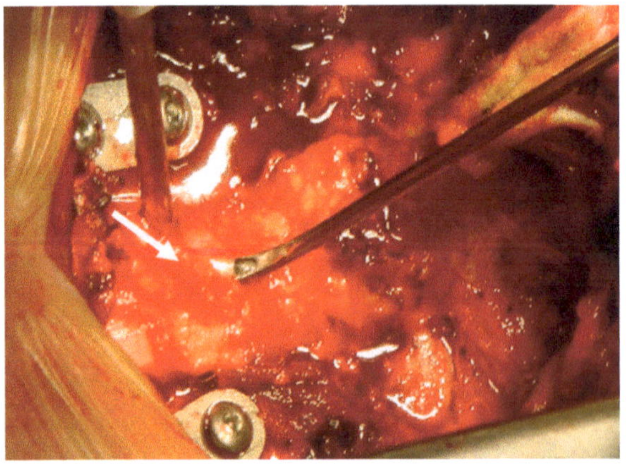

Fig. 10.20 Use of MESNA during flavectomy. The *arrow* indicates the residual yellow ligament, adherent to the dura, and chemically dissected by MESNA

The incidence of spinal cord injury ranges from 0 to 3%, whereas injury to an individual nerve root has been reported as high as 15% [101]. Technical errors, introduction of instruments under the central lamina, as well as ischemic injury due to hypoperfusion or aggressive distraction can lead to irreversible spinal cord injury. Inadvertent coagulation, use of retractors, and sharp instrumentation during surgery is in most cases responsible for direct lesions of the spinal cord and nerve roots. Root paresis is more commonly associated with laminoplasty techniques (see later), but has also been reported in laminectomy patients. In the study of Dai et al. [102], 37/287 patients who underwent cervical laminectomy developed a postoperative radiculopathy. C5 radiculopathy was the most common found, and typically resolved with time.

10.3.1.2 Bleeding from Venous Plexus

In the lateral region of the dural sac, where the emerging nerve roots are encountered, an abundant venous plexus is present. When bleeding in this region occurs, it is better to gently use tampons to coagulate with surgicel and spongostan soaked with tranexamic acid.

10.3.1.3 Lateral Mass Removal

Problems associated with this procedure include both the incomplete removal of the laminae (with persistence of the stenosis), and excessive removal of the laminae and articular apophyses (with consequent instability, especially in patients in whom a stabilization is not performed). The error is to extend the dissection too laterally in the attempt to completely decompress the nerve roots.

To allow a wide decompression of the nerve roots, it is sufficient to remove the posterior wall of the neuroforamen without weakening the lateral mass. This technique is easier and safer if a probe is inserted to protect the nerve root while decompression is performed by using a diamond coated burr (Fig. 10.21). If lateral mass resection is more than 50%, instability most likely occurs; nonetheless, reports of postoperative instability in patients without facetectomy are available [103]. In a comparison of treatment modalities for multilevel spondylotic radiculopathy, Herkowitz [104] noted a 25% incidence of postoperative kyphotic deformities in 2 years in a population operated after cervical laminectomy with bilateral partial facetectomy. For this reason, as we already stated, we support the indication to segmental fixation and fusion after laminectomy procedures. Postlaminectomy kyphosis is more often encountered in the pediatric population. Once occurred, treatment of these deformities is strictly dependent on mobility of the curves on the sagittal plane. When cervical spine is still mobile, a posterior instrumentation and fusion in lordosis is the treatment of choice. In case of patients with stiff cervical and noncorrectable kyphosis (because of retraction of the anterior ligamentous structures and intervertebral disk degeneration) without facet ankylosis, it is necessary to perform an MSC, with wide cord decompression and instrumented fusion in distraction with restoration of the lordosis (this maneuver is possible after having removed the anterior portion of the vertebral bodies and the adherent anterior longitudinal ligament). In patients with sagittal deformity in kyphosis and facet ankylosis, the clinical picture is severe, and a more complex posterior approach with facet osteotomy followed by an anterior approach with corpectomy and fusion and then posterior fixation is required. These operations are performed in one surgical time, with the patient in lateral decubitus (see Chap. 6).

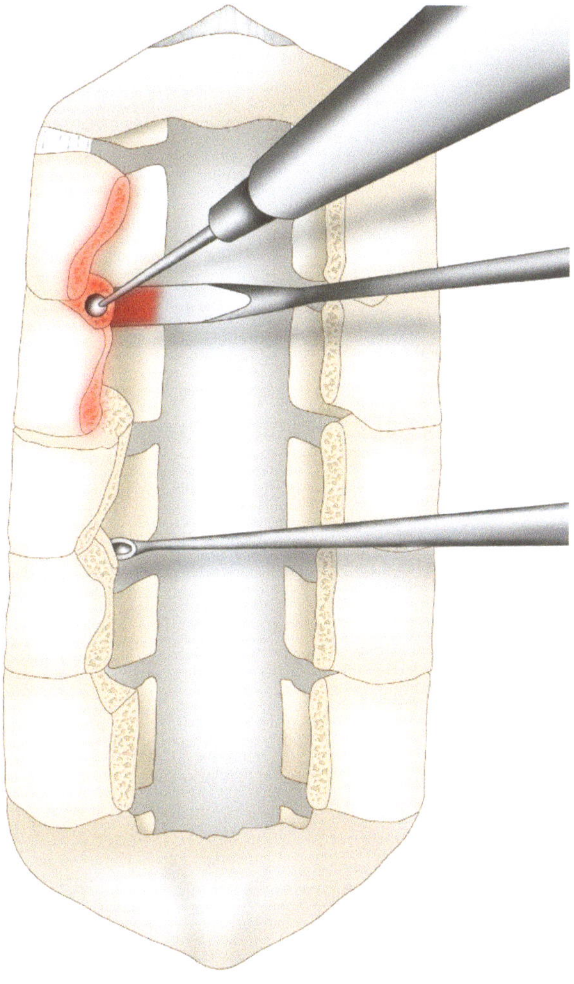

Fig. 10.21 After removal of the laminae and the ligamentum flavum, the roots must be freed laterally to the level of the opening of the root canal. The roots must be protected during this procedure, and this is achieved by placing a spatula in front of the anterior facets and behind the nerve roots and the dural sac. Decompression is achieved with an air drill. Any remnants of ligamentum flavum or bony fragments, which remain on the wall at the inferior facet should be removed with curets

10.3.1.4 General Complications

General complications have been widely reported in patients undergoing laminectomy procedures. These comprehend air embolism, infections, epidural hematoma, cerebellar hemorrhage, and deep venous thrombosis [99]`. General status of the patient should be considered when planning a laminectomy procedure. Age over 70 years, diabetes, coronary artery disease, obstructive pulmonary disease, peripheral vascular disease, stroke, alcoholism and tobacco use are all risk factors for that in most severe cases can contraindicate surgery [105].

10.3.2 Laminoplasty

About 40 years ago, to avoid complications as post-laminectomy kyphosis, swan neck, and instability, occurring after wide posterior noninstrumented decompression, Japanese authors described laminoplasty techniques, which allowed to obtain a wide posterior decompression, and to preserve the range of motion of the cervical spine [106]. These techniques were widely used [107], especially in Japanese population, where a high incidence of OPLL was found [108]. One of the first techniques was described by Hirabayashi in 1987, the so-called expansive open-door laminoplasty [109]. This surgical technique aims at expansion of the cross-sectional area of the stenotic spinal canal and reconstructing the spinal canal osteoplastically. Since then, several modifications and other techniques have been described.

Despite the increased number of techniques described, expansive laminoplastics are divisible into three types: "extensive laminoplasty" (open-door laminoplasty) [109], mid-dorsal laminoplasty, and Z-plasty. There are two modifications of open-door laminoplasty with bone grafting in the opened space, namely, Itoh's modification with wiring [110–112] and Matsuzaki's modification with screws and wiring [112]. Mid-dorsal laminoplasty had Kurokawa's modification with mid-longitudinal or mid-segmental bone graft and wiring. Three types of Z-plasty may be performed: on the lamina using Hattori's method, between each lamina using Sakou's reciprocal method, and between two segmental laminae using the Chiba University technique [107, 112].

At present, unilateral open-door laminoplasty using titanium miniplates or bone graft via a unilateral approach is one of the techniques. Graft materials for laminoplasty either between the bilateral lamina or between lamina and lateral mass include a resected spinous process, or miniplates [113].

The only study comparing laminoplasty vs. laminectomy and fusion has been performed by Heller and co-workers on a matched population of 26 patients affected by cervical myelopathy [114]. In the study population, a greater percentage of patients in the laminoplasty group reported a significant subjective improvement in strength, numbness, pain, and gait. Moreover, two patients in the laminectomy plus fusion group complained of persistent bone graft site discomfort at latest follow-up. Complications were observed only in the laminectomy group, and most were related to the fusion procedure: progression of myelopathy ($n=2$), nonunion ($n=5$), broken hardware (two screws in two patients), adjacent degeneration requiring anterior surgery ($n=1$), postoperative kyphosis ($n=1$), deep infection requiring resurgery and iv antibiotics ($n=1$), and donor site pain ($n=2$), all occurred, but complication rate looks higher with respect to other reports available in literature. No complications were reported in the laminoplasty cohort, and no patient required additional surgery; nonetheless, the same authors report that the overall rate of complications observed at their institution after laminoplasty approximates 8%, a more reproducible result.

Several complications have been reported with each laminoplasty technique, and range from general complications associated with posterior cervical spine surgery, such as postoperative hematoma, spinal cord lesion, and liquoral fistulas, to others strictly related to the laminoplasty procedure itself. In the study of Satomi et al. [115], the incidence of complications after expansive open-door laminoplasty was 10.8% (22/204 patients). Complications included postoperative weakness of the upper extremities in 7.8% (16/204), closure of lamina requiring laminectomy in 1.5% (3/204), and 0.5%, respectively, for deep infection requiring removal of laminar spacers (1/204), pseudomeningocele in which a lumbar drainage has been effective in resolving symptoms (1/204), and death due to pneumonia (1/204).

Complications occurring with the laminoplasty technique are summarized in Table 10.3, and can be divided into:

- Complications related to the laminae or hinge
- Selective paralysis of the C5 nerve root
- Wrong patient selection

10.3.2.1 Complications Related to the Laminae or Hinge

Fracture of the lamina, closure of the lamina ("door") in the follow-up period, fusion of the laminae, postoperative kyphosis, and progressive loss of segmental motion in the postoperative period can all be associated with relapse or new neurological symptoms. Risk is increased in patients with postoperative inversion of cervical lordosis [116, 117]. Fracture or dislocation of the hinge of the laminoplasty in the open-door technique can lead to a migration of the bony fragment up to the spinal canal with potential injury to the spinal cord and nerve roots. This could occur intraoperatively or in the immediate postoperative period. It is then important to evaluate the stability of the hinge that can intraoperatively be reinforced with a minifragment plate, or the technique can be converted to a wide laminectomy associated with a posterior instrumented fusion. When it occurs postoperatively, fracture of a hinge or loss of fixation of the lifted lamina can also cause nerve root or spinal cord palsy, above all in case of migration of the lamina into the spinal canal. Computerized tomography allows for early diagnosis, and patient should be referred for revision surgery. Prevention requires careful preparation of the hinge side; an adequate learning curve is necessary before undertaking the procedure [118].

10.3.2.2 Selective Paralysis of the C5 Root

One of the typical complications of laminoplasty procedures is the selective paralysis of the C5 root, which could occur in 4 up to 13% of patients. This complication usually develops few days after surgery, and affects the "hinge side" nerve root. At this level, nerve palsy affects the deltoid and biceps brachii muscle, being only rarely multisegmental and pluriradicular. Several theories have been proposed to explain the potential injury mechanism of the C5 nerve root, such as a root traction injury secondary to spinal cord backshift in the spinal canal, or sagittal cervical spine imbalance in the postoperative period. None of these hypotheses has been significantly associated with this lesion; conversely, recent studies found an association with a selective myelopathy of the gray matter in the spinal cord at that level. This invalidating complication luckily tends to resolve spontaneously in 1–2 years in most cases [119].

10.3.2.3 Wrong Patient Selection

Despite the advances in surgical techniques, one of the most important factors for a successful laminoplasty remains the selection of the appropriate patient for surgery. Current indications to laminoplasty are cervical spondylotic myelopathy, OPLL disease developmental cervical spinal stenosis, better if without myelopathy. Contraindications are a preoperative alignment in kyphosis, one or two levels myelopathy due to soft or hard disk herniation (requiring an anterior direct decompression), and above all presence of preoperative definite or potential segmental instability such as in rheumatoid arthritis patients [120, 168]. Laminoplasty should not be performed in patients with neutral or kyphotic spines with kyphosis angle exceeding 13° [121]; moreover, it is often required to perform additional procedures such as foraminotomy that can be difficult depending on the chosen laminoplasty technique [101].

10.3.3 Posterior Instrumentation at the Lower Cervical Spine

(lateral mass screws, pedicle screws, laminar hooks) and wiring techniques

Presence or prevention of segmental instability or postoperative deformities are the main indications for instrumentation at the subaxial cervical spine. The main aim of the use of instrumentation in patients affected by multilevel degenerative stenosis of the cervical spine is to allow for proper deformity reduction or maintenance of alignment and rigid stabilization of the affected segment. The use of instrumentation allows for early mobilization in the postoperative period.

Several techniques have been described to obtain a stable fusion with instrumentation at the cervical spine via a posterior approach, and each is related to specific complications. It is fundamental, when planning a surgical decompression via a posterior approach, to evaluate which bony structures will be left for instrumentation anchoring. In particular, the lateral masses represent the safer and most stable fixation point of the lower cervical spine for screw-based instrumentations, introduced at first by Roy–Camille. The insertion point for the screw is the apex of the lateral mass. Screw is inserted perpendicular to the joint plane, and with 15° inclination externally to ensure adequate protection to the vertebral artery, or screw insertion can be performed at the lateral

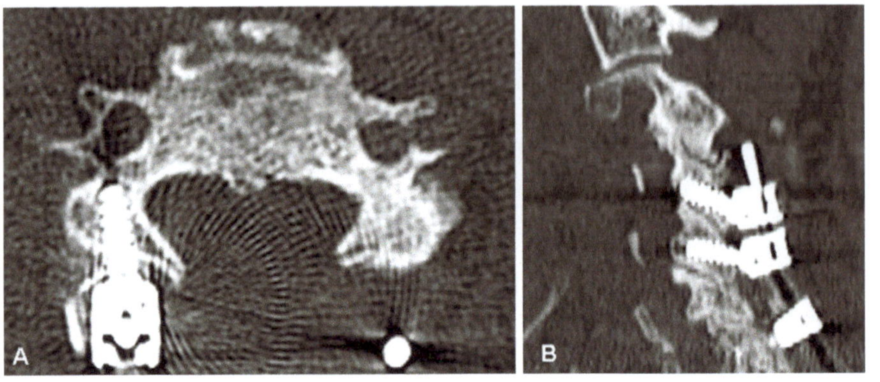

Fig. 10.22 (**a**) The screw is inserted perpendicularly to the lateral mass. A longer screw should have violated the intertrasversarium canal, with damage to the vertebral artery. (**b**) Positioning of the screws onto the articular apophyses with a 45° inclination is easier when using polyaxial screws

masses with a more inferior and medial entry point and 45° of sagittal slope (Fig. 10.22). Instrumentation alone is able to maintain long-lasting fixation, and associated fusion techniques represent a fundamental integration to this surgery. Bone grafting usually requires the use of corticocancellous bone (from local bone from laminae and spinous process removal during laminectomy procedures, iliac crest, or allograft) is posed on the lateral aspect of the lateral masses after adequate preparation of the graft bed to stimulate osteointegration. The fusion bed before stabilization is prepared by careful decortication of the lateral masses, better with the air drill, and by removal of the cartilaginous surfaces of the facet joint by the use of curets (Fig. 10.23). Some authors described the technique of cervical posterior fusion by the use of bone graft ensured to the lateral masses by means of wires, which nowadays is no more performed [122–124]. In this case, bone graft is corticocancellous harvested from the iliac crest (or from donors), whose shape nicely adapts to the physiological lordosis of the cervical spine.

Instrumentation complications (Table 10.4) can be related to:

- Wiring techniques and laminar hooks
- Lateral mass or pedicle screw fixation with plates or longitudinal bars
- Bone graft mobilization

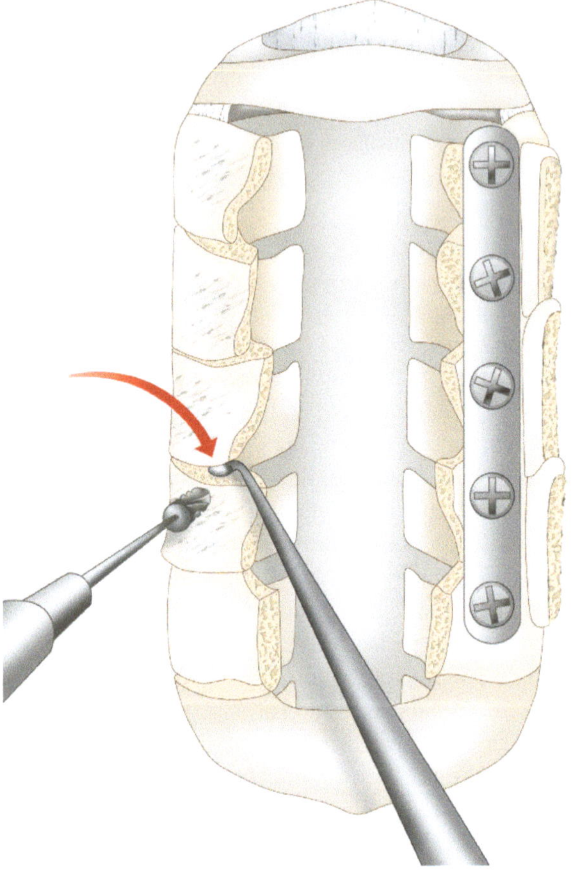

Fig. 10.23 The fusion bed before stabilization is prepared by careful decortication of the lateral masses, better with the air drill, and by removal of the cartilaginous surfaces of the facet joint by the use of curets

10.3.3.1 Wiring Techniques and Laminar Hooks

Wiring techniques have been at first described by Rogers in 1942 [125]; afterwards, other wiring techniques according to Bohlman, Robinson–Southwick have been implemented. Classically, fixation at the cervical spine was performed with wiring techniques, while instrumentation with screw-based systems was considered only for patients with incompetent posterior elements such as in fractures or after laminectomy surgery. After an extended laminectomy procedure, internal fixation is recommended to avoid postoperative destabilization of the bony structures, namely lateral

Table 10.4 Complications of posterior Instrumentation

Implant	Complication	Consequences	Tips/tricks
Lateral masses screws	Screw impingement on the nerve root	Persistent neurological pain	Often need screw repositioning
	Vertebral artery injury	Potential neurological injury and need for ligation	Purchase unicortical fixation or bicortical fixation with lateral screw direction
	Screw loosening	Potential mobilization of the implant	Screw removal and eventual repositioning of implant
Laminar hooks	Hook impingement in the spinal canal	Dural tear, spinal cord compression	Careful dissection and adequate preparation of the laminae
	Laminar fracture		
Wiring techniques	Impingement in the spinal canal	Subdural hematoma Dural tears Spinal cord lesions	Avoid passage of wirings at the level of injury
	Loss of fixation Wire Breakdown Laminar, Lateral Mass, Spinous Process Fracture	Implant failure Recurrence of deformity Need for revision surgery	Possible need to shift to screw-based instrumentation
Pedicle screws	Screw impingement on the nerve root or spinal cord	Persistent pain or neurological deficit New deficit	Often need screw repositioning
	Pedicle fracture	Loss of fixation point Potential spinal cord or root damage	Extend fusion to adjacent level Need for spinal decompression and bone fragments removal
	Vertebral Artery injury	Potential neurological injury	Difficult to control via a posterior approach Rare need for ligation
	Screw loosening	Potential implant mobilization	Screw removal and eventual repositioning of implant

masses and facet joints. These are weakened in case of wide surgical dissection that requires opening of the neuroforamen. As we already stated, in these cases, if instrumentation and proper fusion is not performed, severe iatrogenic complications such as swan neck deformity and developmental segmental instability can occur, leading to a progressive neurological deterioration (sometimes worse than the preoperative picture). At present, in most cases stabilization is performed with the use of instrumentation based on lateral mass screw fixation connected to plates or longitudinal bars, easier when using polyaxial screws.

Generally, stabilization performed by means of hooks and wiring techniques are not indicated because the laminae are removed. However, for laminectomies involving less than three levels, these techniques may be used, anchoring hooks and wires to the laminae above and below the laminectomy.

Complications mainly related to the use of wires are related to the violation of the spinal canal, and associated risk of spinal cord injury or dural tear with CSF fluid leak.

10.3.3.2 Screw-Based Systems

Lateral Mass Screw Fixation

Complications associated with the rigid fixation to the posterior cervical spine are mainly related to the direct conflict between the screw and the nerve root, lesions to the vertebral artery, screw mobilization or breakage, and fracture of the plate or bar [79]. Nonetheless, the procedure of lateral mass screw insertion is generally considered safe and effective in cervical stabilization. In a study on 143 patients in which 1,026 lateral mass screws were implanted, results and complications related to screw insertion were recorded [126]. Screws were part of plate/screw constructs (30.8%) or polyaxial screw-rod constructs. In the study, additional procedures, such as occipito-cervical fusion or anterior decompression and fusion, were performed in some cases. Postoperative CT scan showed bicortical screw fixation in 92.4%. Complications associated with the use of screws were very low. No evidence of vertebral artery injury, neural foramen, or canal violations occurred. Neurological injury after surgery occurred in one patient (0.7%), and consisted of persistent C5 radiculopathy; but authors advocated neurological injury being independent from screw insertion. Screw pullout occurred in three old patients, and occurred with plate–screws constructs. Eight screws at C7 violated the inferior facet joint. Twenty screws out of 1,026 (1.9%) breached the transverse foramen by less than 1 mm. These data support general evidence in literature regarding the low complication rates associated with lateral mass screw fixation procedure; nonetheless, meticulous adherence to surgical technique and adequate training is required to avoid complications.

Conflicts between screw and nerve root are reported in most series in less than 2% of patients [127, 128]. In the studies of Heller et al. [129, 130], a maximum 3.6% incidence of nerve root injury using the Roy–Camille and Magerl trajectories was predicted. When symptomatic, the occurrence of a conflict with the nerve root is not easy to resolve and several rules help to decrease the risk of injury. The use of a unicortical (and not bicortical) screw fixation is associated with a decreased rate of complications, without weakening of the biomechanical validity of the implant [131]. In case of postoperative radiculopathy resistant to pharmacological treatment, a radiographic analysis with multislice CT scan is mandatory (Fig. 10.24). If a conflict is suspected, surgical revision with screw repositioning is required. Screw mobilization is far more frequent in patients with plate–screw systems in which the screw is not anchored to the plate, while is rarer in more

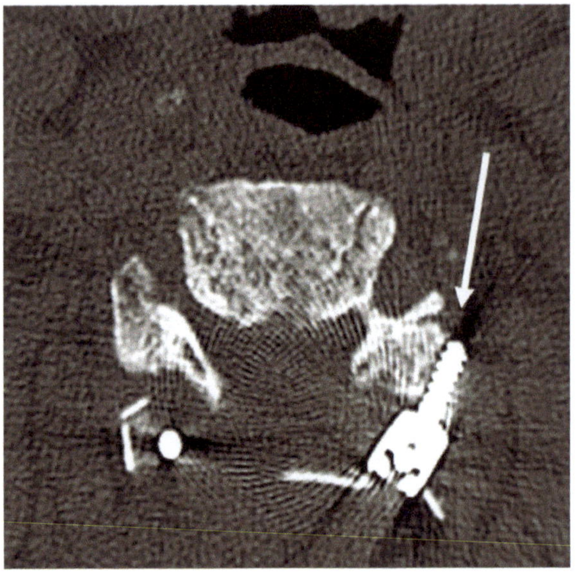

Fig. 10.24 Axial CT scan showing a malpositioned screw at the lateral mass in a patient with postoperative radiculopathy

recent instrumentations of locked plate–screw systems and bar–screw systems [131]. Screw mobilization is asymptomatic in most cases, and often requires just repeated follow-up controls up to the occurrence of fusion. Sometimes, mobilization of screws happens when the bone graft has achieved solid fusion and removal of instrumentation leaves a stable spinal segment (Fig. 10.25). Mobilization of the instrumentation can lead to the loss of surgical correction of spinal deformity, and revision surgery in these patients is

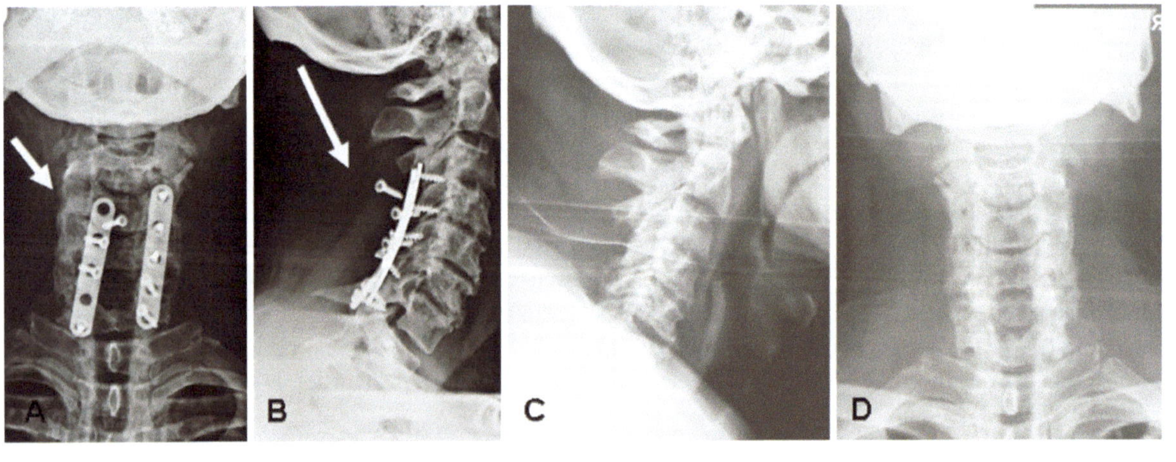

Fig. 10.25 Screw mobilization after multilevel posterior cervical plate fixation as shown by the arrows on anteroposterior and lateral radiographs in a patient undergoing stabilization with hardware without bone graft. The patient underwent revision surgery, consisting in removal of instrumentation. No instrumentation revision was performed because fusion was achieved

required. In case of symptomatic nonunion, revision of the stabilization via a posterior approach is a viable option. Alternatively, an anterior instrumented fusion procedure can be performed. Risk of lesions to the vertebral artery is very scant when proper surgical technique of screw insertion is respected. Nonetheless, in case of direct lesion during drilling, bone wax closure of the drill hole is performed and screw inserted. In the postoperative period, a cervical angiogram should be obtained for damage evaluation, and decide for further arterial exposure and ligation. In one patient with screw insertion in a lateral mass with a long drill tip and incidental lesion of the vertebral artery, anecdotally referred by the same Roy–Camille, he fixed the problem by inserting the screw in the prepared site, without postoperative sequelae.

10.3.3.3 Pedicle Screw Fixation

The diameter and morphology of pedicle screws in the cervical spine exposes to major complications of screw malpositioning, with potential direct damage to neurovascular structures as the spinal cord, nerve roots, and vertebral artery, the latter being at the highest risk for injury [132]. Much more than in the lumbar spine, placement of cervical pedicle screws requires a three-dimensional knowledge of pedicle anatomy, but significant variability of the entrance and angle of the pedicle is common. To solve the problem, computer-based navigation systems have been suggested as a guide for cervical pedicle screw insertion. For these reasons, neurovascular complications are more frequently associated with this procedure. In the study of Abumi et al. [133] on 180 patients treated with cervical pedicle screw placement, vertebral artery injury was reported in one patient, and radiculopathy in three due to excessive reduction. When compared, lateral mass screw fixation is much safer and, with proper technique, is associated with a very low rate of neurovascular damage risk even in case of screw malpositioning [134].

10.3.3.4 Bone Graft Mobilization

We observed as an incidental finding without clinical sequelae the mobilization of a corticocancellous bone graft bar posed laterally with respect to the instrumentation: this translated medially postoperatively posing between the muscular plane and the dura (Fig. 10.26). When corticocancellous bone bars are used, we routinely secure them to the lateral masses or to the metal bars with reabsorbable wires to avoid mobilization.

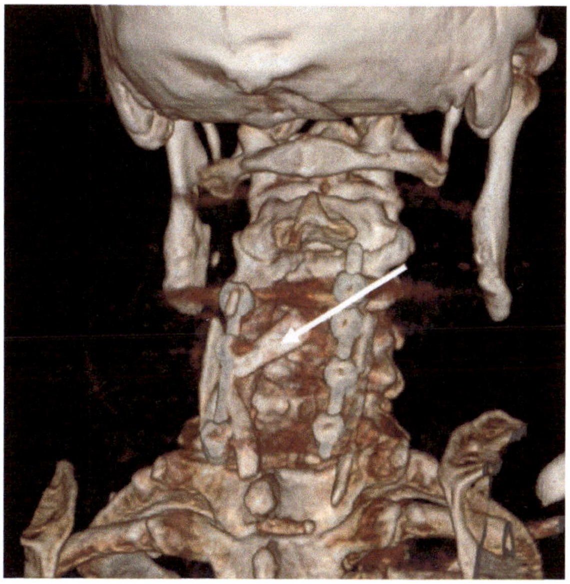

Fig. 10.26 Corticocancellous bone graft that moved medially postoperatively posing between the muscular plane and the dura

10.4 Cervical Spine Arthroplasty

10.4.1 Implants

Despite much research, only few CSA devices have been implanted in humans [135]. The "Cervical Spine Study Group" developed a nomenclature to classify the different devices on the base of different characteristics: articularity, materials, design, type of fixation, and kinematics. Artificial disks can be non-, uni-, and biarticulating. The implant can present a metal-on-metal, a metal-on-polymer (ultra–high molecular-weight polyethylene), ceramic-on-polymer, or ceramic-on-ceramic coupling. The disk is either modular or nonmodular. Artificial disks may be constrained, semi-, or unconstrained [136].

The Bryan™ Cervical Disk (Medtronic Sofamor Danek) is a metal-polyurethane device, and presents a couled motion mechanism with a "shock absorption" similar to the intact disk. The implant consists of two titanium alloy shells, covered with porous titanium, with an internal nucleus in polyurethane. The nucleus is surrounded by a flexible polyurethane membrane.

The implants with metal on polyethylene are Prodisc-C™ (Synthes, Spine), Porous Coated Motion (PCM) (Cervitech), and Active-C (Aesculap). ProDisc-C is similar to lumbar disk replacement device (Prodisc-L). It is made of two endplates of a cobalt–chromium–molybdenum alloy resurfaced in plasma-sprayed titanium, with a metal on polyethylene articular surface posed at the bottom plate. The implant presents a central metallic keel for anchoring to the vertebral body for primary stability. PCM device presents two porous Co–Cr surfaces coated with TiCaP at the endplates with a polyethylene at the bottom endplate. The implant is unconstrained [137].

The Prestige™ (Medtronic Sofamor Danek) is a coupled semi-constrained metal on metal implant [138]. It consists of an ellipsoid at the inferior component articulating with a corresponding surface on the superior component. The implant has been subjected to several design evolutions. The latest version, the PRESTIGE LP (i.e., Low Profile), presents a reduction of the anterior flange that allows a movement similar to the intact mobile spinal segment [139].

10.4.2 Clinical Results

10.4.2.1 Bryan Cervical disk

The Bryan disk is the CSA device with the greatest number of implants, with more than 2 years follow-up data already available in 2004 [140].

Goffin et al. [141] published the first clinical results of a prospective multicenter clinical trial on the Bryan for single-level degenerative disk disease, reporting interesting clinical results, but biased from low patient adhesion at follow-up (of the 97 initial patients, only 60 were followed clinically for 6 months, and 30 were available at the 1 year follow-up). In the study group, segmental range of movement (ROM) was preserved after 1 year in approximately 88% of patients. Reported complications were related to the surgical technique and to migration of the device confirmed in one patient, and suspected in another [142]. The same authors in a following study [141] reported results with longer follow-up, and the first results of double level implants. Motion preservation was comparable with reports of the first study (about 88% in the single implant and 86% in the two-level implant) at 1 year follow-up, and good clinical results were reported. More recently, newer reports on these patients showed satisfactory results in more than 90% of patients at the 2 year follow-up [143]. In the study by Pickett [144] on 14 patients followed for 2 years, implant shell endplate tended to become kyphotic at follow-up, despite the overall Cobb angle being preserved postoperatively. In another study with longer follow-up by the same author [145], an increased overall cervical ROM was observed. The author suggested the increase in ROM being secondary to redistribution and increase of motion in all the other cervical motion segments.

CSA devices have also been used in patients affected by cervical myelopathy. Duggal et al. [146] found no difference between clinical results and overall complications in patients with radiculopathy and myelopathy treated by CSA implant. In the study by LaFuente et al. [147] conversely, patients with radiculopathy undergoing CSA had better results than those with myelopathy. Sekhon [148] presented a case series of 11 patients with 15 implants. In this study, a patient affected by myelopathy who received implant of two devices presented worsening of the clinical picture associated with the development of postoperative segmental kyphosis. The same author suggested careful evaluation of patients as regards preoperative spinal deformity before device implantation.

Recently, Coric reported the results of a multicenter randomized clinical trial comparing patients affected by radiculopathy or myelopathy and undergoing either CSA or anterior interbody fusion with approximately 2 years follow-up. Results showed segmental motion preservation, with comparable clinical results between the two groups [149].

In a prospective study on 115 patients randomized to either receive a Bryan artificial disk replacement or ACDF with allograft plus plate fixation and followed for 2 years, patients in the CSA group compared favorably with ACDF in single-level surgery [84].

10.4.2.2 Prestige

Cummins designed the precursor version of this implant (Cummins/Bristol) and reported results on the treatment of disk degeneration adjacent to a previous fusion or in patients with Klippel–Feil Syndrome [138]. Many of these patients reported clinical improvement, while complications ranged from screw mobilization or breakage, subluxation of the implants, dysphagia, transient palsy (due to drilling lesion), and mobilization of the implant with subsequent revision surgery.

The Prestige implant was developed and investigated in two clinical studies in Europe on savage indications, reporting clinical and radiographic improvement at 2 years follow-up [150]. Then, a prospective randomized multicentric study on single-level degenerative disk disease was performed. Wigfield reported the results of a case control study comparing the CSA vs. spinal fusion to observe the ability to preserve adjacent segment degeneration, but no significant differences were found [150–152].

A multicentric study on 541 patients with radiculopathy from advanced single-level intervertebral disk degeneration compared the PRESTIGE ST cervical disk with anterior discectomy and fusion with a 2 year follow-up. At the end of the study, the group of patients with disk replacement reported maintenance of segmental motion at the prosthetic level, with better neurological outcome and clinical results, and above all, a lower rate of revision surgery with respect to spinal fusion [136].

10.4.2.3 Prodisc-C

One of the first clinical available reports was performed on 27 patients affected by single-level degenerative disk disease treated with this device and followed for 1 year. Patients showed good clinical results, with improvement of NDI and VAS score, and recovery of an average segmental ROM approximating 10°. In the study, no complications related to the surgical technique, use of the implant, allergic reactions, mobilizations or visceral complications related to anterior surgery were reported. Moreover, the author did not report spontaneous fusions at the operated or adjacent levels [7]. Recently, the results of the implant of Prodisc-C compared with ACDF for cervical disk degeneration with 3 years follow-up have been reported. No complications were reported as regards implant use, disk degeneration adjacent to the fused or prosthetic level, and with good clinical results were reported in both groups [153]. Bae reported the results with multilevel implants compared with single-level implants using Prodisc-C device, showing no differences in terms of clinical results between the two groups [154].

A 2 year prospective, randomized, controlled multicenter study compared Prodisc-C vs. ACDF with allograft fusion for single-level cervical disk degeneration. Revision surgeries occurred in 9 out of 106 of ACDF patients (8.5%), and in 2 out of 103 of the CSA group (1.8%); results indicated that the arthroplasty device was superior to ACDF with allograft and plating at the 24 months follow-up [155].

10.4.3 Complications and Revision Surgery

As in other surgeries, most of complications occurring during CSA are due to an error in patient selection and recruitment [141]. Therefore, appropriate selection and adherence to scientific evidence is recommended for both the patient and the surgeon.

Goffin divided complications of cervical arthroplasty surgery into five different classes [141]: wrong indications (facet joint degeneration, preoperative instability, ossification of the posterior longitudinal ligament disease, systemic diseases, myelopathy), intraoperative and immediate complications (similar to anterior discectomy and fusion procedures, malpositioning, sizing of the device, postoperative kyphosis), early postoperative complications (device migration, persisting neurological deficit), intermediate postoperative complications (subsidence, periprosthetic ankylosis and loss of motion, Myelopathy), and long-term postoperative complications (mobilization, implant failure, debris).

In the early reports on CSA implant on small samples of patients, authors reported no complications as regards either surgical approach or cervical disk implants [156]. On the other hand, from a critical review of literature on larger series, a wide range of complications related to CSA surgery was reported [157]. Also, complications are related to the anterior surgical approach, and comprehend CSF leakage, esophageal lesions, wound hematomas, representing approximately 6% of complications per operated level [141]. Despite recent reports suggesting that there is no difference in clinical results between patients affected

Table 10.5 Complications of cervical spine arthroplasty

Complication	Consequences	Tips/tricks
Prevertebral ossification	Loss of segmental motion	Postoperative NSAIDs administrationfor 2–3 weeks No postoperative bracing
Inadequate surgical decompression (nerve roots)	Neurological deficits and/or radicular pain	Sometimes requires surgical revision (even with posterior microforaminotomy)
Postoperative kyphosis	Long-term sagittal deformity and risk of adjacent segment degeneration or implant failure	Check for patients whose cervical spines are straight or kyphotic preoperatively Carefully perform intraoperative preparation of the endplate
Subsidence	Segmental kyphosis implant mobilization	Main risks are osteoporosis and inadequate preparation of the endplate Try to use devices with the largest possible footprint
Mechanical failure, inability to preserve segmental motion and implant mobilization	Loss of segmental movement Dysphagia and spinal cord compression	Revision surgery and subsequent fusion can be required
Implant of adjacent keeled prosthesis	Split sagittal fractures of thevertebral body	Avoid adjacent keeled prosthesis Bracing or posterior surgical revision and fusion can be management options
Wearing (potential complication)	Implant loosening	Revision fusion surgery can be required
Revision Surgery	Problems of loss of bone stock, fibrosis, adherences	Fusion surgery, even leaving in situ the device and performing a posterior approach Revision of implant
Wrong indications	Potential poor results and serious complications	*Carefully check for:* Facet joints degeneration Preoperative instability Systemic diseases (osteoporosis and inflammatory diseases) Previous posterior surgery Advanced age OPLL Myelopathy

by myelopathy (excluding ossification of the posterior longitudinal ligament disease patients) or radiculopathy [158], the same Goffin suggests to distinguish between radiculopathy and myelopathy, which are two distinct diseases. The potential progression of myelopathy should be tentatively interrupted by performing a fusion. In fact, in myelopathy patients, prevention of degeneration at the adjacent segment is secondary with respect to the risk of progression of the disease [141].

Other complications are specifically related to the implant of disk arthroplasty in the cervical spine (Table 10.5):

- Loss of movement following prevertebral ossification. Risk factors have been identified such as preexisting spondylosis or segmental ankylosis, and others directly related to surgical technique or to the device itself. Heller and Goffin indicated how the use of NSAIDs for 2–3 weeks in the postoperative period lessens the tendency to spontaneous ankylosis. In the analysis of lumbar spine arthroplastic surgery results, spontaneous ankylosis has been found in long-term studies in up to 60% implants (32/53) at 17 years, but such long-term results on CSA are not available to date [137].
- Neurological deficits due to the implant of a cervical prosthetic disk are rare. These are most commonly due to inadequate root decompression in the neuroforamen. In the studies on Bryan cervical disk arthroplasty, inadequate decompression has been the cause of failure in a large number of patients.
- In patients whose cervical spines are straight or kyphotic preoperatively, very often worsening of the kyphotic alignment can be observed postopera-

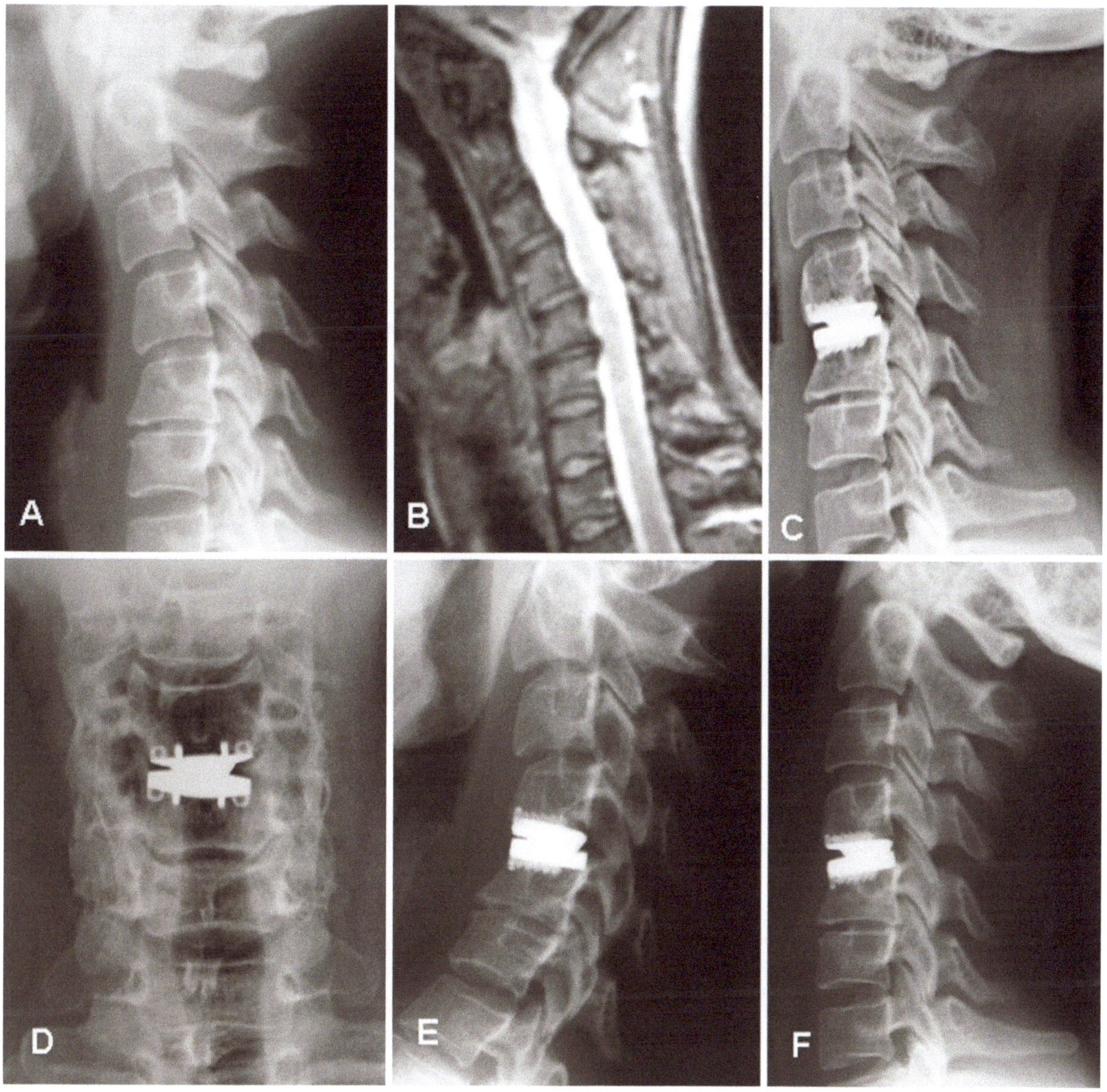

Fig. 10.27 (**a**) Patient with C5–C6 discopathy, and segmental C4–C5 kyphosis. (**b**) The MRI showed a bulging of the intervertebral disk C4–C5. (**c**) The patient underwent C4–C5 cervical disk replacement. The lateral radiograph showed persistence of the segmental kyphosis. (**d**) The anterolateral radiograph showed asymmetry in the arthroplasty positioning. Lateral radiographs in (**e**) flexion, and (**f**) extension showed not reducible segmental kyphosis

tively (Fig. 10.27) [148]. This can be related to the intraoperative preparation of the endplate that influences the angle of insertion of the device [159].

- Subsidence could occur in patients with osteoporosis, and is dependent from the relationship between the device and the endplate, the latter needing adequate preparation. One of the factors mainly influencing the risk of subsidence is the footprint of the device. This should be as large as possible to sustain axial loadings mainly on the peripheral part of the implant and not at the center of the vertebral body.
- Mechanical failure, inability to preserve segmental motion, and implant mobilization have all been reported [159].
- Wearing is the physical process secondary to the sliding of two surfaces. In patients undergoing arthroplasty, the debris can activate an inflammatory reaction due to cytokines (TNF-α1, MMP1, interleukin-1, interleukin-6, and prostaglandin E2),

and loss of surface congruency with subsequent mechanical failure [51]. From the experience in total joint replacement surgery, the inflammatory response can lead to pain, osteolysis, and formation of pannus with subsequent implant loosening [128]. No reports at present are available on the effect of osteolysis on CSA [160].

- As described in lumbar spine arthroplasty [161], the use of keeled devices can lead to split fractures of adjacent vertebral bodies also in the cervical spine [162].
- Other possible complications are strictly related to the need of revision surgery. In fact, revision surgery after implant failure or wearing already represents a major issue in joint replacement surgery and in lumbar disk replacement, and even more in the cervical spine for anatomical and biomechanical factors. Several revision strategies have been reported, but all of these require the conversion of the arthroplasty segment into fusion [136]. At present, only few reports of this procedure are reported, given the small number of removed implants, mainly due to the scant follow-up available up to date. In fact, when considering data on total joint replacement in the young patient (whose age is the same as that of patients who could benefit from a cervical prosthetic disk), implant survival rises up to 89% at 5 years for total hip replacement [163] and 93.7% at 20 years for total knee arthroplasty below the age of 45 [164]. Moreover, as observed in joint replacement, cervical implants undergo osteointegration [165], and when revision surgery is needed the surgeon has to face the problem of loss of bone stock, a critical element when further surgeries at the same level are required.

10.5 Pitfalls Related to Minimally Invasive Cervical Spine Surgery

In the field of minimally invasive techniques, it is necessary to distinguish between percutaneous techniques and minimally invasive techniques. The first are performed under fluoroscopic control with the aim to remove herniae, or posterior osteophytes, and rarely allow a decompression of the myeloradicular structures. On the other hand, minimally invasive techniques are performed with a smaller incision when compared with the standard approach, but with a constant direct visualization of the segment of the spine where surgery is performed using a magnification of the operative field. The latter have an incidence of complications similar to those reported with traditional techniques. More recently, new endoscopic techniques have been developed, with dedicated instrumentation and microscope, which allow to realize precise discectomies and foraminotomies. These systems contain one or two endoscopes, which are mounted on a tubular retractor and the specific characteristics differ on the basis of the different manufacturers. They also contain a camera head, a video integrator system that incorporates camera and xenon light source into one system, and video peripherals. Finest corrections or adjustments of the endoscope tip are possible in three-dimensional space by using the NeuroPilot steering device. For the detailed features of endoscopic techniques, the reader should refer to other publications [166]. These newly developed technologies have specific complications (Table 10.6). Endoscopic techniques, on the one hand, allow early mobilization of the patient, early discharge, and rapid return to activities of daily-living. On the other hand, because of the difficulties in obtaining accurate dissection and wide control of the operative file, one can have higher rates of complications when compared with standard procedures.

Singer [167] reported on 87 patients undergoing microsurgical or endoscopic anterior cervical foraminotomy. One patient had a relapse of radicular pain 2 days after the operation and had to undergo revision surgery. One patient had difficult arterial bleeding, which could be controlled with Tachocomb. Five patients had transient palsy of the recurrent laryngeal nerve. Poor wound healing was observed in three patients. All these minor complications resolved with no untoward effect. One patient, who had previously undergone ACD and fusion at the affected level, experienced a Horner's syndrome.

All the possible complications of the endoscopic access, the preservation of the interverbral disk (which in its lateral part has been violated), the difficult learning curve, leave these techniques to very experienced surgeons with adequate training. The benefit–cost ratio of endoscopic procedures may seem to be favorable. However, the surgeon should take into account all the possible complications, which may occur with this kind of surgery and also consider all the possible medico-legal consequences.

Table 10.6 Complications of minimally invasive techniques at the cervical spine

Technique	Complication	Consequences	Tips/tricks
Anterior foraminotomy	Neurological complications due to direct trauma or inadequate decompression	Mild radicular symptoms to serious neurological complications (hemiparesis, Horner syndrome)	Check for conflict between the sympathetic nerves and self-retractor Convert the procedure for neurological repair Often reintervention required
	Discitis	Infection and segmental fusion kyphotic angulation	Diagnostic tests plus prolonged intravenous antibiotic
	Vertebral artery injury	Risk of dissection and hemorrhage and neurological deficits, or pseudoaneurysm formation	Careful uncovertebral joint drilling Risk of violation of the transverse foramen
	Wrong-level surgery	High risks of medicolegal consequences	Fluoroscopic double check of correct level
	Spinal instability	Segmental Kyphotic Angulation	Need for revision fusion surgery or posterior fusion
	Poor patient selection	Increased risk of postoperative complications and	*Avoid patients with:* Advanced disk degeneration Stiff neck Short neck Surgery at the cervicothoracic junction
Posterior foraminotomy	Intraoperative bleeding	minimally invasive approach often difficult	Perform the surgery in sitting position. In incontrollable bleeding, convert to open surgery
	Dural tears	CSF leak	Gelfoam and lumbar drain
	Neurological damage	Root lesion and new neurological symptoms	Adequate learning curve required
	Air embolism	Related to the sitting position	Continuous Doppler monitoring required
	Poor patient selection	Persisting neurological complaints (wrong indications)	Better results with early surgery

10.5.1 Anterior Approaches

Anterior microforaminotomy was developed to preserve the disk at the intervertebral space as much as possible, while directly eliminating compression at the nerve root [168]. Dedicated instrumentations have been developed to perform this surgery [168, 169]. Anterior microforaminotomy was initially described by Verbeist [170] to address vertebral artery insufficiency and cervical radiculopathy, but it has been limited in its applications for radicular disease of the cervical spine because of concerns regarding potential vertebral artery injury [166].

A consistent risk associated with the minimally invasive techniques is failure to adequately decompress the nerve root. Adequate training with experienced surgeons should be completed before performing this procedure as a surgeon. In case of incomplete neurological decompression, patients could require reoperation.

Other potential complications related to this operation are vertebral artery injury, nerve root injury, wrong-level surgery, epidural hematoma, wound hematoma, spinal instability, and other potential complications that can occur with conventional anterior cervical approaches.

The most feared risk of the procedure is inadvertent lesion to the vertebral artery during uncovertebral joint drilling. The risk of lesion is highest at C6–C7, lateral to the uncinate process, and at the transverse foramen [168]. The C6–C7 high risk for injury is due to the vertebral artery position between the transverse process of C7 and the longus colli muscle. To avoid this injury, splitting of the longus colli muscle at the level of the C6 transverse process is recommended [168]. Then, muscle stump reflection toward the transverse process of C7 fully exposes the vertebral artery. At the uncinate process, injury to the vertebral artery can be avoided by leaving a thin layer of cortical bone during drilling of the uncovertebral joint. The bone is then carefully removed with a small curet and Kerrison punch after drilling. A deep, thin blade retractor can be placed just medial to the vertebral artery to prevent iatrogenic injury [169]. Violation of the transverse foramen during drilling is also associated with vertebral artery injury: often a brisk venous bleeding during drilling indicates violation of the foramen, and represents a lesion to the venous plexus surrounding the vertebral artery in the foramen itself. Injury to the vertebral artery can be serious, and is difficult to repair, above all when minimally invasive approaches are used [171]. In case of lesion, packing with gelfoam or bone wax can stop the bleeding; then, a postoperative angiogram should explore the possibility of dissection or pseudoaneurysm formation. Other authors advocate direct exposure of the vessel in the foramen and repair or clamping, rather than merely packing the bleeding site [16].

Postoperative instability with anterior foraminotomy is extremely rare because the resection of the disk is limited to the most lateral aspect of uncovertebral joint. Patients with asymptomatic contralateral foraminal narrowing at the same level may develop new radicular symptoms contralateral to the anterior cervical foraminotomy. These are most likely caused by some residual hypermobility after the procedure [169].

Additional complications can be related to poor patient selection. Patients with mechanical neck pain do poorly with simple nerve root decompression, and often require fusion. Junctional levels (i.e., cervicothoracic junction and levels adjacent to previous fusions) may worsen neck pain after partial removal of the uncovertebral joint, where pre-existing altered spinal biomechanics is found.

10.5.2 Posterior Approaches

Minimally invasive posterior approaches also aim at motion preservation and sparing of paravertebral muscles from stripping related to standard procedures. Muscle preservation decreases the risk of postoperative complaints such as neck pain, and the risk of kyphotic deformity caused by the extensive surgical muscle dissection if instrumentation is not performed.

An important point is selection of the patient. Patients with long-lasting symptoms and severe neurological deficits are at risk for poor results with this technique [172]. In general, the best candidates for posterior foraminotomy are younger patients with soft lateral disk herniations, and patients not eligible to anterior surgery for short neck or location of the pathology below T1 or above C3 [173]. Tomaras et al. [158] reported the results of 200 out-patients laminoforaminotomies, with 92.8% excellent or good results.

Posterior cervical foraminotomy via an endoscopic approach is associated with minimal postoperative complaints related to soft tissue dissection and risk of kyphosis. Burke et al. [174] used a rigid endoscope to perform the procedure; on the other hand, others advocated the use of an oblique view to provide a clear view of the operating, drilling, and coagulating zones. Another important issue is the type of retraction system. They reported the use of a self-retaining nasal speculum, which is held by the assistant, while other authors used tubular retractors [175].

10.5.2.1 Surgical Technique

The patient can be placed in two possible positions. In young and healthy patients, the best position is the semi-seated position, with the head fixed by a Mayfield head holder. This position minimizes blood loss; however, attention must be paid to possible air embolism and a continuous Doppler monitoring should be used intraoperatively. For older patients, the prone position is suggested.

Lateral fluoroscopy or plain radiography is used to identify the desired surgical level. The starting point is approximately 2–3 cm lateral to the midline. Adjunctive anteroposterior view allows for precise determination for the starting position in the transverse plane. A guide wire is inserted under fluoroscopic monitoring in two perpendicular planes up to the rostral lamina of the facet joint of the desired level. Then, a 2 cm incision is made around the Kirschner-wire and sequential dilators are used down to the posterior spinal elements. Some instrumentations provide a light source connected to the dilator system. Then retractors are used and visualization of the field is undertaken under magnification. The triangular space delimited by the two laminae is identified after proper coagulation. Once this exposure is complete, the foraminotomy is performed.

This approach allows for one to two level foraminotomy. Increase in visual field can require the use of an expandable retractor such as the MAXCESS minimally invasion decompressive system and instruments (NuVasive, San Diego, CA). This device uses a split radiolucent blade design for use in conventional and minimally invasive procedures. Retractor blades are posed in cranial, caudal, and transverse plane (medial or lateral).

Once the exposed facet joint is partially drilled, the nerve root is found on the base of the visual field, and must be manipulated to expose the herniated disk fragment, which lies ventrally to the nerve root. Increasing the visual field can require one to drill down part of the caudal pedicle (2–3 mm). Dorsal retraction of the nerve root allows for disk fragment exposure and removal. Before concluding the procedure, one should check both above and below the nerve root to make sure that all the disk fragments have been adequately removed.

10.5.2.2 Complications

Sitting position decreases intraoperative bleeding. In a series of patients in whom the procedure was performed in the open prone position, or minimally invasive prone or sitting position, this latter showed reduced operative times, estimated blood loss, postoperative length of stay, and pain medication requirements in the sitting position group. The sitting position significantly reduces epidural venous engorgement, and decreases blood loss. In addition, this position allows blood to flow out of the tubular retractor rather than engorge and obstacle the endoscopic view of the operative field.

In 100 patients who underwent posterior cervical minimally invasive foraminotomy, complications were reported in three patients [173]: two cases of dural puncture required no intervention other than Gelfoam, and one case of superficial wound infection. The risk of dural injury can be reduced with experience in performing this technique, since most dural tears were reported early in a surgeon's experience. Patients should be advised of this potential complication and informed that, with appropriate management, dural tears are in most cases not related to severe complications [176].

The Kirschner-wire and the dilators can be inadvertently pushed between the cervical laminae and injure the nerve root or the spinal cord; conversely, lateral displacement of the Kirschner-wire or dilators can result in nerve root or vertebral artery injury: careful adherence to surgical technique and two perpendicular fluoroscopic monitoring are required. The use of the anteroposterior fluoroscopic view also shows the reciprocal relationship of the Kirschner-wire and dilators with respect to the facet joint.

The following complications may occur from a minimally invasive posterior approach: spinal cord injury with resultant quadriplegia, tetraplegia, or paraplegia because of unwarranted attempts to remove disk fragments or osteophytes located along the anterior aspect of the spinal canal and nerve roots, or because of spinal cord compression or contusion resulting from inadvertent penetration of an instrument into the spinal canal, or because of vigorous placement of instruments into the spinal canal during laminotomy/laminectomy; reflex symptomatic dystrophy following partial nerve root or cord injury; instability as a result of a wider than necessary decompression with total facet removal (particularly in the younger patient) leakage of CSF from advertent dural laceration or faulty dural repair; formation of a postoperative meningocele due to inadvertent dural laceration or inadequate dural repair; damage to the vertebral artery as it ascends through the foramen transversarium or over the lateral portions of C1; postoperative compressive hematoma in the subdural or epidural space following closure with poor hemostasis [177].

Core Messages

- Anterior cervical surgery in the degenerative spine is usually related to a good clinical outcome, but when complications occur, they can lead to severe or life-threatening consequences.
- Incomplete decompression, eccentric or too deep drilling, kyphosis and/or loss of lordosis, and vascular and soft tissue lesions are the major determinants of complications of surgical techniques to the anterior cervical spine.
- The use of anterior instrumentation, while providing immediate stabilization, can lead to a wide range of intraoperative and postoperative complications: when these occur, implant failure, screw mobilization, plate rupture, and plate or graft mobilization can lead to often life-threatening complications and require a revision surgery.
- Cages implant should respect strict indications and careful surgical technique: preservation of

the vertebral endplate and correct localization is mandatory to avoid structural collapse and implant subsidence or dislocation.

- When approaching cervical spine diseases from a posterior route, injuries to delicate structures such as meninges, spinal cord, and nerve roots, together with vascular lesions and instrumentation-related injuries (comprehending wiring, hooks and screw based implants) are between the most encountered complications.
- Laminoplasty procedures require appropriate patient selection, and patients with preoperative neutral or kyphotic spine, myelopathy, or segmental instability should not be referred to this surgery. Closure of the lamina, fracture, or dislocation of the hinge and selective paralysis of the C5 nerve root are among the most common complications related to laminoplasty surgery.
- Most complications occurring during CSA are due to an error in patient selection and recruitment, and strict adherence to indications allows for minimization of risks. In patients with myelopathy, the potential progression of disease should be tentatively interrupted by performing a fusion, provided that the aim of prevention of adjacent disk degeneration is secondary with respect to the risk of progression of the myelopathy.
- Wrong device positioning, sizing and subsidence, postoperative kyphosis, implant migration, and persisting neurological deficits are among the most common device-related complications encountered in this surgery. Provided the short follow-up is available, it is expected for spine surgeons to face an increased number of revision surgeries.
- Complications related to anterior microforaminotomy procedures range from incomplete neurological decompression (often requiring reoperation), vertebral artery injury, nerve root injury, wrong-level surgery, epidural hematoma, wound hematoma, and spinal instability.
- In posterior cervical microendoscopic laminoforaminotomy, dural tears with CSF leaks, nerve root or spinal cord injury and, only rarely, vertebral artery lesions, can complicate the procedures.

References

1. Fountas KN, Kapsalaki EZ, Nikolakakos LG et al (2007) Anterior cervical discectomy and fusion associated complications. Spine 32:2310–2317
2. Romano PS, Campa DR, Rainwater JA (1997) Elective cervical discectomy in California: postoperative in-hospital complications and their risk factors. Spine 22:2677–2692
3. Smith GW, Robinson RA (1958) The treatment of certain cervical-spine disorders by anterior removal of the intervertebral disc and interbody fusion. J Bone Joint Surg Am 40-A:607–624
4. Cloward RB (1959) Vertebral body fusion for ruptured cervical discs. Am J Surg 98:722–727
5. Bailey RW, Badgley CE (1960) Stabilization of the cervical spine by anterior fusion. J Bone Joint Surg Am 42-A:565–594
6. Robinson RA (1964) Anterior and posterior cervical spine fusions. Clin Orthop Relat Res 35:34–62
7. Bertalanffy H, Eggert HR (1989) Complications of anterior cervical discectomy without fusion in 450 consecutive patients. Acta Neurochir (Wien) 99:41–50
8. Cloward RB (1971) Complications of anterior cervical disc operation and their treatment. Surgery 69:175–182
9. Boni M, Cherubino P, Denaro V et al (1984) Multiple subtotal somatectomy. Technique and evaluation of a series of 39 cases. Spine 9:358–362
10. Boni M, Denaro V (1982) The cervical stenosis syndrome with a review of 83 patients treated by operation. Int Orthop 6:185–195
11. Denaro E (1991) Stenosis of the cervical spine. Springer, Berlin
12. Denaro V (1994) Surgical management of cervical myelopathy according to the Boni-Denaro technique. In: Kehr P (ed) Rachis cervical dégénératif et traumatique, Cahiers d'enseignement de la SOFCOT, Vol 48. Expansion Scientifique Francaise, Paris, pp 174–182
13. Heidecke V, Rainov NG, Marx T et al (2000) Outcome in Cloward anterior fusion for degenerative cervical spinal disease. Acta Neurochir (Wien) 142:283–291
14. Lesoin F, Bouasakao N, Clarisse J et al (1985) Results of surgical treatment of radiculomyelopathy caused by cervical arthrosis based on 1000 operations. Surg Neurol 23: 350–355
15. Chozick BS, Watson P, Greenblatt SH (1994) Internal carotid artery thrombosis after cervical corpectomy. Spine 19:2230–2232
16. Golfinos JG, Dickman CA, Zabramski JM et al (1994) Repair of vertebral artery injury during anterior cervical decompression. Spine 19:2552–2556
17. Eleraky MA, Llanos C, Sonntag VK (1999) Cervical corpectomy: report of 185 cases and review of the literature. J Neurosurg 90:35–41
18. Daentzer D, Deinsberger W, Boker DK (2003) Vertebral artery complications in anterior approaches to the cervical spine: report of two cases and review of literature. Surg Neurol 59:300–309; discussion 309
19. Neo M, Fujibayashi S, Miyata M et al (2008) Vertebral artery injury during cervical spine surgery: a survey of more than 5600 operations. Spine 33:779–785
20. Hoshino Y (1987) Enlargement of spinal canal by the sagittal splitting of spinal processes. Shujutsu 41:489–497

21. Curylo LJ, Mason HC, Bohlman HH et al (2000) Tortuous course of the vertebral artery and anterior cervical decompression: a cadaveric and clinical case study. Spine 25:2860–2864
22. Jamjoom ZA (1997) Pharyngo-cutaneous fistula following anterior cervical fusion. Br J Neurosurg 11:69–74
23. Orlando ER, Caroli E, Ferrante L (2003) Management of the cervical esophagus and hypofarinx perforations complicating anterior cervical spine surgery. Spine 28:E290–E295
24. Brown JA, Havel P, Ebraheim N et al (1988) Cervical stabilization by plate and bone fusion. Spine 13:236–240
25. Goldstein LA, Thompson WR (1982) Esophageal perforations: a 15 year experience. Am J Surg 143:495–503
26. Mayr MT, Subach BR, Comey CH et al (2002) Cervical spinal stenosis: outcome after anterior corpectomy, allograft reconstruction, and instrumentation. J Neurosurg 96: 10–16
27. Zdeblick TA, Bohlman HH (1989) Cervical kyphosis and myelopathy. Treatment by anterior corpectomy and strut-grafting. J Bone Joint Surg Am 71:170–182
28. Winslow CP, Winslow TJ, Wax MK (2001) Dysphonia and dysphagia following the anterior approach to the cervical spine. Arch Otolaryngol Head Neck Surg 127:51–55
29. Hoshino Y, Kurokawa T, Nakamura K et al (1996) A report on the safety of unilateral vertebral artery ligation during cervical spine surgery. Spine 21:1454–1457
30. Leelamanit V, Limsakul C, Geater A (2002) Synchronized electrical stimulation in treating pharyngeal dysphagia. Laryngoscope 112:2204–2210
31. Logemann JA (2007) Oropharyngeal dysphagia and nutritional management. Curr Opin Clin Nutr Metab Care 10: 611–614
32. Kahraman S, Sirin S, Erdogan E et al (2007) Is dysphonia permanent or temporary after anterior cervical approach? Eur Spine J 16:2092–2095
33. Hannallah D, Lee J, Khan M et al (2008) Cerebrospinal fluid leaks following cervical spine surgery. J Bone Joint Surg Am 90:1101–1105
34. Riew KD, Cheng I, Pimenta L et al (2007) Posterior cervical spine surgery for radiculopathy. Neurosurgery 60:S57–S63
35. Kitchel SH, Eismont FJ, Green BA (1989) Closed subarachnoid drainage for management of cerebrospinal fluid leakage after an operation on the spine. J Bone Joint Surg Am 71:984–987
36. Wheeler DL, Enneking WF (2005) Allograft bone decreases in strength in vivo over time. Clin Orthop Relat Res 435:36–42
37. Boni M, Di Guglielmo L, Denaro V (1987) CT evaluation of the multiple subtotal somatectomy results. In: Kehr P, Weidner A (eds) Cervical spine. Springer, Austria, pp 124–130
38. Vadala G, Di Martino A, Tirindelli MC et al (2008) Use of autologous bone marrow cells concentrate enriched with platelet-rich fibrin on corticocancellous bone allograft for posterolateral multilevel cervical fusion. J Tissue Eng Regen Med 2:515–520
39. Jones J, Yoo J, Hart R (2006) Delayed fracture of fibular strut allograft following multilevel anterior cervical spine corpectomy and fusion. Spine 31:E595–E599
40. Hughes SS, Pringle T, Phillips F et al (2006) Settling of fibula strut grafts following multilevel anterior cervical corpectomy: a radiographic evaluation. Spine 31:1911–1915
41. Denaro V, Di Martino A, Longo UG et al (2008) Effectiveness of a mucolythic agent as a local adjuvant in revision lumbar spine surgery. Eur Spine J 17:1752–1756
42. Denaro V, Kehr P (eds) (1989) Infected cervical spine in five cases. In: Cervical spine II. Springer, Vienna, pp131–138
43. Eck JC, Humphreys SC, Lim TH et al (2002) Biomechanical study on the effect of cervical spine fusion on adjacent-level intradiscal pressure and segmental motion. Spine 27:2431–2434
44. Kaiser MG, Haid RW Jr, Subach BR et al (2002) Anterior cervical plating enhances arthrodesis after discectomy and fusion with cortical allograft. Neurosurgery 50:229–236; discussion 236–228
45. Reitman CA, Hipp JA, Nguyen L et al (2004) Changes in segmental intervertebral motion adjacent to cervical arthrodesis: a prospective study. Spine 29:E221–E226
46. Fuller DA, Kirkpatrick JS, Emery SE et al (1998) A kinematic study of the cervical spine before and after segmental arthrodesis. Spine 23:1649–1656
47. Goffin J, Geusens E, Vantomme N (2004) Long-term follow-up after interbody fusion of the cervical spine. J Spinal Disord Tech 17:79–85
48. Stabler A, Eck J, Penning R et al (2001) Cervical spine: postmortem assessment of accident injuries–comparison of radiographic, MR imaging, anatomic, and pathologic findings. Radiology 221:340–346
49. Boni M, Denaro V (1982) Surgical treatment of cervical arthrosis. Follow-up review (2–13 years) of the 1st 100 cases operated on by anterior approach. Rev Chir Orthop Reparatrice Appar Mot 68:269–280
50. Hilibrand AS, Carlson GD, Palumbo MA et al (1999) Radiculopathy and myelopathy at segments adjacent to the site of a previous anterior cervical arthrodesis. J Bone Joint Surg Am 81:519–528
51. Gonzalez O, Smith RL, Goodman SB (1996) Effect of size, concentration, surface area, and volume of polymethylmethacrylate particles on human macrophages in vitro. J Biomed Mater Res 30:463–473
52. Denaro V, Gulino G, Denaro L (1998) Sovraccarichi funzionali dopo artrodesi della colonna cervicale. Giornale Italiano di Ortopedia e Traumatologia 24:473S–479S
53. Grubb MR, Currier BL, Shih JS et al (1998) Biomechanical evaluation of anterior cervical spine stabilization. Spine 23:886–892
54. Jackson RP, McManus AC (1994) Radiographic analysis of sagittal plane alignment and balance in standing volunteers and patients with low back pain matched for age, sex, and size. A prospective controlled clinical study. Spine 19:1611–1618
55. Oda I, Cunningham BW, Buckley RA et al (1999) Does spinal kyphotic deformity influence the biomechanical characteristics of the adjacent motion segments? An in vivo animal model. Spine 24:2139–2146
56. Stokes IA, Wilder DG, Frymoyer JW et al (1981) 1980 Volvo award in clinical sciences. Assessment of patients with low-back pain by biplanar radiographic measurement of intervertebral motion. Spine 6:233–240
57. Katsuura A, Hukuda S, Saruhashi Y et al (2001) Kyphotic malalignment after anterior cervical fusion is one of the factors promoting the degenerative process in adjacent intervertebral levels. Eur Spine J 10:320–324

58. Wright IP, Eisenstein SM (2007) Anterior cervical discectomy and fusion without instrumentation. Spine 32:772–774; discussion 775
59. Samartzis D, Shen FH, Lyon C et al (2004) Does rigid instrumentation increase the fusion rate in one-level anterior cervical discectomy and fusion? Spine J 4:636–643
60. Samartzis D, Shen FH, Matthews DK et al (2003) Comparison of allograft to autograft in multilevel anterior cervical discectomy and fusion with rigid plate fixation. Spine J 3:451–459
61. Rapoff AJ, Conrad BP, Johnson WM et al (2003) Load sharing in premier and zephir anterior cervical plates. Spine 28:2648–2650; discussion 2651
62. Greene DL, Crawford NR, Chamberlain RH et al (2003) Biomechanical comparison of cervical interbody cage versus structural bone graft. Spine J 3:262–269
63. Spivak JM, Chen D, Kummer FJ (1999) The effect of locking fixation screws on the stability of anterior cervical plating. Spine 24:334–338
64. DuBois CM, Bolt PM, Todd AG et al (2007) Static versus dynamic plating for multilevel anterior cervical discectomy and fusion. Spine J 7:188–193
65. Bose B (2003) Anterior cervical arthrodesis using DOC dynamic stabilization implant for improvement in sagittal angulation and controlled settling. J Neurosurg 98:8–13
66. Epstein NE (2003) Anterior cervical dynamic ABC plating with single level corpectomy and fusion in forty-two patients. Spinal Cord 41:153–158
67. Park JB, Cho YS, Riew KD (2005) Development of adjacent-level ossification in patients with an anterior cervical plate. J Bone Joint Surg Am 87:558–563
68. Steinmetz MP, Warbel A, Whitfield M et al (2002) Preliminary experience with the DOC dynamic cervical implant for the treatment of multilevel cervical spondylosis. J Neurosurg 97:330–336
69. Epstein NE (2007) Complication avoidance in 116 dynamic-plated single-level anterior corpectomy and fusion. J Spinal Disord Tech 20:347–351
70. Ipsen BJ, Kim DH, Jenis LG et al (2007) Effect of plate position on clinical outcome after anterior cervical spine surgery. Spine J 7:637–642
71. Bose B (1998) Anterior cervical fusion using Caspar plating: analysis of results and review of the literature. Surg Neurol 49:25–31
72. Connolly PJ, Esses SI, Kostuik JP (1996) Anterior cervical fusion: outcome analysis of patients fused with and without anterior cervical plates. J Spinal Disord 9:202–206
73. Gassman J, Seligson D (1983) The anterior cervical plate. Spine 8:700–707
74. Geisler FH, Caspar W, Pitzen T et al (1998) Reoperation in patients after anterior cervical plate stabilization in degenerative disease. Spine 23:911–920
75. Heidecke V, Rainov NG, Burkert W (1998) Anterior cervical fusion with the Orion locking plate system. Spine 23:1796–1802; discussion 1803
76. Lowery GL, McDonough RF (1998) The significance of hardware failure in anterior cervical plate fixation. Patients with 2- to 7-year follow-up. Spine 23:181–186; discussion 186–187
77. Tye GW, Graham RS, Broaddus WC et al (2002) Graft subsidence after instrument-assisted anterior cervical fusion. J Neurosurg 97:186–192
78. Kostuik JP, Connolly PJ, Esses SI et al (1993) Anterior cervical plate fixation with the titanium hollow screw plate system. Spine 18:1273–1278
79. McCullen GM, Garfin SR (2000) Spine update: cervical spine internal fixation using screw and screw-plate constructs. Spine 25:643–652
80. Sahjpaul RL (2007) Esophageal perforation from anterior cervical screw migration. Surg Neurol 68:205–209; discussion 209–210
81. Panjabi MM, Isomi T, Wang JL (1999) Loosening at the screw-vertebra junction in multilevel anterior cervical plate constructs. Spine 24:2383–2388
82. Mourning D, Reitman CA, Heggeness MH et al (2007) Initial intervertebral stability after anterior cervical discectomy and fusion with plating. Spine J 7:643–646
83. Ning X, Wen Y, Xiao-Jian Y et al (2008) Anterior cervical locking plate-related complications; prevention and treatment recommendations. Int Orthop 32:649–655
84. Sasso RC, Smucker JD, Hacker RJ et al (2007) Artificial disc versus fusion: a prospective, randomized study with 2-year follow-up on 99 patients. Spine 32:2933–2940; discussion 2941–2932
85. Papadopoulos EC, Huang RC, Girardi FP et al (2006) Three-level anterior cervical discectomy and fusion with plate fixation: radiographic and clinical results. Spine 31:897–902
86. Singh K, Vaccaro AR, Kim J et al (2003) Biomechanical comparison of cervical spine reconstructive techniques after a multilevel corpectomy of the cervical spine. Spine 28:2352–2358; discussion 2358
87. Singh K, Vaccaro AR, Kim J et al (2004) Enhancement of stability following anterior cervical corpectomy: a biomechanical study. Spine 29:845–849
88. Hacker RJ, Cauthen JC, Gilbert TJ et al (2000) A prospective randomized multicenter clinical evaluation of an anterior cervical fusion cage. Spine 25:2646–2654; discussion 2655
89. Vaidya R, Carp J, Sethi A et al (2007) Complications of anterior cervical discectomy and fusion using recombinant human bone morphogenetic protein-2. Eur Spine J 16:1257–1265
90. Cauthen JC, Theis RP, Allen AT (2003) Anterior cervical fusion: a comparison of cage, dowel and dowel-plate constructs. Spine J 3:106–117; discussion 117
91. Kanayama M, Hashimoto T, Shigenobu K et al (2003) Pitfalls of anterior cervical fusion using titanium mesh and local autograft. J Spinal Disord Tech 16:513–518
92. Hasegawa K, Abe M, Washio T et al (2001) An experimental study on the interface strength between titanium mesh cage and vertebra in reference to vertebral bone mineral density. Spine 26:957–963
93. Dorai Z, Morgan H, Coimbra C (2003) Titanium cage reconstruction after cervical corpectomy. J Neurosurg 99:3–7
94. Hee HT, Majd ME, Holt RT et al (2003) Complications of multilevel cervical corpectomies and reconstruction with titanium cages and anterior plating. J Spinal Disord Tech 16:1–8; discussion 8–9
95. Das K, Couldwell WT, Sava G et al (2001) Use of cylindrical titanium mesh and locking plates in anterior cervical fusion. Technical note. J Neurosurg 94:174–178
96. Cho DY, Lee WY, Sheu PC (2004) Treatment of multilevel cervical fusion with cages. Surg Neurol 62:378–385; discussion 385–376

97. Cho DY, Liau WR, Lee WY et al (2002) Preliminary experience using a polyetheretherketone (PEEK) cage in the treatment of cervical disc disease. Neurosurgery 51:1343–1349; discussion 1349–1350
98. Vaccaro AR, Robbins MM, Madigan L et al (2004) Early findings in a pilot study of anterior cervical fusion in which bioabsorbable interbody spacers were used in the treatment of cervical degenerative disease. Neurosurg Focus 16:E7
99. Wiggins GC, Shaffrey CI (2007) Dorsal surgery for myelopathy and myeloradiculopathy. Neurosurgery 60:S71–S81
100. Rao RD, Currier BL, Albert TJ et al (2007) Degenerative cervical spondylosis: clinical syndromes, pathogenesis, and management. J Bone Joint Surg Am 89:1360–1378
101. Yonenobu K, Hosono N, Iwasaki M et al (1991) Neurologic complications of surgery for cervical compression myelopathy. Spine 16:1277–1282
102. Dai L, Ni B, Yuan W et al (1998) Radiculopathy after laminectomy for cervical compression myelopathy. J Bone Joint Surg Br 80:846–849
103. Yonenobu K, Okada K, Fuji T et al (1986) Causes of neurologic deterioration following surgical treatment of cervical myelopathy. Spine 11:818–823
104. Herkowitz HN (1988) A comparison of anterior cervical fusion, cervical laminectomy, and cervical laminoplasty for the surgical management of multiple level spondylotic radiculopathy. Spine 13:774–780
105. Komotar RJ, Mocco J, Kaiser MG (2006) Surgical management of cervical myelopathy: indications and techniques for laminectomy and fusion. Spine J 6:252S–267S
106. Kaminsky SB, Clark CR, Traynelis VC (2004) Operative treatment of cervical spondylotic myelopathy and radiculopathy. A comparison of laminectomy and laminoplasty at five year average follow-up. Iowa Orthop J 24:95–105
107. Miyazaki K, Kirita Y (1986) Extensive simultaneous multisegment laminectomy for myelopathy due to the ossification of the posterior longitudinal ligament in the cervical region. Spine 11:531–542
108. Mizuno J, Nakagawa H (2006) Ossified posterior longitudinal ligament: management strategies and outcomes. Spine J 6:282S–288S
109. Hirabayashi K, Watanabe K, Wakano K et al (1983) Expansive open-door laminoplasty for cervical spinal stenotic myelopathy. Spine 8:693–699
110. Itoh T (1986) Clinical studies on the significance of en bloc laminoplasty for cervical compressive myelopathy. Nippon Seikeigeka Gakkai Zasshi 60:1109–1123
111. Itoh T, Tsuji H (1985) Technical improvements and results of laminoplasty for compressive myelopathy in the cervical spine. Spine 10:729–736
112. Tomita K, Nomura S, Umeda S et al (1988) Cervical laminoplasty to enlarge the spinal canal in multilevel ossification of the posterior longitudinal ligament with myelopathy. Arch Orthop Trauma Surg 107:148–153
113. O'Brien MF, Peterson D, Casey AT et al (1996) A novel technique for laminoplasty augmentation of spinal canal area using titanium miniplate stabilization. A computerized morphometric analysis. Spine 21:474–483; discussion 484
114. Heller JG, Edwards CC II, Murakami H et al (2001) Laminoplasty versus laminectomy and fusion for multilevel cervical myelopathy: an independent matched cohort analysis. Spine 26:1330–1336
115. Satomi K, Ogawa J, Ishii Y et al (2001) Short-term complications and long-term results of expansive open-door laminoplasty for cervical stenotic myelopathy. Spine J 1: 26–30
116. Maeda T, Arizono T, Saito T et al (2002) Cervical alignment, range of motion, and instability after cervical laminoplasty. Clin Orthop Relat Res 401:132–138
117. Ratliff JK, Cooper PR (2003) Cervical laminoplasty: a critical review. J Neurosurg 98:230–238
118. Yonenobu K, Oda T (2003) Posterior approach to the degenerative cervical spine. Eur Spine J 12(Suppl 2): S195–S201
119. Sakaura H, Hosono N, Mukai Y et al (2003) C5 palsy after decompression surgery for cervical myelopathy: review of the literature. Spine 28:2447–2451
120. Mukai Y, Hosono N, Sakaura H et al (2004) Laminoplasty for cervical myelopathy caused by subaxial lesions in rheumatoid arthritis. J Neurosurg 100:7–12
121. Suda K, Abumi K, Ito M et al (2003) Local kyphosis reduces surgical outcomes of expansive open-door laminoplasty for cervical spondylotic myelopathy. Spine 28: 1258–1262
122. Callahan RA, Johnson RM, Margolis RN et al (1977) Cervical facet fusion for control of instability following laminectomy. J Bone Joint Surg Am 59:991–1002
123. Sim FH, Svien HJ, Bickel WH et al (1974) Swan-neck deformity following extensive cervical laminectomy. A review of twenty-one cases. J Bone Joint Surg Am 56:564–580
124. Stauffer ES, Kelly EG (1977) Fracture-dislocations of the cervical spine. Instability and recurrent deformity following treatment by anterior interbody fusion. J Bone Joint Surg Am 59:45–48
125. Rogers W (1942) Treatment of fractures and dislocations of the cervical spine. J Bone Joint Surg Am 24:145–248
126. Sekhon LH (2005) Posterior cervical lateral mass screw fixation: analysis of 1026 consecutive screws in 143 patients. J Spinal Disord Tech 18:297–303
127. Deen HG, Birch BD, Wharen RE et al (2003) Lateral mass screw-rod fixation of the cervical spine: a prospective clinical series with 1-year follow-up. Spine J 3:489–495
128. Goodman SB, Huie P, Song Y et al (1998) Cellular profile and cytokine production at prosthetic interfaces. Study of tissues retrieved from revised hip and knee replacements. J Bone Joint Surg Br 80:531–539
129. Heller JG, Carlson GD, Abitbol JJ et al (1991) Anatomic comparison of the Roy-Camille and Magerl techniques for screw placement in the lower cervical spine. Spine 16:S552–S557
130. Heller JG, Silcox DH III, Sutterlin CE 3rd (1995) Complications of posterior cervical plating. Spine 20:2442–2448
131. Ebraheim NA, Rupp RE, Savolaine ER et al (1995) Posterior plating of the cervical spine. J Spinal Disord 8: 111–115
132. Ludwig SC, Kramer DL, Vaccaro AR et al (1999) Transpedicle screw fixation of the cervical spine. Clin Orthop Relat Res 359:77–88
133. Abumi K, Shono Y, Ito M et al (2000) Complications of pedicle screw fixation in reconstructive surgery of the cervical spine. Spine 25:962–969

134. Wertheim SB, Bohlman HH (1987) Occipitocervical fusion. Indications, technique, and long-term results in thirteen patients. J Bone Joint Surg Am 69:833–836
135. Denaro V, Papalia R, Denaro L et al (2009) Cervical spinal disc replacement. J Bone Joint Surg Br 91:713–719
136. Mummaneni PV, Burkus JK, Haid RW et al (2007) Clinical and radiographic analysis of cervical disc arthroplasty compared with allograft fusion: a randomized controlled clinical trial. J Neurosurg Spine 6:198–209
137. Putzier M, Funk JF, Schneider SV et al (2006) Charite total disc replacement–clinical and radiographical results after an average follow-up of 17 years. Eur Spine J 15:183–195
138. Cummins BH, Robertson JT, Gill SS (1998) Surgical experience with an implanted artificial cervical joint. J Neurosurg 88:943–948
139. Mummaneni PV, Haid RW (2004) The future in the care of the cervical spine: interbody fusion and arthroplasty. Invited submission from the joint section meeting on disorders of the spine and peripheral nerves, March 2004. J Neurosurg Spine 1:155–159
140. Boden SD, Balderston RA, Heller JG et al (2004) An AOA critical issue. Disc replacements: this time will we really cure low-back and neck pain? J Bone Joint Surg Am 86-A:411–422
141. Goffin J, Van Calenbergh F, van Loon J et al (2003) Intermediate follow-up after treatment of degenerative disc disease with the Bryan cervical disc prosthesis: single-level and bi-level. Spine 28:2673–2678
142. Goffin J, Casey A, Kehr P (2002) Preliminary clinical experience with the Bryan cervical disc prosthesis. Neurosurgery 51:840–845
143. Anderson PA, Rouleau JP, Bryan VE et al (2003) Wear analysis of the Bryan cervical disc prosthesis. Spine 28:S186–S194
144. Pickett GE, Mitsis DK, Sekhon LH et al (2004) Effects of a cervical disc prosthesis on segmental and cervical spine alignment. Neurosurg Focus 17:E5
145. Pickett GE, Rouleau JP, Duggal N (2005) Kinematic analysis of the cervical spine following implantation of an artificial cervical disc. Spine 30:1949–1954
146. Duggal N, Pickett GE, Mitsis DK et al (2004) Early clinical and biomechanical results following cervical arthroplasty. Neurosurg Focus 17:E9
147. Lafuente J, Casey AT, Petzold A et al (2005) The Bryan cervical disc prosthesis as an alternative to arthrodesis in the treatment of cervical spondylosis: 46 consecutive cases. J Bone Joint Surg Br 87:508–512
148. Sekhon LH (2004) Cervical arthroplasty in the management of spondylotic myelopathy: 18-month results. Neurosurg Focus 17:E8
149. Coric D, Finger F, Boltes P (2006) Prospective randomized controlled study of the Bryan cervical disc: early clinical results from a single investigational site. J Neurosurg Spine 4:31–35
150. Wigfield CC, Gill SS, Nelson RJ et al (2002) The new Frenchay artificial cervical joint: results from a two-year pilot study. Spine 27:2446–2452
151. Traynelis VC (2002) Spinal arthroplasty. Neurosurg Focus 13:E10
152. Wigfield C, Gill S, Nelson R et al (2002) Influence of an artificial cervical joint compared with fusion on adjacent-level motion in the treatment of degenerative cervical disc disease. J Neurosurg 96:17–21
153. Delamarter RB (2006) Cervical disc replacement: over 3 year prospective randomized clinical outcomes and range of motion follow-up with the prodisc-C prosthesis (Paper #16). Presented at the 34th Cervical Spine Research Society, The Breakers – Palm Beach, FL
154. Bae HW (2006) 1 versus 2 versus 3 -level cervical artificial disc replacements: a prospective report of clinical outcomes with the prodisc-C (paper #19). Presented at the 34th Cervical Spine Research Society, The Breakers – Palm Beach, FL
155. Murrey D, Janssen M, Delamarter R et al (2009) Results of the prospective, randomized, controlled multicenter Food and Drug Administration investigational device exemption study of the ProDisc-C total disc replacement versus anterior discectomy and fusion for the treatment of 1-level symptomatic cervical disc disease. Spine J 9:275–286
156. Bertagnoli R, Zigler J, Karg A et al (2005) Complications and strategies for revision surgery in total disc replacement. Orthop Clin North Am 36:389–395
157. Bazaz R, Lee MJ, Yoo JU (2002) Incidence of dysphagia after anterior cervical spine surgery: a prospective study. Spine 27:2453–2458
158. Tomaras CR, Blacklock JB, Parker WD et al (1997) Outpatient surgical treatment of cervical radiculopathy. J Neurosurg 87:41–43
159. Pickett GE, Sekhon LH, Sears WR et al (2006) Complications with cervical arthroplasty. J Neurosurg Spine 4:98–105
160. Cunningham BW, Orbegoso CM, Dmitriev AE et al (2002) The effect of titanium particulate on development and maintenance of a posterolateral spinal arthrodesis: an in vivo rabbit model. Spine 27:1971–1981
161. Bertagnoli R, Duggal N, Pickett GE et al (2005) Cervical total disc replacement, part two: clinical results. Orthop Clin North Am 36:355–362
162. Datta JC, Janssen ME, Beckham R et al (2007) Sagittal split fractures in multilevel cervical arthroplasty using a keeled prosthesis. J Spinal Disord Tech 20:89–92
163. Rubinstein RA Jr, Beals RK (1993) The results of treatment of posttraumatic avascular necrosis of the femoral head in young adults: report of 31 patients. Contemp Orthop 27:527–532
164. Crowder AR, Duffy GP, Trousdale RT (2005) Long-term results of total knee arthroplasty in young patients with rheumatoid arthritis. J Arthroplasty 20:12–16
165. Jensen WK, Anderson PA, Nel L et al (2005) Bone ingrowth in retrieved Bryan cervical disc prostheses. Spine 30:2497–2502
166. Jho HD, Kim MH, Kim WK (2002) Anterior cervical microforaminotomy for spondylotic cervical myelopathy: part 2. Neurosurgery 51:S54–S59
167. Saringer WF (2006) Anterior cervical foraminotomy (microsurgical and endoscopic). In: Mayer HM (ed) Minimally invasive spine surgery. Springer, Berlin, pp 82–91
168. Jho HD (1996) Microsurgical anterior cervical foraminotomy for radiculopathy: a new approach to cervical disc herniation. J Neurosurg 84:155–160
169. Johnson JP, Filler AG, McBride DQ et al (2000) Anterior cervical foraminotomy for unilateral radicular disease. Spine 25:905–909
170. Verbiest H (1968) A lateral approach to the cervical spine: technique and indications. J Neurosurg 28:191–203

171. Cosgrove GR, Theron J (1987) Vertebral arteriovenous fistula following anterior cervical spine surgery. Report of two cases. J Neurosurg 66:297–299
172. Woertgen C, Holzschuh M, Rothoerl RD et al (1997) Prognostic factors of posterior cervical disc surgery: a prospective, consecutive study of 54 patients. Neurosurgery 40:724–728; discussion 728–729
173. Adamson TE (2001) Microendoscopic posterior cervical laminoforaminotomy for unilateral radiculopathy: results of a new technique in 100 cases. J Neurosurg 95:51–57
174. Burke TG, Caputy A (2000) Microendoscopic posterior cervical foraminotomy: a cadaveric model and clinical application for cervical radiculopathy. J Neurosurg 93:126–129
175. Roh SW, Kim DH, Cardoso AC et al (2000) Endoscopic foraminotomy using MED system in cadaveric specimens. Spine 25:260–264
176. Wang JC, Bohlman HH, Riew KD (1998) Dural tears secondary to operations on the lumbar spine. Management and results after a two-year-minimum follow-up of eighty-eight patients. J Bone Joint Surg Am 80:1728–1732
177. Young PH, Young JP, Young JC (2006) Microsurgical posterior approaches to the cervical spine. In: Mayer HM (ed) Minimally invasive spine surgery. Springer, Berlin, pp 107–117

Cervical Spine Bone Tumor Surgery

11

Luca Denaro, Alberto Di Martino, Umile Giuseppe Longo, and Vincenzo Denaro

Contents

11.1 General Considerations in Cervical Spine Tumor Surgery

The management of tumors of the cervical spine has undergone considerable advances in the last few years. Together with the advances of chemotherapy, radiotherapy, and immunotherapy, new techniques and combined surgical approaches have been developed. New generations of instrumentation are available to decompress, reconstruct, and stabilize the cervical spine, contributing to improve the prognosis of patients [2, 5, 9, 12, 15, 18]. The reoperation rate for local relapse and failure of surgery is directly related to the patient survival [41]. Nowadays, diagnostic imaging studies (volumetric spiral CT, MRI, angio-MRI) are a useful tool to stage the extent and location of the tumor. Combined management strategies also allow for a better prognosis in several patients. A biopsy should be performed in patients with suspected spinal tumor to establish a definitive histological diagnosis, unless a primary tumor is known or local tumor relapse is suspected [8, 14]. Percutaneous needle radiographic or CT-guided tumor biopsy in most instances will allow one to formulate a preoperative diagnosis. The needle biopsy can be easily performed through a transoral approach under local anesthesia when lesions are located in the anterior portion of C1 and C2, and the antero-superior portion of C3. An anterolateral presternocleidomastoid approach is indicated for lesions located in the anterior portion of the vertebrae C3–C7. The biopsy is performed after the identification of the neurovascular bundle (the vagus nerve, the common carotid artery, and the internal jugular vein), which is protected during the procedure under the fingers of the surgeon. A posterior approach allows to perform

L. Denaro (✉)
Department of Neuroscience, University of Padua, Via Giustiniani 5, 35128 Padua, Italy
e-mail: lucadenaro@hotmail.com

L. Denaro et al. (eds.), *Pitfalls in Cervical Spine Surgery*,
DOI: 10.1007/978-3-540-85019-9_11, © Springer-Verlag Berlin Heidelberg 2010

biopsies on the posterior portion of the vertebrae. Biopsy can be performed during surgery in patients in whom a fine needle biopsy does not allow to formulate a diagnosis, or in patients with a structural collapse and neurological damage requiring immediate surgical decompression and stabilization [25].

Surgery in the treatment of tumors of cervical spine (either primary or metastatic) is not easy to standardize [11]. The experience of the surgeon in dealing with these patients is paramount, because it is often difficult to generalize or standardize the type of surgical procedures for tumor removal. In most cases, after tumor removal, the surgeon must stabilize the operated segments. Bone grafting procedures and instrumentation are used to restore spinal stability. The surgeon will need to adapt the surgical procedure to the individual requirements. Therefore, the surgical approach, type of fixation, and management must be specifically adapted to the single patient. In patients with neurological deficits, surgery represents the best option to maximize the chances of recovery [21, 27, 29, 32, 38].

Corticosteroid therapy is the first-line therapy in most of these patients, before the definitive surgical management. Both high- and low-dose corticosteroid regimens have been used [33], but, to date, the exact dose has not been proven [37]. Common sense suggests administration of high dosage corticosteroid therapy in nonambulating patients, while dose can be decreased in patients with incomplete neurological lesion to balance drug-related complications [7, 37].

Adjuvant and neoadjuvant therapy (including chemotherapy, radiation therapy, and hormone therapy) can be administered before or after surgery in relation to the type of tumor.

In a trial on 121 patients with spinal metastasis and spinal cord compression, patients were randomized to surgery followed by radiotherapy ($n=50$) or radiotherapy alone ($n=51$) [28]. Surgical treatment resulted in significant better maintenance of bladder continence, muscle strength, functional ability, and survival when compared with patients receiving radiotherapy alone. In particular, 84% (42/50) patients were able to walk after surgery when compared with 57% (29/51) in the radiotherapy group. Direct surgery plus postoperative radiotherapy is superior to radiotherapy alone for patients with spinal cord compression from metastatic cancer.

11.1.1 Indications

Cervical spinal tumor surgery may be associated with a high degree of difficulty in reaching and removing the tumor, and may require combined approaches. In the cervical spine, the surgeon has to be constantly aware of the various vascular and neurological structures encountered during the approach. A tumor at this level of the spine, even if completely benign histologically may produce compression of the structures within the canal, and require complete removal followed by segmental stabilization. Therefore, even benign tumors may have an overall good prognosis quoad vitam, but poor quoad valetudinem.

En bloc resection of the mass is required for both primitive and secondary tumors with very good prognosis, although this can result in more aggressive surgery [36]. As already stated, the complete excision of the tumor may require more complex surgery and combined surgical approaches, and may determine complications on the neighboring vascular, myeloradicular, and visceral structures [3, 23, 35].

In general, surgical treatment of cervical spine tumors may involve two contrasting surgical strategies: palliative surgery (with neural decompression and spine stabilization) or curative surgery (consisting of en bloc tumor radical resection and stabilization).

Palliative surgery aims at the decrease of local pain, segmental stabilization, and prevention of further neurological damage. It is the treatment of choice in most patients with spinal metastases, especially those with tumors with worst prognosis (i.e., lung cancer, visceral or brain metastasis) and pathologic fracture.

As a general rule, patients with osteoblastic metastatic tumors at the cervical spine, in the absence of neurological deficits can be treated conservatively (orthoses, chemotherapy, radiation therapy). When osteolythic lesions occur, surgery can prevent acute or worsening neurological deficits from vertebral pathologic fractures [14]. Metastatic tumor excision followed by reconstruction of the bone loss and segmental stabilization is a good therapeutic option (Fig. 11.1) [8, 31].

Bone loss can be filled with either allograft, titanium or carbonium fiber mesh cages filled with homologous bone graft or, rarely, with acrylic cement. Titanium plates and screws anteriorly, and plates or longitudinal bars and lateral mass screws posteriorly can be used. Often, circumferential fusion via a

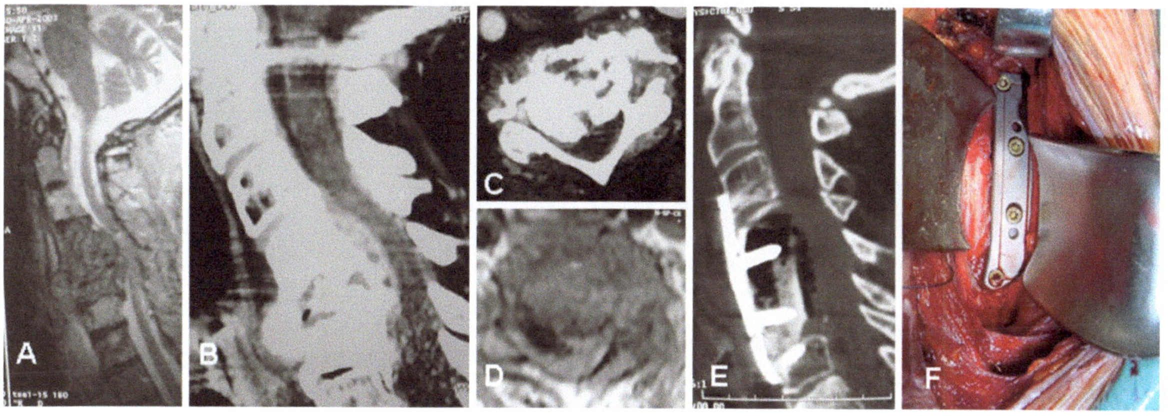

Fig. 11.1 Colon tumor metastatic to the cervical spine. Preoperative (**a**), (**b**) CT scan, and (**c**, **d**) MRI showing C4–C6 vertebral involvement with tumor tissue compressing the spinal cord and also extending anteriorly. (**e**, **f**) Surgery consisted in C3–C7 anterior decompression and fusion with bone allograft and plate fixation. Two days postoperatively, the patient had a vascular stress of the spinal cord after the wide decompression recovering functions in 15 days

combined anterior and posterior approach is required to restore the segment stability [39]. In patients with poor prognosis, conservative treatment should be considered first. In selected patients with poor prognosis but good general status, we described a type of stabilization surgery with the aim to realize an "internal bracing," consisting of a system of metal wiring stabilized with acrylic cement. The main advantages of this surgery are the reduced surgical times and the low perioperative morbidity [13].

11.2 Complications

Complications occurring in these patients are mainly surgical lesions: (1) vascular lesions (carotid artery, vertebral artery, jugular vein), (2) lesions of visceral structures (pharynx, esophagus), (3) neurological lesions both in the neck (vagus nerve, phrenic nerve, recurrent laryngeal nerves, cervical plexus, and brachial plexus, mainly to the primary trunks near to the intervertebral foramina), and in the spinal cord canal (lesions to the spinal cord, nerve roots, and dura mater), (4) related to the use of devices (breakage, mobilization, and migration), (5) related to bone graft (rupture, collapse, and resorbtion) (See Chap. 17), (6) general complications (pulmonary, urological, cardiocirculatory, deep vein thrombosis.) (See Chap. 1), and (7) infections. (Table 11.1).

Moreover, several factors can increase the risk of intra or postoperative complications, including prolonged chemiotherapy, radiotherapy in the week before surgery, malnutrition, and chronic use of steroids [16, 26]. Often, patients with tumors (especially with metastases) of the cervical spine are in poor general status.

In the literature, several complications are reported in these patients, despite relatively few papers are available on the topic.

On a population of 76 patients with spinal metastases [39], involvement of the cervical spine occurred in 7% of patients. The overall complication rate was 19% (not separated between spinal levels), and included neurological deterioration ($n=4$), mortality ($n=2$), massive intraoperative bleeding ($n=2$), dislodgement of titanium mesh cage ($n=2$), deep wound healing defect ($n=2$), deep vein thrombosis ($n=2$), liquoral fistula ($n=1$), iatrogenic spinal compression ($n=1$), inadequate stabilization ($n=1$), paravertebral hematoma ($n=1$), renal failure ($n=1$), and stress ulcer bleeding ($n=1$).

In the study of Wise et al. [41], complications occurred in 25% (20/80) of patients. Postoperative wound infection and urinary tract infections were between the most common complications. Five of 80 (5.7%) patients died for causes related to surgical complications in the postoperative period. Preoperative neurological status was also related to the occurrence of complications, with a higher Frankel grade associated with an increased risk of complications.

Table 11.1 Complications of tumors surgery: rifare in base allelenco del PROF

Injury site	Consequences	Tips/tricks
Vertebral artery (C1–C2 or C3–C7)	Hemorrhage Neurological deficits midolari ed encefalici	Perform preop arteriography and embolization If need to perform en bloc excision with the tumor, need to ligate above and below
Neck soft tissues (pharinx esophageal) lesions	Esophageal fistula due to esophageal wall necrosis or tears for incaute dissection use self-retractors Mediastinitis and sepsis	Methylene blue swallowing for an early diagnosis Position a nasogastric tube after surgical repair Wide spectrum antibiotics
Dura, spinal cord,and nerve roots (plus neoplastic aracnoiditis)	Mechanical or vascular neurological lesions Paradoxical infarction of the spinal cord CSF fluid leak	Careful decompression Start corticosteroid therapy at decompression Repair of dural tears plus eventual CSF lumbar drain
Vertebral body collapse and failure of bone gap reconstruction and instrumentation	Subsequent segmental kyphosis and structural loss Graft collapse or mobilization	Often due to incomplete surgery Fixation of bone graft or meshnotin distraction Inadequate postoperative immobilization
Intra and extradural hematomas	Progressive neurological deficits	Coagulative screening preoperatively Anticothrombotic drugs after surgery Check for hepatic metastases Careful intraop hemostasis *Rapidly evolving deficits:*immediate surgical revision *Slow progressive deficits:*angyoMRI, arteriography, and eventual embolization before surgical revision

In a multicentric study of 223 patients operated for spinal metastasis [19], the overall surgical perioperative mortality rate was 5.8%, and both minor and major morbidity occurred in 21% of patients. Implant failure occurred in 2.2% and wound complications developed in 4% of patients. Medical complications such as pneumonia, deep vein thrombosis, and urinary tract infection occurred in 7.6%, and surgical complications including cerebrospinal fluid leakage, thoracic duct injury, and dysphagia occurred in 7.2%. Complications occurred mainly in patients undergoing less aggressive surgery, provided that these patients were generally in worse general status. Surgery was effective in improving the quality of life by enabling better pain control, helping patients to regain or maintain mobility, and improving sphincter control.

11.2.1 Vascular Complications

The most important vascular complications involve the vertebral artery, which may be damaged during the excision of the tumor as a consequence of its close relationship with the vertebral body. Lesions of these structures may occur in patients with a large extravertebral extension of the tumor and direct invasion of the vessels. Lesions can also occur during the initial stages of surgery (See Chap. 7) for the inappropriate use of retractors, or when a large surgical exposition is required, especially to the jugular vein. This is the reason why the jugular vein is excised en bloc with the sternocleidomastoid muscle in the presence of proliferative lymph node lesions given the difficult dissection.

Particular attention must be reserved to the thyroid vessels and to the thyreolinguofacial trunk during the approaches to the high cervical spine.

11.2.1.1 Vertebral Artery Lesions

Preoperative arteriography and embolization are mandatory. Arteriography allows to evaluate the vascularization and invasivity of the tumor and the boundaries of the mass in relation to the neighboring anatomical structures. All these preoperative data allow the surgeon to plan a detailed preoperative surgical strategy. Preoperative embolization is particularly helpful in patients in whom an en bloc resection is planned, as it produces a relatively bloodless field from which the tumor can be completely excised. Embolization allows to better locate the surgical cleavage plane [4]. Vertebral artery injury is encountered mainly when resecting C1–C2 lesions. At that level, the vertebral artery is particularly vulnerable posteriorly where, out of the traverse foramen of C2, it curves to reach the posterior arch of C1 in the foramen magnum [1, 6].

Preoperative arteriography can show a vertebral artery occluded by a thrombus. In these instances, when an en bloc removal of the tumor mass is needed, the surgeon must perform an artery ligation cephalad and caudal to the tumor mass, attempting to preserve the neighboring neurological structures. Once the tumor mass is gently separated from the vertebral plane, preserving the paravertebral sympathetic chain (risk of Claude-Bernard-Horner syndrome), the anterior portion of the transverse foramen can be opened and vertebral artery ligation performed, even with metallic clips [24].

In our experience, in locally aggressive tumors (Enneking stage III) such as some osteoblastomas, the tumor mass after embolization had a cleavage on the vertebral artery, and was removed without vessel lesion or need for ligation [10].

Vascular lesions involving the carotid artery and the jugular vein may occur both during the surgical approaches, and as a consequence of extraskeletal tumors, which may dislocate and invade the anatomical structures of the neck, with alteration of their normal anatomical relationship.

11.2.2 Lesions of the Deep Structures of the Neck

Lesions to soft tissues mainly involve the pharynx and esophagus. As reported in the surgical approach section, these lesions mainly result from the mechanical action (excessive distraction and compression) of the surgical retractors (mainly self-retractors) that cause local ischemia with necrosis of the wall, formation of scar tissue and eventual fistulization after 1 or 2 weeks from surgery [20]. These lesions are more frequent in tumor surgery because longer surgical times are usually required. We prefer to use manual retraction during anterior surgery to periodically decrease the traction of the retraction blades [8]. Lesions of the deep structures of the neck can also occur during surgical dissection of the tumor mass, during dissection of tumoral masses with extraskeletal development and visceral involvement, and such lesions should be evaluated intraoperatively and immediately repaired [17]. In the upper surgical approach, this event is far less frequent because the pharyngeal wall is less adherent to the deep planes and much more mobile when compared with the distal portion. In the occurrence of necrosis of the esophageal wall, usually diagnosis is performed when the esophageal fistula is already formed, a few days or 1–2 weeks after surgery. In the first few days, if the patient is still fasting, fistulization shows the loss of saliva from the wound, which is often thought to be a septic drainage. The diagnosis is then performed by making the patient swallow methylene blue, which will exit the wound after few minutes (see Chap. 7). This is extremely dramatic, and requires application of a nasogastric tube after surgical repair, starving, and administration of drugs to block saliva production (i.e., atropine, etc.).

11.2.3 Neurological Complications

11.2.3.1 Myeloradicular Lesions and Liquoral Fistulas

Lesions to neural structures can occur when attempting wide excision of destructive tumors invading the spinal canal and neural structures. The slow invasion of the peridural space leads to the occurrence of neoplastic pachymeningitis (Fig. 11.2) over the dura mater and nerve roots, a difficult surgical cleavage mainly when the posterior longitudinal ligament is also infiltrated. Neurological lesions can be due in the majority of patients to direct damage to the spinal cord and to the nerve roots during the excision of the mass, and less frequently to medullar ischemia caused by traumatic obliteration, or in the attempt to perform hemostasis of the blood vessels distributing to the spinal cord (radicular arteries).

Moreover, decompression of the ischemic spinal cord can lead to paradoxical infarction of the medulla (Fig. 11.3) [40]. Dural tears are difficult to repair,

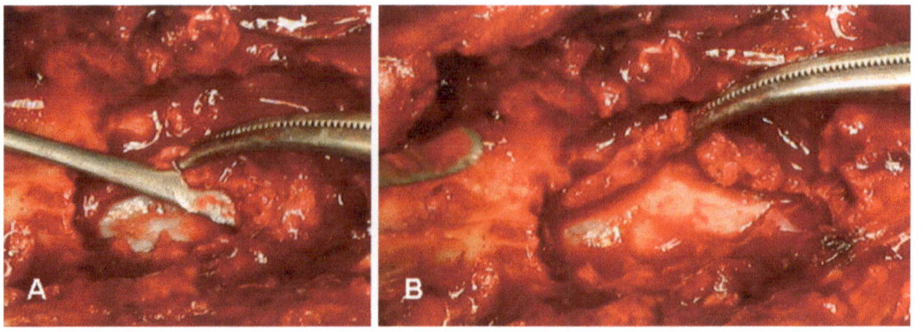

Fig. 11.2 (**a**, **b**) Intraoperative findings of neoplastic pachymeningitis enveloping the dura mater and nerve roots. Decompression maneuver is associated with increased risk of dural tears and spinal cord lesions. Only the removal of the neoplastic pachymeningitis can guarantee an adequate decompression after laminectomy. The use of MESNA facilitated the chemical dissection of the surgical planes

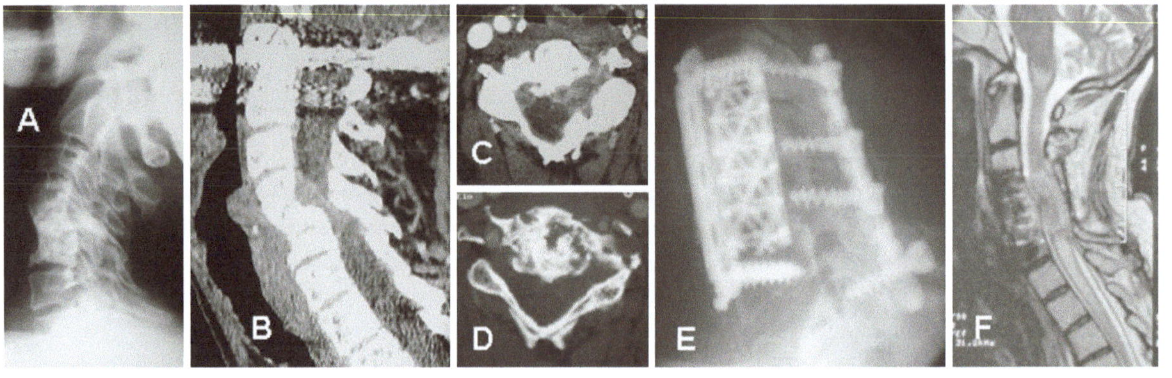

Fig. 11.3 Patient with metastatic thyroid tumor to the cervical spine. (**a**) Preoperative radiograph showing C4–C5 vertebral collapse with segmental kyphosis. (**b**) Sagittal and (**c**, **d**) Axial CT scan showing the extension of the tumor mass and involvement of the spinal canal. (**e**) Surgery consisted in two stage: posterior decompression and plate fixation followed by anterior decompression and fusion with a titanium mesh cage and plate fixation. (**f**) Few hours postoperatively, the patient developed complete tetraplegia. Postoperative MRI showed paradoxical spinal cord infarction after decompression. In this patient, the surgical indication and the surgical procedure were correct. The infarct was not predictable, even though the patient had been consented for this potential complication

especially in the distal portion of the dura. In such instances, repair is possible through the use of synthetic patch grafts and fibrin glue, associated with a lumbar subarachnoid drain and prophylactic antibiotics [22, 30].

11.2.3.2 Intradural and Extradural Hematoma

Intradural and extradural hematoma are mainly postoperative complications and are often encountered in patients undergoing cervical tumor surgery (5%), and are associated with developing neurological deficits. A careful clinical monitoring in awake patients and electrophysiological monitoring (SEP/MEP) intraoperatively and in the postoperative period in intensive care units patients should be routinely performed. In the management of these patients, it is important to remember that:

1. Screening and prophylaxis of coagulative disorders preoperatively and beginning of antithrombotic drugs after surgery. Often, coagulation disorders arise from hepatic involvement by the primary tumor.
2. Careful intraoperative hemostasis, mainly during surgical decompression of those patients with neoplastic pachymeningitis. In these patients, cleavage and removal of the tumor mass is difficult and dangerous for the risk of intradural hemorrhages and liquoral fistulae.
3. Immediate surgical revision once worsening of the neurological picture occurs in a progressive fashion.

In case of nonrapidly progressive postoperative neurological deficit, MRI, arteriography, and eventual urgent segmental embolization can be performed before surgical revision.

11.2.4 Extracanalar Neurological Lesions

Extracanalar neurological lesions may involve all the neurological structures of the neck. They include:

- Nerve fibers of the cervical and the brachial plexus out of the intervertebral foramina. Sometimes the primary trunks can be infiltrated by the tumor, and it can be necessary to sacrifice them to perform the excision of the mass.
- Cervical sympathetic chain, with consequent Bernard–Horner syndrome, when the tumor involves the lateral portion of the vertebral bodies.
- All the nerves of the neck (i.e., vagus, phrenic, hypoglossal) when the tumor has an extracanalar extension.

11.2.5 Reconstruction Failures

After excision of the tumor, several factors may determine failure of the reconstruction (performed with bone graft and mesh, cages, or plate and screws). They include:

1. Errors of evaluation of the boundaries between the tumor mass and the healthy vertebral body.

This is an insidious pitfall when the preoperative study of the patient does not include the systematic use of magnetic resonance imaging with paramagnetic contrast media, volumetric spiral computed tomography, and bone scan. Imaging, in fact, may allow the surgeon to better identify the lesion and plan the resection. As stated earlier, preoperative arteriography and embolization are mandatory. Preoperative embolization is particularly helpful to produce a relatively bloodless field, from which the tumor can be completely excised, and to help the surgeon to identify the boundaries of the tumor. In patients in whom preoperative embolization is not possible, the surgeon must be sure to position the hardware (mesh, cage, and screws) in the healthy portion of the vertebra. Sometimes, the intervertebral disc resists to tumor invasion. This can mislead the surgeon to an underestimation of the extension of the tumor mass, because the tumor could skip the disc space and involve the adjacent vertebral body, leading the surgeon to apply devices (mesh, cage, and screws) in tumor tissue (Fig. 11.4).

In tumors with prevalently anterior body involvement and sparing of the posterior elements, we undertook a posterior approach first to stabilize the cervical segment and give stability to the posterior aspect of the spine, followed by excision of the mass via an anterior

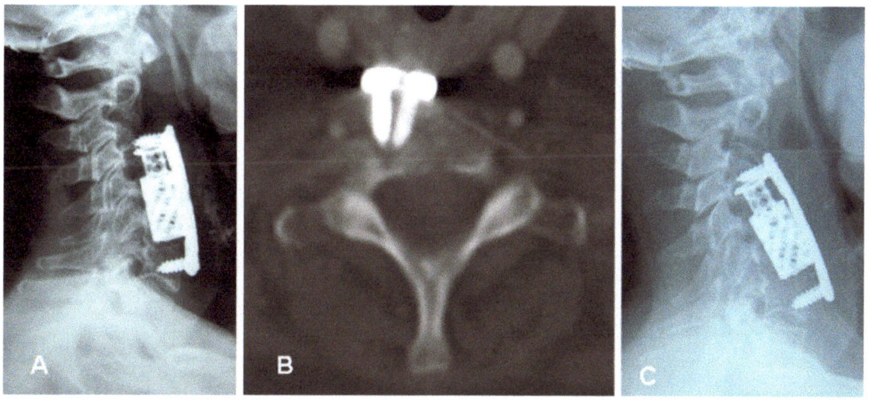

Fig. 11.4 Early failure of a reconstruction with stabilization for a metastasis to the cervical spine of a nonsmall cell lung tumor. The screws were positioned into the vertebral bodies damaged by the tumor. The surgeon should have extended the stabilization to the healthy vertebral bodies. (**a**) Postoperative lateral radiograph, (**b**) axial CT scan showing the screws inserted into the tumoral tissue. (**c**) Mobilization of the hardware

approach at the same operative time, or some days after the index procedure (Fig. 11.3).

In tumors in the posterior aspect of the vertebra, which generally involve only one side of the articular apophyses and laminae, we stabilize the side not involved by the tumor with plates and screws (and bone graft), and reconstruct the affected side after the excision of the mass with bone graft to fill the bony gap following the excision, and fixed to the proximal and distal healthy articular joints.

2. Inadequate hardware to allow stability.

Several devices currently available, if well implanted, guarantee immediate stability of the operated segment. However, if a mechanic reconstruction of the segment is not associated, the applied devices can fail. As general consideration, even though several devices can represent an adequate option in patients with fractures, their use alone is not able to provide stability if mechanic reconstruction of the segment is not performed.

In the past, we observed the use of biomechanically inadequate hardware, such as plates applied into the spinous processes, which broke the latter and mobilized itself.

3. Inadequate postoperative immobilization of the cervical spine

In tumoral surgery, even in patients in whom all the above principles are applied (i.e., adequate fixation), and screws are positioned in the healthy portion of a vertebra, the portions of a vertebra close to the tumor have always inferior mechanical proprieties because of the surrounding hypervascular tissue. Therefore, the hardware is not able to resist to the stresses, especially in rotation, when long stabilization are performed.

It is important to apply an adequate orthosis, depending on the type and localization of surgery (See Chap. 19) to allow an adequate immobilization of the operated segment. The choice of orthosis is guided by biomechanical requirements. When a rigid fixation of the cervical spine is required, a good option is represented by the Halo fixator, which provides the most rigid immobilization of any currently available orthoses. In patients with less severe pathology, other rigid or semirigid orthoses may be sufficient. In tumors with better prognosis, stabilization is performed with bone graft, and immobilization is mandatory to obtain healing.

4. Inadequate adjuvant therapy (CT and RT) in relation to the type of tumor

In this condition, the tumor may continue to invade the surrounding tissues and cause loss of stability.

11.2.5.1 General Complications

In patients with both primary and secondary tumors of the cervical spine, an impairment of the health status of the patient, with possible general complications, is always present.

Length of surgery and complex surgical options may also compromise the respiratory functions of the patient, who may be constricted to rest at bed and to wear orthosis for long periods. This may determine more frequently bronco-pneumonia in the portions of the lung near to the operated segment. The neurological damages, often incomplete, may cause transient gastrointestinal and urological pareses, with sepsis and hyperthermia being challengingly managed.

All these complications are described more thoroughly in Chaps. 1–3.

Core Messages

- Surgery in the management of cervical spine tumors (either primary or metastatic) is not easy to standardize with regard to surgical steps, which are related to tumor histology and localization.
- The need for aggressive surgery, often required in cervical tumor management is associated to a high difficulty in reaching and resetting the tumor and can require multiple approaches, being constantly aware of the various vascular and neurological structures during the approach.
- Preoperative identification of patients at potentially good prognosis is of paramount importance to select those who could benefit from more aggressive surgical treatments.
- Radiotherapy, malnutrition, and chronic use of steroids contribute significantly to increase the risk of intra or postoperative complications.

> Lesions to the vertebral artery at either C1–C2 and C3–C7, lesions to hollow viscuses in the neck (mainly esophageal perforations), spinal cord, and root lesions, CSF fluid leak and fistulas, vertebral body collapse, failure of instrumentation or bone graft, and intra/extradural hematomas are often encountered in this surgery and can lead to life-threatening complications in this fragile patient population.

References

1. An HS, Cooper M (1998) Cervical spine instrumentation. In: An HS (ed) Principles and techniques of spine surgery. Williams and Wilkins, Philadelphia, pp 65–73
2. Bauer H (1997) Posterior decompression and stabilization for spinal metastases: analysis of Sixty-seven consecutive patients. J Bone Joint Surg Am 79A:514–522
3. Bauer HCF, Wedin R (1995) Survival after surgery for spinal and extradural metastases. Prognostication in 241 patients. Acta Orthop Scand 66:143–146
4. Berenstein A, Lasjaunias P (1992) Surgical neuroangiography: endovascular treatment of benign tumors of the spinal column. Springer, New York, NY, pp 119–130
5. Bilsky MH, Boakye M, Collignon F, Kraus D, Boland P (2005) Operative management of metastatic and malignant primary subaxial cervical tumors. J Neurosurg Spine 2:256–264
6. Brislin BT, Hilibrand AS, Taylor BA (2002) Complications of anterior and posterior cervical instrumentation. In: Vaccaro AR, Betz RR, Zeidman SM (eds) Principles and practice of spine surgery. C.V. Mosby, St. Louis
7. Cole JS, Patchell RA (2008) Metastatic epidural spinal cord compression. Lancet Neurol 7:459–466
8. Denaro E (1991) Stenosis of the cervical spine causes, diagnosis and treatment. Springer, Berlin
9. Denaro V, Denaro L, Papalia R, Marinozzi A, Di Martino A (2007) Surgical management of cervical spine osteoblastomas. Clin Orthop Rel Res 455:190–195
10. Denaro V, Di Martino A, Ippolito M, Papalia R (2006) Surgical team in the management of bone metastasis. Supp Pall Cancer Care (2 Suppl):17–23
11. Denaro V, Di Martino A, Ippolito M, Pappietro N (2006) Tumori Primitivi del Rachide Cervicale. Giornale Italiano di Ortopedia e Traumatologia 10:S244–S248
12. Denaro V, Gulino G, Papapietro N, Denaro L (1998) Treatment of metastasis of the cervical spine. Chir Organi Mov 83:127–137
13. Denaro V (1988) Treatment of metastases and systemic tumors of the cervical spine. Neuroorthopedics 6:101–110
14. Fourney DR, York JE, Cohen ZR, Suki D, Rhines LD, Gokaslan ZL (2003) Management of atlantoaxial metastases with posterior occipitocervical stabilization. J Neurosurg (Spine 2) 98:165–170
15. Ghogawalw Z, Mansfield FL, Borges LF (2001) Spinal radiation before surgical decompression adversely affects outcomes of surgery for symptomatic metastatic spinal cord compression. Spine 26:818–824
16. Goldstain LA, Thompson WR (1982). Esphageal perforations: a 15 year experience. Am J Surg143:495–502
17. Hertlein H, Mittlmeier T, Schurmann M et al (1994) Posterior stabilization of C2 metastases by combination of atlantoaxial screw fixation and hook plate. Eur Spine J 3:52–55
18. Ibrahim A, Crockard A, Antonietti P et al (2008) Does spinal surgery improve the quality of life for those with extradural (spinal) osseous metastases? An international multicenter prospective observational study of 223 patients. J Neurosurg Spine 8:271–278
19. Jamjoom ZAB (1997) Pharyngo-cutaneous fistula following anterior cervical fusion. Br J Neurosurg 11:69–74
20. Jones DC, Hayter JP, Vaughan ED et al (1998) Oropharyngeal morbidity following transoral approaches to the upper cervical spine. Int J Oral Maxillofac Surg 27:295–298
21. Kitchel SH, Eismont FJ, Green BA (1989) Closet subarachnoid drainage for management of cerebrospinal fluid leakage after an operation to the spine. J Bone Joitn Surg (Am) 71:984–987
22. Kocialkowski A, Webb JK (1992) Metastatic spinal tumors: survival after surgery. Eur Spine J 1:43–48
23. Landreneau RJ, Weigelt JA, Meier DE et al (1995) The anterior operative approach to the cervical vertebral artery. J Am Coll Surg 180:475–480
24. Mazel C, Balabaud L, Bennis S, Hansen S (2009) Cervical and thoracic spine tumor management: surgical indications, techniques, and outcomes. Orthop Clin N Am 40:75–92
25. McPhee IB, Williams RP, Swanson CE (1998) Factors influencing wound healing after surgery for metastatic disease of the spine. Spine 23:726–732
26. Neo M, Fujibayashi S, Miyata M et al (2008) Vertebral artery injury during cervical spine surgery. a survey of more than 5600 operations. Spine 33:779–785
27. Patchell RA, Tibbs PA, Regine WF et al (2005) Direct decompressive surgical resection in the treatment of spinal cord compression caused by metastatic cancer: a randomized trial. Lancet 366:643–648
28. Piper JG, Menezes AH (1996) Management strategies for tumors of the axis vertebra. J Neurosurg 84:543–551
29. Riew DK, Khanna N (2002) Treatment of cerebrospinal fluid leaks. In: Vaccaro AR, Betz RR, Zeidman SM (eds) Principles and practice of spine surgery. C.V. Mosby, St. Louis, MO, pp 727–743
30. Roy-Camille R, Judet Th, Saillant G., et al (1982) Tumeurs du Rachis. Encicl Med-CHir Techniquee Chirurgicales, Orthopedie 11: 44–165
31. Shin H, Barrenechea IJ, Lesser J et al (2006) Occipitocervical fusion after resection of craniovertebral junction tumors. J Neurosurg Spine 4:137–144
32. Sorenson PS, Helweg-Larsen S, Mouridsen H et al (1994) Effect of high-dose dexamethasone in carcinomatous metastatic spinal cord compression treated with radiotherapy: a randomized trial. Eur J Cancer 30A:22–27
33. Sundaresan N, Rosen G, Boriani S (2009) Primary malignant tumors of the spine. Orthop Clin N Am 40:21–36

34. Sundaresan N, Rothman A, Manhart K et al (2002) Surgery for solitary metastases of the spine. Rationale and results of treatment. Spine 27:1802–1806
35. Tokuhashi Y, Matsuzaki H, Toriyama S et al (1990) Scoring system for the preoperative evaluation of metastatic spine tumor prognosis. Spine 15:1110–1113
36. Vecht CJ, Haaxma-Reiche H, van Putten WLJ et al (1989) Initial bouls of conventional versus high-dose dexamethasone in metastatic spinal cord compression. Neurology 39:1255–1257
37. Vieweg U, Meyer B, Schramm J (2001) Tumour surgery of the upper cervical spine – a retrospective study of 13 cases. Acta Neurochir 143:217–225
38. Weigel B, Maghsudi M, Neumann C et al (1999) Surgical management of symptomatic spinal metastases. Postoperative outcome and quality of life. Spine 24:2240–2246
39. Whitecloud T (1978) Complications of anterior cervical fusion. Instr Course Lect 30:411–424
40. Wise JJ, Fischgrund JSA, Herkowitz HN et al (1999) Complications, survival rates, and risk factors of surgery for metastatic disease of the spine. Spine 24:1943–1951
41. Yazawa Y, Frassica FJ, Chao EYS et al (1990) Metastatic bone disease. A study of the surgical treatment of 166 pathologic humeral and femoral fractures. Clin Orthop Rel Res 251:213–219

Cervical Spine Traumas

12

Luca Denaro, Umile Giuseppe Longo, Alberto Di Martino, and Vincenzo Denaro

Contents

12.1 Introduction

The cervical spine is involved in more than half of all the patients with traumatic spine injuries. To discuss about the most frequent complications occurring in the management of patients with cervical spine injury, it is necessary to briefly introduce some aspects of the methodological approach, therapeutic options, surgical indications and techniques. The main goals of management of patients with cervical spine injuries are decompression, alignment, stabilization, and, if necessary, reconstruction, to prevent further neurological damage and to promote neurological and functional recovery. An adequate management of cervical spine fractures starts from a proper classification of the injury type and assessment of stability of the affected segment [1].

Cervical spine fractures can be classified as "stable" or "unstable". Moreover, lesions can be distinguished on the basis of spinal cord compromise. Lesions with spinal cord involvement are severe and unstable and require surgical management. On the other hand, lesions without spinal cord involvement can evolve toward a stable or unstable lesion [2].

Stability is a crucial key point to determine the choice of management, and it is determined by the integrity of the anatomical structures constituting the cervical spine. Fractures, dislocations, or fracture-dislocations can determine instability because they compromise the continuity of the osteoligamentous systems [3–5]. Conservative management is a reasonable option in patients with stable lesions, while surgery is indicated in patients with unstable lesions.

White and Panjabi defined instability as "the loss of the ability of the spine under physiological loads to maintain relationships between vertebrae in such a way that the spinal cord or nerve roots are not damaged or irritated and deformity or pain does not develop".

L. Denaro (✉)
Department of Neuroscience, University of Padua, Via Giustiniani 5, 35128 Padua, Italy
e-mail: lucadenaro@hotmail.com

L. Denaro et al. (eds.), *Pitfalls in Cervical Spine Surgery*,
DOI: 10.1007/978-3-540-85019-9_12, © Springer-Verlag Berlin Heidelberg 2010

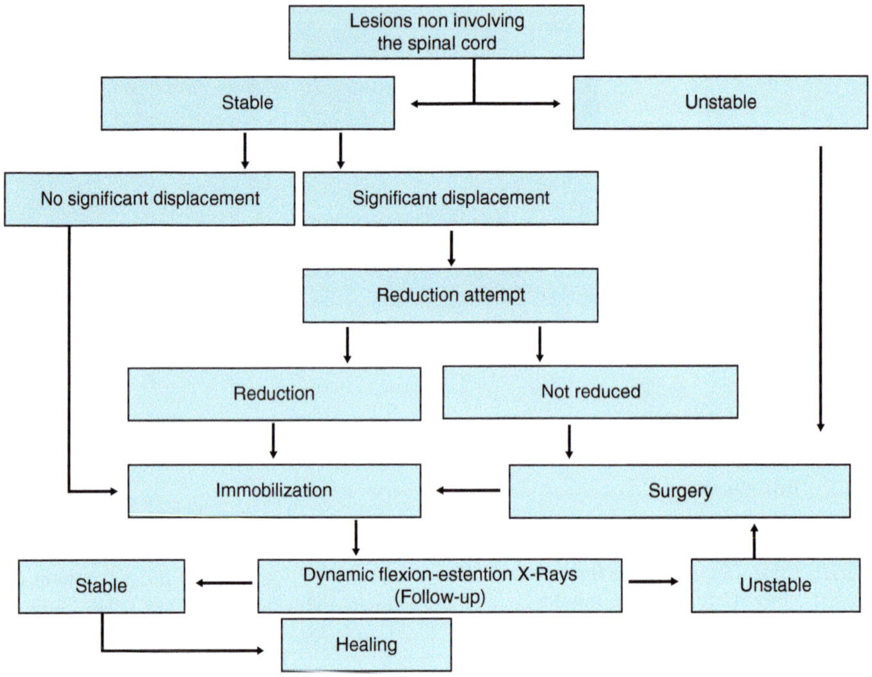

Fig. 12.1 Flowchart for the management of cervical spine trauma patients with lesions not involving the spinal cord

A distinction between bony and ligamentous lesions must be pointed out. Lesions that mainly involve bone structures may determine temporary instability. Successful fracture healing (with bony callus formation) and subsequent stabilization of these lesions may be obtained with reduction and immobilization. On the other hand, ligamentous or osteo-ligamentous lesions may cause irreversible instability with secondary dislocation. At the atlanto-axial level, a dislocation cannot occur if the transverse ligament is intact. If the transverse ligament is ruptured and the alar ligaments remain intact, the dislocation of the anterior arch of the atlas with respect to the dens varies from 3 to 5 mm. If both the transverse and alar ligaments are ruptured, then the dislocation exceeds 5 mm. In the lower cervical spine, stability depends on the integrity of the anterior longitudinal ligament, the intervertebral disc, the posterior longitudinal ligament, the apophyseal joints, the ligamenta flava, and the interspinous ligaments. The greatest degree of stabilization is provided by the posterior longitudinal ligament where it is fused to the intervertebral disc. In ligamentous lesions, the functional unit is stable if this system remains intact. Therefore, when the posterior disco-ligamentous complex is injured, progressive loss of physiological relationships between the adjacent vertebrae occurs [6].

In general, high potential instability lesions, such as cervical spine fractures-dislocations and dislocations associated with progressive neurological deficits, should be reduced and fixed as soon as possible [7].

On the basis of these concepts, our criteria to guide management are the following:

- Lesions without spinal cord involvement (Fig. 12.1):

Stable lesions that do not require reduction are immobilized with brace (Minerva cast, Halo, SOMI-brace). Lesions with significant displacement must be reduced by traction (halo traction), before immobilization (halo jacket or halo cast). If reduction is unsuccessful, the residual deformity may cause secondary neurological syndromes and posttraumatic stenosis. In these cases, surgical reduction followed by immobilization in an orthopedic brace is necessary. After the required period of immobilization, fusion and stability must be checked radiologically in both static and dynamic conditions.

The dynamic tests are always performed on the conscious patient in the presence of the surgeon, because the patient must actively participate in flexion, extension, rotation, and lateral flexion.

The radiographic signs of ligamentous instability are as follows:

(a) At C1–C2 level, the signs of instability are:
   - In lateral view: the relationship between the anterior arch of the atlas and the dens of the axis. A separation greater than 3 mm of C1 on

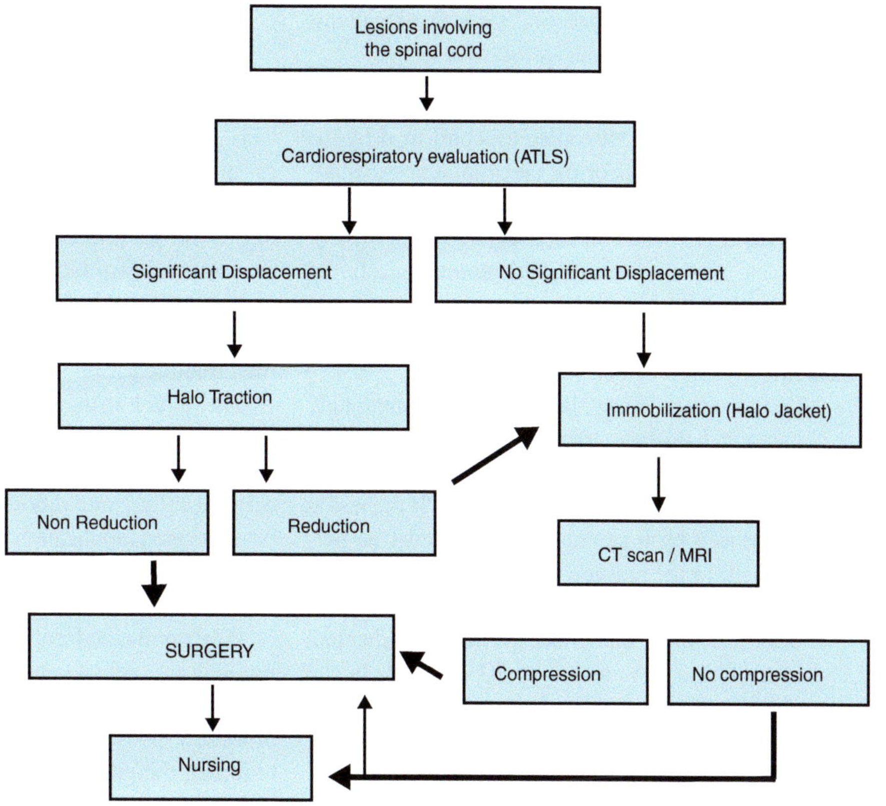

Fig. 12.2 Flowchart for the management of cervical spine trauma patients with lesions involving the spinal cord

C2 in adults indicates instability, while in children, a diastasis of 5 mm should be considered as normal.

- In the antero-posterior view, a separation between the dens of the axis and the lateral masses of the atlas greater than 7 mm suggests instability.

(b) At C3–C7 level, the signs of instability are as follows:

- Abnormal separation of the spinous processes
- Upward sliding of the articular facets
- Anterior kyphosis of an intervertebral disc, while the others are in lordosis
- Horizontal shift exceeding 3.5 mm of one vertebra on another. In 20% of children aged 7–8 years, there is a diastasis of several mm between C2 and C3, which is considered to be physiological [1].

• Lesions with spinal cord involvement:

Lesions with spinal cord involvement are unstable by definition and require surgical management. The decisional algorithm of these patients is shown in Fig. 12.2. The first step is to reduce the dislocation, to decompress the spinal cord and nerve roots (especially in case of neurological lesion because of bone or disc fragments) [1, 2]. Successively, the fractured vertebral bodies must be stabilized to allow repair [2]. The surgical indications must consider morphological criteria (type and level of lesion, degree of dislocation, and stability), clinical criteria (complete or incomplete lesion), and chronological criteria (to establish the best timing for surgery), in relation to the time between injury and admission, the initial treatment, and the patient's cardio-respiratory condition. The therapeutic possibilities and prognosis depend on collaboration between the intensive care physician and the surgeon. After stabilization of respiratory, cardiovascular, thermal, and electrolyte disorders, the orthopedist must evaluate the clinical findings and determine the proper timing for surgery. Because of their possible influence on the final prognosis, the patient's respiratory and cardiovascular conditions must be carefully evaluated [5]. The prognosis is better in patients with preoperative current volume (C.V.) greater than 700 mL/m^2, even though immediate surgery is required in patients with complete or incomplete tetraplegia.

On the basis of these concepts, we manage patients with spinal cord involvement as follows:

1. Incomplete medullary lesions (tetraplegia, incomplete paraplegia, or monoplegia), confirmed by the neurological findings or by electrodiagnostic studies (evoked potentials). Early decompression provides the best chance for recovery.
2. Complete medullary lesions. Patients must be referred to specialized centers, and managed in intensive care units, where appropriate radiological and neurological investigations can be performed.
   - Displacement must be reduced immediately using a halo-type traction device under local anesthesia. Immediate surgery is required if the lesion cannot be reduced by traction. If the lesion is reduced by traction, a CT scan must be performed. In the presence of cord compression by disc or bony fragments, immediate surgical decompression and stabilization is indicated, even with a C.V. less than 700 mL/m^2. In the absence of compression, immediate surgical stabilization is advisable, but only with C.V. greater than 700 mL/m^2. When the patient's C.V. is less than 700 mL/m^2, the prognosis is very poor, and treatment should be limited to an orthopedic brace with halo traction and nursing care.
   - Simple fractures should be immediately immobilized with an orthosis. If compression of the spinal cord is detected at imaging, surgery is indicated. In the absence of compression, surgery can be deferred until cardiorespiratory recovery, and the patient managed with kinesitherapy.

This therapeutic strategy applies to patients referred to specialized centers within 24–36 h from injury. Otherwise, the management must be modified according to the general condition of the patient. From our experience, two factors influence the prognosis of patients affected by cervical spine fractures with spinal cord injury (SCI), namely the time between injury and final treatment, and the type of initial treatment.

The initial management of cervical spine injuries with or without spinal cord involvement is similar. Patients with C1 or C2 fractures must be left in a hard cervical collar, until more definitive immobilization can be performed (application of a halo). Patients with lower cervical fractures should remain in a hard cervical collar until a definitive diagnosis of the fracture is made.

Polytraumatized patients with cervical spine fracture require special handling during the evaluation and early phase of the management. During the emergency procedure phase of management, when a reduction is required, the patient must be kept in traction to determine if other procedures are required, such as laparotomy, thoracotomy, or stabilization of femur or pelvis. Obviously, this influences the choice of anesthetic technique, avoiding manipulating the neck (See Chap. 5).

One of the most common pitfalls in patients with cervical spine injury is missed or delayed diagnosis of

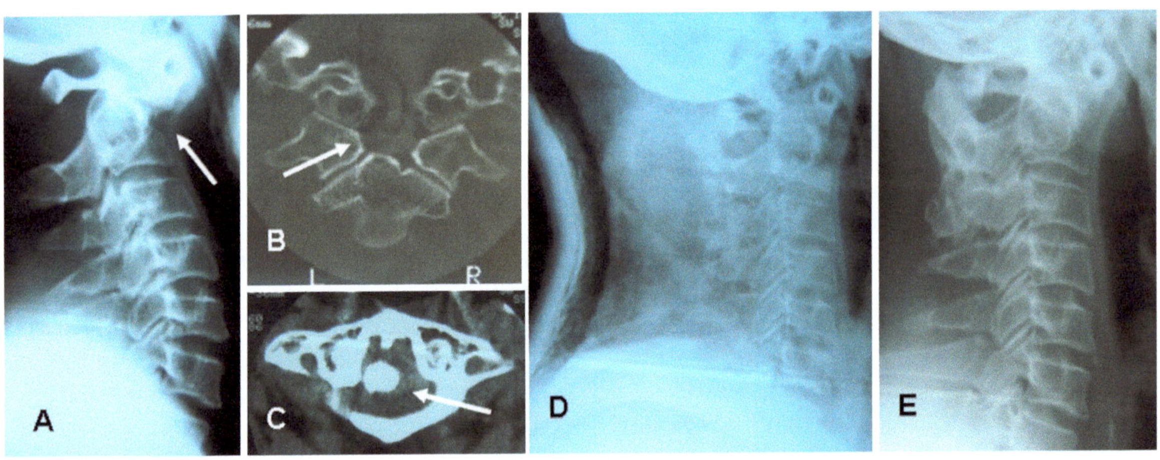

Fig. 12.3 (**a**) Lateral radiograph of a patient with asymptomatic odontoid fracture with anterior subluxation of the complex atlas-dens of the axis following a trauma. (**b**, **c**) On the basis of the CT scan, a congenital pseudoarthrosis was diagnosed. The patient was managed conservatively. One year after the trauma, the patient started to complain of progressive neurological deficits. The patient underwent surgery, which consisted of reduction and fixation with bone graft and C1–C2 fusion with nonreabsorbable wires, followed by the application of a Minerva cast. (**d**, **e**) Three months postoperative radiograph showing solid fusion that extended down to C3

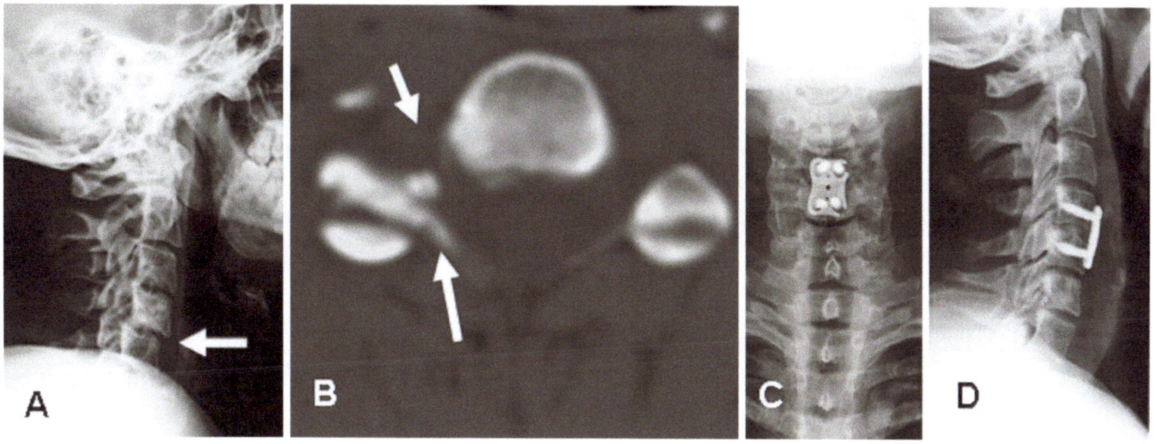

Fig. 12.4 (**a**) C4–C5 fracture-dislocation conservatively managed with application of brace. The patient complained of a late deltoid progressive paralysis. (**b**) Axial CT scan showing facet fracture-dislocation with a bony fragment into the right foramen and associated disc herniation. (**c, d**) Surgery consisted of anterior reduction, decompression, and fusion with plate fixation. The complication in this patient was the inadequate diagnosis, and the choice of a conservative management

cervical spine injury at trauma centers, which occurs at a rate of 1–4.6% (Figs. 12.3 and 12.4). The most frequent reasons for missed injuries are inadequate radiographs (44%) and misinterpretation of adequate radiographs (47%). Up to 71% of patients with missed injuries or delayed diagnosis do not suffer adverse consequences. However, severe complications, ranging from death (20%) to quadriplegia (40%) or other new neurologic deficit (40%) have been reported in the remaining (29%) patients who deteriorate from a missed injury.

12.2 Classification and Surgical Indications

Evaluation of the cervical spine in the trauma setting requires a dedicated trauma team and multiple specialists. Extensive diagnostic evaluation allows adequate morphology pattern evaluation and address surgeon's requirement for patient management and surgical treatment.

Trauma to the cervical spine can be generally classified as fractures, dislocations, fractures-dislocations, and sprains. According to the localization of trauma, they can be divided into upper and lower cervical spine injuries.

12.2.1 Upper Cervical Spine Injuries

The upper cervical spine consists of atlas, axis, and skull base. The latter, although technically not a part of the cervical spine, plays a fundamental role in the normal functional alignment of the two upper cervical vertebrae. Therefore, the upper cervical spine includes all osseous and ligamentous structures between the skull base surrounding the foramen magnum and the cranial side of the C-3 vertebral segment. The integrity of the upper cervical spine is essential for survival and function, because of the neurovascular structures contained within its bony elements. At the level of the upper cervical spine, there is the transition from brainstem to spinal cord, and the upper cervical spine protects the enclosed neural elements, allowing at the same time, a substantial portion of the head motion. Atlas and axis have particular anatomico-physiological and biomechanical aspects. Small ligaments extending between the skull base and the third cervical segment allow the upper vertebral spine to maintain its appropriate anatomic relationship. Injuries to osteoligamentous components at this level may compromise structural integrity of the upper cervical spine. Obviously, osteoligamentous lesions at this level have clinical pictures and neurological risks different from those of the lower cervical vertebrae.

Common complications of upper cervical spine trauma include damages to vessels, neurological structures, esophagus, and trachea. All these complications will be described in detail in the following paragraph. A brief description of the vascular complications is now reported. Vascular injuries can occur in patients with upper cervical spine trauma. Vertebral artery disruption may occur in any distractive upper cervical spine injury (such as atlantoaxial dissociation or type III or IV atlantoaxial rotary subluxation), or in any displaced fracture involving the transverse foramen. Fractures to the atlas ring have not been described to be commonly associated with local vertebral artery trauma, despite the vertebral artery running in close proximity to the rostral lamina of the posterior ring of the atlas. Forced hyperflexion injuries (anteriorly displaced type III odontoid fractures) can determine thrombosis of the carotid arteries. Management of vascular injuries is described in detail in Chap. 8.

Upper cervical spine injuries include occipital condyle fractures, occipito-cervical dissociation and instability, and fractures of the atlas and the axis. Complications of the most common upper cervical spine trauma surgery are reported in Table 12.1.

- *Occipital condyle fractures:* Occipital condyle fractures seem to be rare, and exact incidence is unknown. Many patients are unconscious on admission, and diagnosis is often incidental during a head CT scan [8]. In polytraumatized patients, the diagnosis is often missed, and the autopsy allows the diagnosis. The most commonly used classification is that of Anderson and Montesano [9]. A Type-I fracture is a comminuted impaction fracture resulting from axial loading and it is considered to be stable; Type II is a condylar fracture with extension into the base of the skull, and it is also considered stable, except in patients in whom the entire condyle has been separated from the occiput. Type III is an avulsion-type fracture at the insertion of the alar ligament and is considered to be unstable. These injuries are likely to be unstable and may represent the bony component of the craniocervical dissociation. In the presence of a unilateral bony injury to an occipitocervical joint, the contralateral side should be scrutinized for any signs of bony or ligamentous injury. Neurological examination is often normal in these patients, even though fatal brainstem injuries, respiratory-dependent quadriplegia, mild degrees of SCI, and cranial nerve injuries have been reported. Treatment depends on segment stability and integrity of alar ligaments. As a general role, stable fractures (unilateral Type I and Type II fractures) should be managed conservatively with a halo fixator. Unstable Type III injuries associated with atlanto-occipital instability are managed with surgery. Obviously, the presence of displaced skull fractures, chest wall trauma, and injuries to other structures, will change the therapeutic plan. A common pitfall of occipital condyle fractures is to miss the diagnosis. Also, these injuries may represent the presentation of patients with atlanto-occipital dissociation. Therefore, serious neurologic sequelae may result when the diagnosis of occipital condyle fractures is missed. Late complications of isolated occipital condyle fractures include posttraumatic arthritis, neck pain, occipital headaches, and limited neck motion. Lower cranial nerve deficits have been reported in up to 31% of patients with occipital condyle fractures [10]. Pitfalls of the management of patients with occipital condyle fractures include those of the halo fixator for the conservative management, and those related to intra or postoperative complications in patients undergoing surgical management. General complications of the halo fixator are described in detail in Chap. 19. Briefly, they include dural pin invasion (around 1% of patients), pin loosening (around 18% of patients), pin tract infection (around 20% of patients), pain at the pin site (around 18% of patients), disfiguring scarring (around 9% of patients), propagation of a skull fracture, occipital decubitus formation, loss of reduction (up to 46% of patients), and pressure sores (around 11% of patients). Anticoagulation drugs for prevention of thromboembolism in patients with acute spine fracture are associated with an increased risk of epidural hematoma formation. The use of halo fixator in older patients is also associated with an increased risk of pulmonary complications and aspiration. Specific complications of the use of halo fixator in these patients are the nonunion and mal-union, with painful deformity from deficit of articulation of the bony segments. On the other hand, the most insidious complications of patients undergoing surgery include the nonunion, vascular and neurological lesions when positioning the screws, and breaking of the hardware (especially when a biological fusion

Table 12.1 Complications of upper cervical spine trauma surgery

Technique	Complication	Consequences	Tips/tricks
Posterior wiring – hooks	Impingement in the spinal canal Loss of fixation Wire breakdown laminar, lateral mass, spinous process fracture Hook impingement in the spinal canal Laminar fracture	Subdural hematoma Dural tears Spinal cord lesions Implant failure Recurrence of deformity Need for revision surgery Dural tear, spinal cord compression	Avoid passage of wirings at the level of injury Possible need to shift to screw-based instrumentation Careful dissection and adequate preparation of the laminae
Transarticular screw fixation	Screw malpositioning	Vertebral artery injury greater occipital nerve and C2 root injury Nonunion Dural tears with liquoral fistulas Spinal cord lesions	Avoid patients with facet or lateral masses C2 degeneration or thoracic kyphosis Use of a k-wire to retract soft tissues and greater occipital nerve Proper fusion technique
Harms and Melcher C1–C2 fixation	C1 lateral mass screw malpositioning C2 pedicle screw misplacement	Vertebral artery lesion C2 nerve root lesion Spinal cord lesion Vertebral artery lesion Dural tears Pedicle fracture	Visualization of the C1 lateral mass after retraction of the C2 dorsal root ganglion Correct entry point visualization of the C1 lateral mass can be impossible Palpate the medial wall of the pedicle during screw insertion Accurate preoperative CT study Avoid too medial screw placement If needed, convert the procedure to a laminar hook – wiring technique or extend fixation to C3
Anterior odontoid screw fixation	Nonunion Inadequate reduction and loss of correction at the fracture site Malpositioning of the screws Screw migration or breakage	Segmental instability and pain Neurovascular injury Loss of reduction Loss of correction, instability, hollow viscus lesions	Adherence to indications Preoperative CT scans to study the reciprocal positioning of bony fragments Revision surgery from a posterior route often required Carefully check on fluoroscopy during screw placement Often requiring surgical revision, new reduction,and posterior approach

does not occur). This risk is increased when the internal fixation is not associated with an adequate bone graft, capable of increasing the chances of bony union.

- *Occipito-cervical dislocation and instability:* Occipito-cervical dissociative injuries are uncommon. They have a high mortality rate. These injuries are usually associated with high cervical cord injury followed by death, and in autopsy studies, represent 5–12% of identified cervical injuries. Survivors of occipito-cervical dissociative injuries have neurological deficits, such as the Brown–Sequard syndrome, central cord syndrome, cervicomedullary syndrome, and cranial nerve injuries. As for occipital condyle fractures, a common pitfall of these injuries, estimated to occur in 50–60% of the patients, is the misdiagnosis, frequently associated with neurological deterioration [11]. After emergent resuscitation and airway management, a halo fixator should be applied. However, it can be contraindicated in patients with associated displaced skull fracture or unstable chest wall.
- *Fractures of the atlas.* Three primary types of fractures of the ring of C1 are generally described: posterior arch fracture, usually occurring at the junction of the posterior arch and the lateral mass; lateral mass fracture, usually occurring on one side only with the fracture line passing either through the articular surface; and burst fracture (Jefferson fracture), characterized by four fractures, two in the

posterior arch and two in the anterior arch [12]. Most fractures of the atlas can be managed with immobilization in halo. Complications of the management of these patients are those described for the halo fixator. Surgical management should be reserved for patients with nonunion and persisting pain. Complications of fractures of the atlas include posttraumatic osteoarthritis as a consequence of a displaced lateral mass fracture. Instability of the atlantoaxial articulation (as demonstrated on flexion-extension radiographs) can result from a disruption of the transverse ligament. C1–2 fusion can be an option for patients with atlantoaxial instability or painful atlantoaxial arthritis. The management of nonunion and severe mal-union of unstable atlas fracture resulting in painful torticollis is an occiput to C-2 fusion [10].

- *Odontoid Fractures:* Odontoid fractures are classically divided according to the Anderson and D'Alonzo system [13] based on the anatomic level of the fracture: Type I fractures occur at the tip of the odontoid process, are generally stable, and can be managed conservatively. Type II fractures occur at the junction between the base of the odontoid process and the body of the axis. These are unstable and often require surgery [14]. Patients with nondisplaced or minimally displaced fractures that are easily reduced can be treated with halo fixator. A significant morbidity and even mortality is associated with odontoid fractures. The most common causes of complications are missed injuries and nonunion [10]. Secondary neurologic deterioration may occur as a consequence of nonunion of a Type II odontoid fracture, defined as the absence of fracture site bridging after 4 months of treatment. Type I injuries are rarely encountered. The risk of nonunion after Type II fractures of the odontoid is 100% in patients managed without immobilization, and from 15 to 85% in patients managed with the application of halo. Absence of any distraction and maintenance of a nearly anatomic fracture reduction are essential points for a successful conservative management. Risk factors for nonunion of Type II odontoid fractures are more than 20% translation, as seen on open-mouth or lateral radiograph, fracture displacement of greater than 5 mm, age above 60 years, and fracture angulation of more than 9°. The rate of nonunion in patients with Type III odontoid fractures range from 9 to 13%, although in patients with fracture displacement of more than 5 mm or angulation exceeding 10°, the nonunion rates are from 22 to 40%. Surgical options for odontoid fractures are dens screw fixation or C1–2 fusion. Anterior approach technique requires the patient being in a supine position on a radiotransparent table. The patient should be intubated with a nasotracheal tube while awake to avoid neurological lesions during intubation maneuvers [15]. A Mayfield head holder can be used (see Chap. 6) and connected to the operative table. When fracture reduction is needed, this should be performed with the patient awake, controlling the neurological examination before intubation. The technique requires the use of fluoroscopy with two perpendicular lateral and transoral views [16]. The use of two independent perpendicular fluoroscopic views is important to correctly visualize the kirschner wire and screw advancement, avoiding complications related to kirschner wire or screw mal-positioning. Incision is performed at the C5–C6 level, by using a standard anteromedial approach. Once below, on the deep cervical space, the tubercle of the axis is identified in a blunt fashion. Using a small drill sleeve, a 1–2 mm kirschner wire is inserted from the antero-inferior margin of the C2 vertebral body under fluoroscopic guidance and directed toward the posterior apex of the dens; a second kirschner wire can be used to avoid distal fragment rotation during screw insertion. Screw insertion requires a cannulated screw of 3.5–4 mm diameter advanced under fluoroscopic guidance. Final position should be checked fluoroscopically in the two perpendicular planes. Use of retractors and guides is recommended during drilling and screw insertion to avoid damage to the soft tissues. The complication most often encountered with this technique is nonunion, reported in a range of cases from 8 to 27%, mainly in the older population. Other reported complications are screws mal-positioning, inadequate reduction and loss of correction at the fracture site, screw migration, and reduction of segmental motion. The procedure is associated with potential neurological damage and serious life-threatening complications, such as injuries of the spinal cord, carotid and vertebral artery, upper airway, and esophageal perforations. To prevent the above-mentioned complications, strict adherence to surgical indications and adequate preoperative radiological study of the reciprocal positioning of

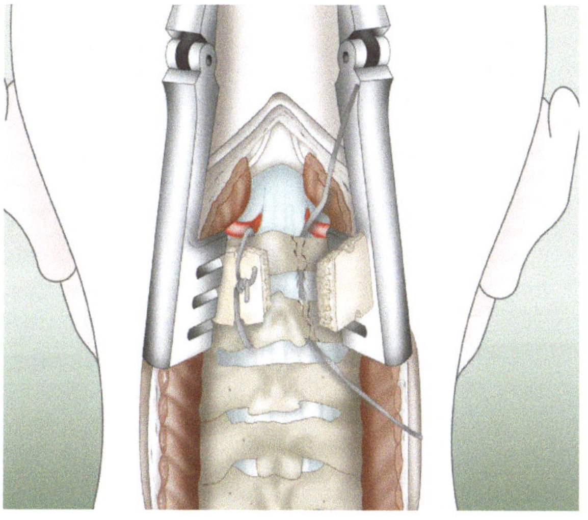

Fig. 12.5 Complications related to the use of wires are related to the violation of the spinal canal as well as the associated risk of SCI or dural tear with CSF fluid leak, and bony fracture

the bony fragments (better with spiral CT scans with sagittal reconstructions to ascertain the real direction of the fracture line) are required. A common cause of early implant failure is the inadequate placement of the hardware within the narrow trajectory of the vertebral body of the axis to the tip of the odontoid [10].

- During the posterior approach, wiring techniques with properly shaped bone graft provide a solid anchoring. The top of the graft is shaped in such a way as to interlock with the posterior arch of the atlas, while its lower portion "sits astride" the spinous process of C2. When two cortico-trabecular grafts are used, these are locked on either side of the midline onto the atlas and axis, obviously with two wires one for each of the grafts. One of the most critical factors to prevent complications in wiring surgery at the C1–C2 level, is strict respect of indications, together with adequate postoperative immobilization (halo fixator) and precise bone graft contouring to maximize bony contact and bone healing. Moreover, the space available in the spinal canal for passing the wires should be taken into consideration before planning wire passage, to avoid damages to the dura mater and spinal cord (Figs. 12.5 and 12.6).
- One of the available screw fixation technique of C1–C2 is the transarticular stabilization technique described by Magerl et al. [17]. This is performed after the identification and exposure of the posterior wall of the facet joints of C1 and C2. Magerl recommends the use of a kirschner wire to retract the adjacent soft tissues and greater occipital nerve. By keeping the joint under visual control, screws are inserted at the base of the articular process of C2 in an oblique fashion to reach the lateral masses of the atlas. The use of fluoroscopy is fundamental to assess the correct positioning and length of the screws. Once the screws are in place, fusion with properly shaped and wired bone graft represent a fundamental surgical time to achieve long-term segmental stabilization. This demanding technique carries an elevated risk of direct lesions to the vertebral artery, the greater occipital nerve and the surrounding venous plexus, lesions to the C2 nerve root, and postoperative nonunion. Moreover, a malpositioned screw can lead to major complications such as dural tears, liquoral fistulas, and, rarely, also

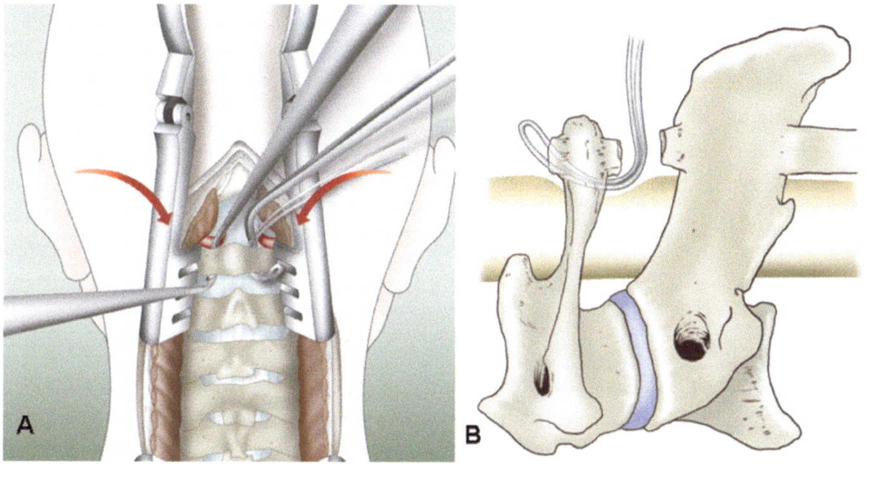

Fig. 12.6 (**a**, **b**) The use of type Songer cable helps to reduce the incidence of spinal cord injury and bony fracture

to direct spinal cord lesions. Another option is to perform transarticular fixation according to the Barbour technique [18].

- Harms and Melcher described a new technique for the stabilization of the C1–C2 joint [19]. The technique they described requires screws inserted in the lateral masses of C1 and C2 pedicle connected by longitudinal bars. Screw positioning at the lateral masses of C1 presents some peculiar problems. Once the posterior arch of C1 is exposed, the lateral mass is visualized by gentle retraction above the dorsal root ganglion of the C2 nerve root. The entry point of the C1 screw is at the center of the lateral mass. A drill is used to prepare the screw entry point, and then the screw is tapped and inserted. Screw insertion follows 20° inclination upward and 15° inclination antero-medially on the transversal plane. It is not a simple procedure due to the difficult exposition of the C1 lateral mass, which sometimes can be impossible. With regard to the C2 pedicle screw, direct palpation of the medial wall of the pedicle is performed; the screw is inserted with 10–25° medial inclination and 25° cephalic with an entry point at the supero-internal part of the lateral mass. After drilling, tapping is suggested before screw insertion. It is important to palpate the medial wall during screw insertion to check for pedicle infraction. An accurate CT preoperative study allows for proper visualization and adequate study of local anatomy, especially vertebral artery position, extremely variable in its passage in the foramen of C1 and in the tract above the C1 posterior arch. Pedicle fracture represents one of the most feared and serious complication of C2 pedicle screw insertion. In case of excessive medial screw insertion, an increased risk of dural tear with cerebrospinal fluid (CSF) leakage can occur. In case of a lesion, a new screw trajectory can be pursued (with less medial inclination), the procedure can be converted to a laminar hook or wiring technique at that level, or instrumentation can be extended down to the C3 lateral masses. Insufficient space for screw placement in the isthmus of C2 and anomalous course of the vertebral artery can complicate positioning of C1–C2 trans-articular screws. Odontoid fractures may determine ventral compression of the spinal chord with progressive neurological damage. It is therefore important to realign the spine before posterior fusion. Patients with Os odontoideum should not undergo anterior screw fixation because of the low chances of fusion.
- Nonunion has been reported in up to 10% of patients after odontoid screws and in around 4% or less percentage of patients undergoing C1–2 fusions using either wire constructs or transarticular screw fixation. Primary neurologic injury is not common in patients with odontoid fracture, but it can be severe, ranging from cranial nerve injuries to quadriplegia. Type II odontoid fracture is the most common fracture associated with neurologic involvement (up to 18–25% of patients). Odontoid fracture also carries a risk of mortality, which is higher in elderly patients. Early surgical stabilization has been proposed in these patients to reduce the risk of death.
- *Bipedicular fractures of the axis with spondylolisthesis ("Hangman's fracture")* (Fig. 12.7): The classification system for this injury was first described by Effendi et al. [20], and later modified by Levine and Edwards [21]. The classification is based on translation and angulation between C2 and C3.
  - Type I injuries are bilateral pars fractures with translation less than 3 mm and without angulation. CT may show a fracture line into the vertebral body, up to the transverse foramen, potentially injuring the vertebral artery. These lesions are better managed with halo. Type IA or atypical traumatic spondylolistesis of the axis is similar to standard Type I fractures, with associated angulations or translations [21].
  - In Type II fractures, the C2–C3 disc and posterior longitudinal ligament are injured, resulting in translation of more than 3 mm and marked angulation. Fractures with oblique fracture line and minimal translation (but significant angulation) are classified as Type IIA. Closed reduction and external immobilization is often able to achieve healing.
  - Type III injuries are a combination of pars fracture with dislocation of the C2–C3 facet joints. These injuries are very unstable, and can be associated with neurological deficits. They require open reduction and internal fixation via a posterior approach, or rarely, anterior C2–C3 fixation.
  - Neurological deficits are more common in Type II and Type III injuries. Patients with Type III injuries frequently have quadriplegia with poor long-term prognosis. One of the most important complications of the management of patients

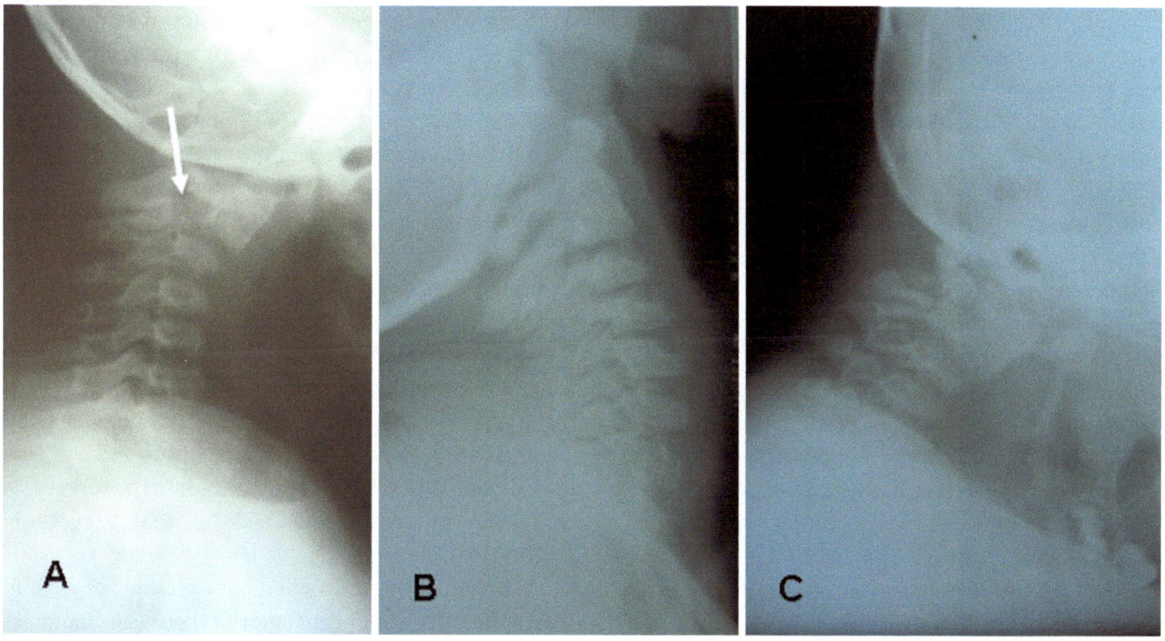

Fig. 12.7 (**a**) Ten-year-old patient affected by bilateral pars fracture of the axis (*arrow*). See anterior slippage of the dens with respect to the body of C3 resulting in segmental kyphosis. Patient was treated conservatively by reduction and application of a halo jacket and healed nicely, which was demonstrated by the 3-month postoperative flexion-extension radiographs (**b**, **c**). The complication in this patient was the mobilization of the anterior pins of the halo, managed with replacement of the halo with a Minerva cast

with these fractures is nonunion, which can be managed by osteosynthesis. In patients managed with halo fixator, successful fracture healing of traumatic spondylolisthesis of C2 occurs in around 95%, even in the presence of displacement of the pars interarticularis. The formation of a painless ptosic pedicle may lead to successful healing. Today, surgical indications for C1–C3 stabilization are very limited, as they are not able to provide an immediate stabilization and may evolve in nonunion. In patients with nonunion, surgery consists of transpedicular fixation. Navigated systems are available to reduce vascular and neurological complications during screw insertion.

- Historically, Hangman's fracture has been closely associated with death in the context of judicial hanging. Today, acute postadmission mortality of Hangman's fractures is 2–3%. Neurologic sequelae are present in 3–10% of this group of patients, and up to 33% in patients with atypical traumatic C-2 spondylolisthesis fractures of the Type Ia subtype.

12.2.2 Lower Cervical Spine Injuries

Several classification systems are available to classify lower cervical spine injuries. An ideal system should include identification and terminology, injury and management, characterization, neurologic factors, grading, and prognosis. To date, none of the available classification systems satisfy these requirements. In fact, the unique anatomic morphology of the cervical spine and the complex loading patterns in real-life injuries limit the generalizability of biomechanical observations into broad statements relating to injury mechanisms and injury patterns [22]. However, some general principles can help to guide systematic evaluation of injuries. Lower cervical spine injuries can be classified into "phylogenies", based on a common mechanism of injury, which emphasizes the orderly sequence of injury progression. Six categories of injury are included: compressive flexion, vertical compression, distractive flexion, compressive extension, distractive extension, and lateral compression. The risk and severity of neurological injury is increased in relation to the injury stage.

In general, flexion injuries of the lower cervical spine can be mechanistically classified with higher stages representing unstable lesions [23]. More severe lesions are associated with high rates of neurological injury. Cervical orthoses may be sufficient in patients with little deformity or flexion sprains without frank facet incongruity. Higher grade lesions require surgery. Obviously, these are general principles, as every patient needs an individualized therapeutic strategy [24]. Distraction injuries are the most unstable injury patterns, with essentially complete loss of continuity of the cervical spine, and they are often associated with severe neurologic deficits, vascular disruption, and stroke. Patients with these injuries are susceptible to further injury and potentially catastrophic deterioration during physical transfers and extreme caution is needed. Complications of lower cervical spine injuries are presented at the end of the following descriptive paragraph and in Table 12.2.

12.2.2.1 Compression Flexion

Compressive flexion injuries are classified into five stages. Stage 1: rounded shape to the anterior superior vertebral body without posterior ligamentous disruption. Stage 2: "beached" appearance of the anterior vertebral body with the loss of anterior height because of compression failure. Stage 3: oblique fracture line from the anterior superior vertebral body to the inferior end plate. Stage 4: up to 3 mm of posterior translation of the posterior vertebral body into the neural canal. Stage 5: more than a 3 mm posterior translation of the posterior vertebral body into the neural canal.

Sagittal body fractures and posterior lamina fractures are commonly associated with compression flexion injuries. In Stage 1 and 2 injuries, the posterior annulus and posterior ligamentous structures remain intact and the majority of patients can be managed with a rigid cervical orthosis. Patients must be monitored by radiographs. Abnormal motion in flexion-extension lateral radiographs can be an indication to arthrodesis. Stage 3 injuries (tear drop fragment without subluxation) are potentially unstable. MRI is needed to assess injuries to the intervertebral disc and posterior ligament [16]. In the absence of injury to these structures, the patient can be managed with a halo fixator. In patients in whom there is also associated posterior ligamentous injury, surgery is required to avoid the risk of late kyphotic deformity.

When neurological deficits are present, especially when there is a significant anterior thecal sac compression from retropulsed bone or extruded disc fragment, surgery is required.

Stage 4 lesions are more unstable, and immobilization in halo fixator is needed. In the presence of a subluxation greater than 3 mm (Stage 5), surgery is required.

12.2.2.2 Vertical Compression

Vertical compressions are classified into three stages. Stage 1: failure of either the superior or inferior end plates. Stage 2: failure of both the end plates with cupping deformity. Stage 3: comminution of the vertebral body with radial displacement of the fragments.

Table 12.2 Complications of anterior sub-axial cervical spine trauma surgery

Lesion	Consequences	Tips/tricks
Myeloradicular injuries	Persisting or worsening of neurological deficits	Correct positioning of the patient Deformity Reduction Use air drills
Deep structures of the neck	Esophageal lesions at the time of trauma	Preoperative evaluation for fragment potentially injuring the esophageal wall
Vascular lesions	Vertebral artery: Hemorrhage, neurological deficits, need for ligation	Bony dissection not lateral to the unci Careful use of curets in the neuroforamen Preoperative angiographies or angio-MRI for the presence of thrombi or aberrant loops
Inadequate postoperative immobilization (see Chap. 19)	Nonunion Graft collapse or mobilization Postsurgical deformity	Correct use of instrumentation Prolonged use postoperative bracing in older patients

12.2.2.3 Distractive Flexion Injuries

Distractive flexion injuries are classified into four stages. Stage 1: forward subluxation of the upper facet in the motion segment with widening of the space between spinous process, resulting in a stretch injury to the posterior ligamentous complex. In Stage 1 (flexion sprain), there is a variable degree of disruption of the posterior ligaments and facet capsules without damage to the vertebral disc. Stage 2: unilateral facet dislocation up to 25% forward subluxation of the vertebral body in the motion segment. Stage 3: bilateral facet dislocation with approximately 50% anterior subluxation of the upper vertebra in the motion segment. Stage 4: gross anterior displacement of the upper vertebra on the lower vertebra in the motion segment (floating vertebra).

In Stage 1 injuries, application of a rigid orthosis can be a good therapeutic option. The exact length of the treatment depends on the symptoms and radiographic signs of stability on flexion-extension views. Unilateral facet dislocation (Stage 2) must be promptly reduced with traction. Many patients heal with halo fixator or another rigid orthotic immobilization, although other patients may require surgery. Patients with Stage 3 and 4 injuries commonly have neurological involvement and must be managed with prompt surgical reduction. Immobilization of these unstable lesions with halo fixator often results in recurrent subluxation or dislocation; therefore, reduction is followed by surgery. One of the reasons for failure of closed reduction can be the presence of a large disc herniation. In the presence of a frank disc herniation at the dislocated segment, anterior discectomy and arthrodesis must be considered.

12.2.2.4 Compressive Extensions

Compressive extensions injuries are classified into five stages. Stage 1: unilateral vertebral arch fracture (pedicle, facet, and/or lamina) with or without rotational displacement of the vertebral body. Stage 2: bilateral laminar fracture without evidence of soft-tissue failure. Stage 3: bilateral disruption of the articular pillars (pedicle, facet ,and/or lamina) without displacement. Stage 4: bilateral disruption of the articular pillars with partial forward subluxation of the fractured vertebra on the vertebra below. Stage 5: bilateral arch fracture with full vertebral body width displacement of the fractured vertebra on the vertebra below. Stage 5: injuries have high incidence of partial or complete spinal chord sparing.

In patients with Stage 1 injuries, hard collar or halo fixator are good therapeutic options. In patients with Stage 2 injuries, there are rarely associated neurological injuries, and immobilization in hard collar or halo fixator is usually sufficient. In patients with neurological involvement, surgery is required.

12.2.2.5 Distractive Extension

Distractive extension injuries are classified into two stages. Stage 1: failure of the anterior longitudinal ligament and annulus fibrosus with widening of the intervertebral disc space anteriorly on radiographs. Stage 2: same findings of Stage 1 injuries with associated posterior displacement of the upper vertebra in the motion segment [25].

Patients with Stage 1 injuries with a large bony involvement may be managed with halo fixator, while patients with lesions involving purely ligamentous structure can be managed with early surgery, because ligaments often do not heal. Patients with Stage 2 injuries are managed with surgery.

12.2.2.6 Lateral Compression

Lateral compression injuries are classified into two stages. Stage 1: asymmetric compression failure of the vertebral body with an ipsilateral, undisplaced vertebral arch fracture. Stage 2: displacement of the vertebral arch fracture or widening of the contralateral articular processes. Fractures of the articular processes, dislocations, or fracture-dislocations are commonly surgically managed via a posterior approach, because it is possible to reduce and stabilize the fracture onto the articular processes. Fractures involving the vertebral body are usually managed via an anterior approach.

12.2.2.7 Complications

Complications associated with surgical techniques in patients with trauma of the lower cervical spine include:

- Myeloradicular injuries
- Vascular lesions
- Lesions to the deep structures of the neck
- Complications related to bone graft and hardware
- Myeloradicular injuries

The spinal cord fills about 35% of the canal at the level of the atlas and approximately 50% of the canal in the remaining portion of the cervical spine (C2–C7). CSF, epidural fat, and meninges fill the remainder of the canal. Up to 5% of patients with a cervical SCI deteriorate neurologically in the early peritrauma period. Around 50% of these cases are iatrogenic. Myeloradicular structures may be damaged following manipulation of an unstable cervical spine with cord edema. To avoid adverse surgical manipulation of the myeloradicular structures, delayed surgery has been proposed in patients with symptomaticneurologiccompression.Electrophysiologic techniques (i.e. somatosensory-evoked or motor-evoked potentials) may monitor neurological integrity in the operating room [26]. Central necrosis of the gray matter with resultant syrinx formation may result from the initial injury or continued microtrauma to the myeloradicular structures, resulting in late ascending paralysis [27].

Myeloradicular injuries may also result from errors during surgery. During the anterior approach, they can arise from use of excessively long screws, which penetrate the posterior cortex and directly injure the dura and underlying neurologic structures, especially when attempting bicortical screw fixation or during the drilling process [28]. It is therefore important to use a drill guide with fixed depth that prevents inadvertent posterior cortex penetration. Bicortical screw fixation can also lead to hematomas in the spinal canal owing to lesions of the venous plexus surrounding the spinal cord, which is located beyond the posterior vertebral wall. When bicortical fixation is performed, dural tear with consequent liquoral leak and fistulae can be encountered. Bicortical screw insertion can be avoided with the use of screws wider than 4 mm diameter with large thread, associated with the use of plates allowing for 10–15° divergent screw insertion on both the sagittal and horizontal planes that improve implant stability and anchoring even with monocortical fixation.

During techniques with a posterior approach to the lower cervical spine, inadvertent penetration into the ligamentum flavum and the spinal canal can occur if careful subperiosteal dissection is not performed. Dural penetration can also occur during the passage of wires too close to the dura. The most common complication associated with wiring procedures in the cervical spine is the loss of fixation and subsequent recurrence of deformity, the latter often being secondary to inadequate postoperative external support. Passage of laminar wirings or the use of laminar hooks should be avoided at the level of injury, where the spinal cord has already been injured by edema or mechanical compression, because a high risk of dural tears and cord lesions at that level can occur.

(a) Vascular lesions

Vascular injuries can arise from the mechanism of trauma, or from the maneuvers of reduction. Carotid artery damage may occur especially during the anterolateral surgical approach. The vertebral artery is the structure most likely at risk for injury with pedicle screw placement (see Chap. 8). The strict anatomic relationship between the vertebral artery and the vertebrae, especially in the lateral portion of the vertebra (foramen transversarium, uncovertebral joints) is a risk factor for injuries to the vertebral artery. Typical vertebral lesions that can involve the vertebral artery are represented by those of the posterior joints, which may determine a damage on the artery. The same may occur for dislocation of the vertebral body. Even though lesions in the vertebral artery can result in decreased flow to the Willis' circle, the majority of the cases are asymptomatic and the lesions are discovered at angiography or angio-MRI. The injury to the vertebral artery act as an alarm for the surgeon during the surgical maneuvers to reduce the fragments of the fractures, and the surgeon must be ready to clamp the artery above and below. In the case of intraoperative bleeding, the artery must be clamped in the intertransversary space, with care to avoid clamping of the nerve roots that are close to the vessel. When it is possible, it is simpler to open above and below the intertransversary foramina to expose the vessel and the adjacent nerve root.

(b) Lesions to the deep structures of the neck

Lesions to the deep structures of the neck are mainly related to the surgical approach and have been extensively treated in another section (see Chap. 8). A peculiar complication of patients with multiple fragments fracture (i.e. tear drop fractures) is the esophageal fistula. This is secondary to a direct trauma over the wall of the esophagus leading to a tear and local necrosis,

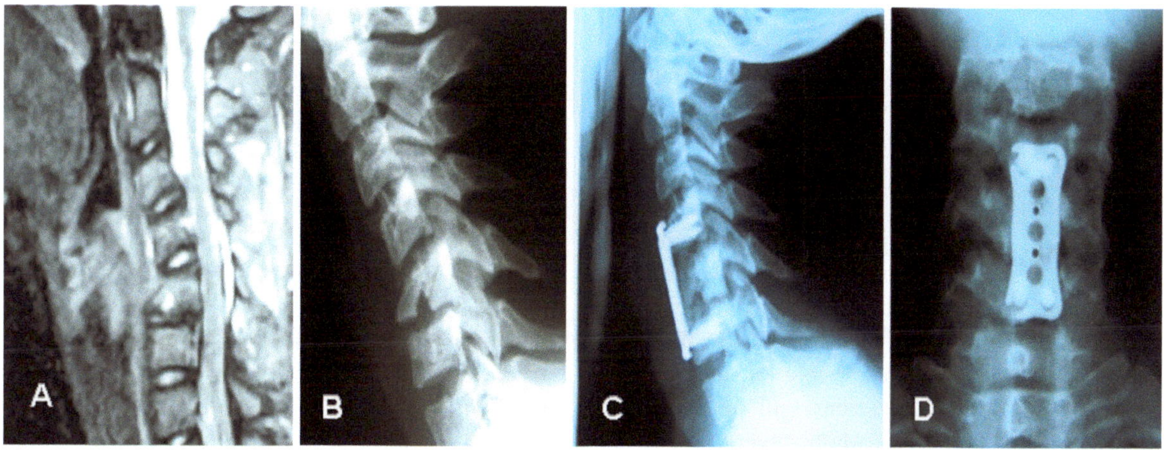

Fig. 12.8 (**a**) MRI scan and (**b**) Lateral radiograph of a patient with a classical tear-drop fracture with anterior bony displaced fragment that impinges over the adjacent soft tissues. (**c, d**) Surgery consisted in reduction of the halo and then anterior decompression and fusion with plate fixation

eventually evolving into a fistula. If these lesions are mainly related to unstable fractures with anterior dislocated fragments (Fig. 12.8), then the surgeon should suspect this in advance and treat lesions intraoperatively.

(c) Complications related to instrumentation fixation and/or failure

Serious complication associated with anterior instrumentation of the cervical spine is hardware loosening and subsequent injury to the surrounding structures. Factors leading to this complication are mainly inadequate postoperative immobilization of the patient (See Chap. 20) and the use of inappropriate instrumentation. Screw or plate mobilization can impinge on the adjacent esophageal wall and evolve up to esophageal perforation with screw expulsion from the mouth or swallowing. To decrease this occurrence, plates with screw retention can be used. In these cases, when mobilization occurs, the conflict with the whole instrumentation leads to immediate dysphagia and allow for early recognition and treatment. Hardware loosening may be the result of osteoporosis with insufficient bony purchase, or being secondary to technical challenges when multiple attempts at screw insertion have led to inadequate purchase. Use of screws with small diameter (less than 3 mm) and low thread do not allow for adequate fixation in the trabecular bone of the vertebral body. Bone quality is another factor related to screw pull-out and is dependent on bone loss or osteoporosis secondary to systemic diseases or pharmacological therapy (see Chap. 1). The plate should be properly molded in lordosis to follow the physiological contour of the cervical spine. The place for the plate position should be adequately prepared by careful anterior osteophyte or fracture fragment removal. If plate contour does not match the anterior aspect of the cervical spine, screws cannot be inserted completely, and a lever arm is created, which favors implant mobilization.

An additional and relatively common complication of anterior cervical plating is misplacement of the screws into the adjacent disc spaces. This complication can be recognized intraoperatively by fluoroscopy obtained after screw placement for confirmation. When screw penetration of the disc space occurs, a high risk of screw-loosening occurs because of movement of the motion segment across the disc space, and the screw should be removed and redirected to a safe bony area. Prevention of screw misplacement can take advantage of proper plate-sizing. It is critical that the chosen plate extends only from the mid-portion of the vertebral bodies above and below the decompressed segment.

During posterior approach, lateral mass screw complications are often related to pass pointing of the drill bit during drilling, screw misplacement, or an oversized screw (too long). The risk of screw placement increases with bicortical screw placement. Other complications associated with screw insertion include screw pullout, iatrogenic foraminal stenosis, facet joint violation, implant failure, and adjacent segment degeneration.

Core Messages

- When treating injuries at the cervical spine, the main goals are spine realignment and stability, and prevention of further neurological damage while promoting neurological and functional recovery.
- Cervical spine injury patients are also divided based on the neurological involvement: patients with SCI will be considered as unstable in any case, while neurologically intact patients can be either stable or unstable. Patients with stable lesions will be treated mainly conservatively, while surgery is indicated in most patients with unstable fractures.
- Patients with SCI should be referred for early surgery of decompression, stabilization, and instrumented fusion.
- Most common complications encountered in this surgery are myeloradicular injuries, hollow viscus and vascular lesions, and complications related to instrumentation fixation and/or failure.
- Anterior odontoid screw fixation need an adequate training and should be performed with respect to strict surgical indications. Patients who are not candidates can benefit from posterior surgical reduction and fusion strategies.
- The halo fixator continues to be an important tool for cervical spine fracture management, and preoperatively, halo fixation may be used to achieve gradual correction of spinal deformity.

References

1. Boni M, Cherubino P, Denaro V (1983) The surgical treatment of fractures of the cervical spine. Ital J Orthop Traumatol 9(Suppl):107–126
2. Boni M, Denaro V (1980) Surgical treatment of traumatic lesions of the middle and lower cervical spine (C3–C7). Ital J Orthop Traumatol 6:305–320
3. Roy-Camille R, Saillant G, Judet T, de Botton G, Michel G (1980) Factors of severity in the fractures of the odontoid process (author's transl). Rev Chir Orthop Reparatrice Appar Mot 66:183–186
4. Roy-Camille R, Saillant G, Laville C, Benazet JP (1992) Treatment of lower cervical spinal injuries–C3 to C7. Spine 17:S442–S446
5. Senegas J, Gauzere JM (1977) Unstable fractures of the spine. IV. Stabilization methods and their results. B. Surgical methods. 6. Treatment of cervical lesions by anterior approach. Rev Chir Orthop Reparatrice Appar Mot 63:466–469
6. Roy-Camille R, Saillant G, Judet T, Mammoudy P (1982) Recent trauma of the lower 5 cervical vertebrae (with or without neurological complications). Ann Chir 36:735–744
7. Roy-Camille R, Saillant G, Judet T, Mammoudy P (1983) Recent injuries of the last 5 cervical vertebrae in the adult (with and without neurologic complications). Sem Hop 59:1479–1488
8. Alcelik I, Manik KS, Sian PS, Khoshneviszadeh SE (2006) Occipital condylar fractures. Review of the literature and case report. J Bone Joint Surg Br 88:665–669
9. Anderson PA, Montesano PX (1988) Morphology and treatment of occipital condyle fractures. Spine 13:731–736
10. Bellabarba C, Mirza SK, Chapman JR (2006) Injuries of the Craniocervical Junction. In: Bucholz RW, Heckman JD, Court-Brown CM (eds) Rockwood & Green's fractures in adults, 6th edn. Lippincott Williams & Wilkins, Philadelphia, pp 1544–1585
11. Anderson PA, Sohail KM, Chapman JR (2004) Injuries to the atlantooccipital articulation. In: Clark CR (ed) The cervical spine, 4th edn. Lippincott Williams & Wilkins, Philadelphia, pp 587–607
12. Hasharoni A, Thomas E (2004) Transverse ligament injury. In: Clark CR (ed) The cervical spine, 4th edn. Lippincott Williams & Wilkins, Philadelphia, pp 608–613
13. Anderson LD, D'Alonzo RT (1974) Fractures of the odontoid process of the axis. J Bone Joint Surg Am 56:1663–1674
14. Rao G, Apfelbaum RI (2004) Dens fracture. In: Clark CR (ed) The cervical spine, 4th edn. Lippincott Williams & Wilkins, Philadelphia, pp 614–628
15. Denaro V (ed) (1991) Surgical approaches in stenosis of the cervical spine. Springer, Berlin, pp 81–138
16. Denaro V (ed) (1991) Imaging in stenosis of the cervical spine. Springer, Berlin, pp 51–62
17. Magerl F, Seemann PS (1985) Stable posterior fusion of the atlas and axis by transarticular screw fixation. In: Kehr P, Weidner A (eds) Cervical spine. Springer Wien, New York, pp 322–327
18. Barbour JR (1971) Screw fixation and fractures of the odontoid process. S Austral Clin 5:20–24
19. Harms J, Melcher RP (2001) Posterior C1–C2 fusion with polyaxial screw and rod fixation. Spine 26:2467–2471
20. Effendi B, Roy D, Cornish B, Dussault RG, Laurin CA (1981) Fractures of the ring of the axis: a classification based on the analysis of 131 cases. J Bone Joint Surg Br 63: 319–327
21. Levine AM, Dacre A (2004) Traumatic spondylolisthesis of the axis: "Hangman's fracture". In: Clark CR (ed) The cervical spine, 4th edn. Lippincott Williams & Wilkins, Philadelphia, pp 629–650
22. Anderson DG, Vaccaro AR (2004) Classification of lower cervical spine injuries, Chapter 47. In: Clark CR (ed) The cervical spine, 4th edn. Lippincott Williams & Wilkins, Philadelphia, pp 651–659
23. Vives MJ (2004) Flexion injuries, Chapter 48. In: Clark CR (ed) The cervical spine, 4th edn. Lippincott Williams & Wilkins, Philadelphia, pp 660-670
24. Mekhail AO, Steinmetz MP, Benzel EC (2004) Subaxial cervical spine burst fracture, Chapter 50. In: Clark CR (ed) The cervical spine, 4th edn. Lippincott Williams & Wilkins, Philadelphia, pp 683–695

25. Vives MJ, Garfin SR (2004) Extension injuries, Chapter 49. In: Clark CR (ed) The cervical spine, 4th edn. Lippincott Williams & Wilkins, Philadelphia, pp 671–682
26. Denaro V, D'Alpa F, Grasso A (1991) Neurophysiological studies in cervical stenosis. In: Denaro V (eds) Stenosis of the cervical spine. Springer, Brelin, pp 71–80
27. Bono CM (2006) Fractures and dislocations of the lower cervical spine. In: Bucholz RW, Heckman JD, Court-Brown CM (eds) Rockwood & Green's fractures in adults, 6th edn. Lippincott Williams & Wilkins, Philadelphia, pp 1498–1543
28. Denaro V (ed) (1991) Surgical techniques in stenosis of the cervical spine. Springer, Berlin, pp 139–278

Infections of the Cervical Spine

13

Luca Denaro, Umile Giuseppe Longo, and Vincenzo Denaro

Contents

L. Denaro (✉)
Department of Neuroscience, University of Padua,
Via Giustiniani 5, 35128 Padua, Italy
e-mail: lucadenaro@hotmail.com

13.1 Introduction

Spinal infections are relatively rare, accounting for only 2–4% of all osteomyelitis infections, and are located preferentially in the thoracic and lumbar segments. Although the cervical segment is the less common spine localization, cervical spinal infections present the highest incidence of neurological involvement [6].

Recent advances in diagnosis and management – with the introduction of antibiotics and more aggressive surgery – greatly improved the prognosis of patients with cervical spinal infection [6].

Spinal infections have a highly variable outcome [6], with dramatic consequences in some patients. Mortality is estimated around 1–20%, depending on the infecting agent and the general health status of the patient. The incidence of paralysis because of direct cord involvement is up to 50%, depending on the patient population and the involved spinal segment.

Cervical spine infections remain a therapeutic challenge. In the suspicion of cervical spine infection, prompt diagnosis and management are a must. Accurate diagnosis and treatment of osteomyelitis in a timely manner is critical for preventing severe neurological injury [1]. Delay in diagnosis, the long recovery period, and the great cost of managing such infections remain unsolved problems.

Reconstructive surgery for cervical spinal infection has become more aggressive after the development of chemotherapeutic drugs. Radical surgical excision and antibiotic therapy are today regarded as the cornerstone of the management of such infections. Internal fixation is frequently used to stabilize the operated segment. Chemotherapeutics provide ancillary support for excision procedure in the majority of the patients.

L. Denaro et al. (eds.), *Pitfalls in Cervical Spine Surgery*,
DOI: 10.1007/978-3-540-85019-9_13, © Springer-Verlag Berlin Heidelberg 2010

Generally, osteomyelitis can be classified as acute, subacute, or chronic, depending on the duration of the symptoms. Osteomyelitis can also be classified as pyogenic or nonpyogenic. The mechanism of infection can be classified as exogenous or hematogenous. Exogenous osteomyelitis can occur by direct infection (through surgical manipulation or trauma), or by local spread from contiguous infected local structures.

Hematogenous osteomyelitis of the cervical spine can be the consequence of any condition determining bacteremia, including urinary, respiratory tract, and soft-tissue infections. The incidence of hematogenous infection of the cervical spine is about 6% of the patients with vertebral osteomyelitis. Many risk factors are involved in the development of a cervical spinal infection (see also Chap. 1), including elderly, history of drug abuse (alcohol/drug users), immunosuppressive conditions (HIV, steroid users, diabetes), tumors, renal failure, septicemia, concurrent infections, and smoking. In addition, all these conditions complicate treatment and limit the ability of the host to fight infection.

The vast majority of bacteria cause pyogenic infections, but some families of bacteria produce chronic granulomatous infections. Pyogenic infections may result from iatrogenic contamination, from traumatic injuries or blood dissemination in any condition determining bacteremia. The most common infectious organism is *Staphylococcus aureus.* Today, it accounts for 50% of all spinal osteomyelitis, but in the past, it was responsible for almost all the cases of spinal infections. *Pseudomonas aeruginosa*, *Escherichia coli*, and *Proteus* are the most common gram-negative pathogens causing cervical spinal infections. *Pseudomonas aeruginosa* is frequently responsible for osteomyelitis in heroin abusers. Anaerobic infections are uncommon [8].

Fungi, spirochetes, and certain bacteria (Mycobacteriaceae, Actinomycetales, and Nocardiaceae) may cause granulomatous infections. Among the various granulomatous infections, the most common one worldwide is tuberculosis. All the granulomatous infections determine similar clinical pictures, and have similar surgical management. The antibiotic drugs to be used in these patients vary according to the infecting pathogens, and often require the help of an infectious-disease specialist.

The starting area of spinal infection is controversial. The intervertebral disc is considered as the primary starting area only for infections resulting from direct inoculation. The metaphyses and cartilaginous endplates are regarded as the starting areas for hematogenous infections.

The incidence of tuberculous spondylitis is variable worldwide, and depends on the quality of the available public health services. The diagnosis of tuberculous spondylitis is often delayed as a result of the rarity of the pathology, and therefore a high index of suspicion is required to avoid misdiagnosis.

In this chapter, we give an overview of the postoperative cervical spine infections.

13.2 Iatrogenic Infections

Although the use of perioperative antibiotics and advances in sterility and surgical technique greatly improved the outcome of patients with postoperative infections after cervical spinal surgery, the latter remain as one of the most troublesome pitfalls after cervical spine surgery with potentially devastating sequelae.

As stated earlier, the rate of infection after cervical spine surgery is variable and depends on many intrinsic and extrinsic factors, including the immunological and nutrition state of the patient [6], choice of surgical approach, and use of internal devices (plates, cage, etc.).

13.2.1 Intrinsic Risk Factors

Higher rate of infection has been reported in immunocompromised patients.

Genetic disorders carry a high risk of complications. Down's syndrome, the result of trisomy of chromosome 21, remains the most common human chromosomal abnormality. Approximately 20% of all patients with Down's syndrome experience orthopedic problems. Most are related to hypotonia, joint hypermobility, and ligamentous laxity. Upper cervical spine instability associated with atlanto-occipital and atlantoaxial hypermobility, and bony anomalies of the cervical spine is common in patient with Down's syndrome. Since it was first reported by Spitzer in 1961 [18], the high potential for morbidity, particularly infection and wound-healing problems, has been a major concern [14]. Postoperative infections in patients with Down's syndrome range between 15 and 30% [5].

Diabetes, corticosteroid therapy, previous spinal surgery, obesity, chronic infection and smoking, extended preoperative hospitalization, prolonged operation duration, and high blood loss have been showed to be the risk factors for postoperative infection in a retrospective survey of 850 spinal procedures [22].

The presence of diabetes mellitus has deleterious effects on the outcome following spine surgery. Patients with high preoperative glucose levels undergoing elective surgery should be differed, as uncontrolled preoperative glucose levels may increase the infection risk.

Patients with rheumatoid arthritis are generally immunocompromised, because of the systemic pathology and the prolonged regime of therapy (steroid therapy is per se a known risk factor) [6].

Patients undergoing organ transplant has been traditionally considered at high risk of infection after surgery. With the enormous advances in the field of organ transplantation, a growing number of transplant patients present for a variety of surgical procedures. The most disconcerting issue in these patients is the chronic immunosuppressive therapy. Hence, broad-spectrum coverage should be considered.

Human immunodeficiency virus (HIV) infection has become a chronic illness requiring continuing medical care and patient self-management education to prevent acute complications and to reduce the risk of long-term complications. Orthopedic surgeons practicing in areas with a high prevalence of HIV infection may expect that up to 10% of their patients who undergo emergent procedures and 1–3% of those who undergo elective surgery will be HIV-positive [11].

Although basic science studies have demonstrated impairment of defenses to routine orthopedic pathogens as well as to opportunistic organisms, clinical studies have demonstrated that this impairment has not resulted in an increased incidence of postoperative infections or failure of wound healing in the asymptomatic HIV-positive patients. Current medical management seems adequate to prevent increased risk of early postoperative infection in the symptomatic HIV-positive patients undergoing orthopedic procedures. The HIV-positive patient with a cervical spine implant may be at increased risk for late hematogenous implant infection as the host defenses diminish. Even though no studies addressed the specific issue of postoperative complications in patients with HIV, regular medical attention, prophylactic antibiotic therapy before invasive procedures, and early evaluation and management of possible infections are regarded as good prophylactic measures. Decisions regarding elective surgery should be made on a risk–benefit basis. It should be kept in mind that infections occurring in HIV patients can have devastating effects, with a mortality rate exceeding 20% [16]. Because the risk of infective surgical complications increases with progression of the disease, guidelines for elective surgery should include an assessment of the HIV-positive patient's immune status, including the CD4 lymphocyte count, history of opportunistic infection, serum albumin level, the presence of skin allergy, and the state of nutrition and general health.

13.2.2 Extrinsic Risk Factors

Many intraoperative factors have been associated with a higher incidence of postoperative spine infections. They include the increased invasiveness and length of surgical procedures, the use of a single glove, the use of additional intraoperative equipment, and a high number of personnel in the operating room. Double gloving, limiting traffic and conversation in the operative room, handling tissues carefully, and periodically releasing self-retaining retractors to allow reperfusion of muscles are measures that decrease the incidence of intraoperative infections.

The invasive nature of surgery, with its increased exposure to blood, means that during surgery there is a high risk of transfer of pathogens [20]. Pathogens can be transferred through surgical contact between the patients and the surgical team, resulting in postoperative or blood-borne infections in patients or blood-borne infections in the surgical team. Both patients and the surgical team need to be protected from this risk, which can be reduced by implementing protective barriers such as wearing surgical gloves.

Wearing two pairs of surgical gloves, triple gloves, glove liners, or cloth outer gloves, as opposed to one pair, is considered to provide an additional barrier and further reduce the risk of contamination. A systematic review conducted by Tanner and Parkinson [20] showed that, to date, the addition of a second pair of surgical gloves significantly reduces perforations to innermost gloves. Triple gloving, knitted outer gloves, and glove liners also significantly reduce perforations to the innermost glove. Perforation indicator systems result in significantly more innermost glove perforations being detected during surgery.

Intraoperative fluoroscopy is used routinely in the operating room for many spinal procedures because it allows the surgeon to confirm the correct operative levels, assess the alignment in multiple planes, and monitor fracture reduction and instrumentation placement. Several different intraoperative fluoroscopy devices are commercially available. All of them are commonly referred to as "C-arms." The portion of the machine over or near the operative field is covered with a sterile drape and care is taken throughout the entire duration of the surgical procedure to ensure maintenance of sterility. Nevertheless, the risk of bacterial contamination exists with any sterile equipment that is employed in an operating room setting.

Biswas et al. [3] conducted a prospective study to evaluate the sterility of 25 C-arm drapes after their use during spine surgery. They concluded that the upper portions of the C-arm exhibited the greatest rates of contamination during spinal procedures, most likely occurring when the undraped portions of the C-arm were rotated to acquire lateral images. The top portion of the C-arm drape should not be considered as sterile in these situations, and avoiding contact with these areas may probably decrease the risks of intraoperative contamination and possibly postoperative infections.

The traffic in and out of the operative room should be kept to a minimum. Self-retaining retractors should be periodically removed or released, and the wound should be irrigated with saline solution.

Operative wounds are frequently contaminated by bacteria originating from the patients' own skin, surgeons' gloves, and dust particles in the atmosphere of the operating theater. Contamination occurs even when careful attention has been paid to theater airflow systems and skin preparation. The contaminating bacterial load is roughly proportional to the length of the time a wound remains open. As a consequence, major operative procedures, such as those involving extensive and prolonged exposure of the spinal structures, are at increased risk of being complicated by surgical site infections [4]. Although in literature there is a lack of adequate-powered, well-designed and conducted randomized controlled trials, in our settings, we usually perform antimicrobial prophylaxis, and copious multiple wound irrigations to prevent infections during cervical spinal surgery.

Each surgical approach carries different risks that must be recognized in an attempt to avoid infection.

Transoral surgeries have been historically related to a greater incidence of infections, upto 66% [6] (see Chap. 7). Despite the initial negative experiences, after the introduction of the operating microscope, operative magnification, and micro-instrumentation [6], the improvement of preoperative imaging with more definite localization of pathology [7], availability of antibiotics, and new devices and techniques to manage dural tears, the transoral approach has gained its well-deserved place in the orthopedic armamentarium [13]. The incidence of infections after transoral surgery currently rates between 0 and 3% [6], similar to anterolateral or posterior approaches [6].

In the anterolateral approach, perforation of the esophagus may lead to life-threatening infections, because of the risk of sequelae from mediastinitis, purulent spondylitis, meningitis, or septicemia [15]. Any tear of the esophagus should be immediately detected and managed to reduce the risk of infection [6] (see Chap. 8).

Respiratory sequelae in spinal cord injured patients have been shown to directly affect the length of the stay in the acute setting and hospital costs [23]. Early tracheostomy has been shown to increase patient's comfort, decrease the need for sedation, improve patient's communication, and reduce weaning time and respiratory morbidity in intensive care unit. In patients with acute cervical spine trauma undergoing anterior cervical stabilization, the optimal timing of tracheostomy after anterior cervical spine surgery remains controversial because of the potential for cross-contamination and deep infection due to the proximity of the surgical wound to the tracheostomy site. Currently, however, there is poor evidence to indicate the safe timing of tracheostomy in these patients.

Berney et al. [2], in a retrospective study, compared the infection rates in patients requiring tracheostomy undergoing anterior vs. posterior cervical spine surgery, and reported the timing of tracheostomy tube placement in such patients. Seventy-one patients with a diagnosis of acute cervical spine injury were included in the study. Tracheostomy was performed on an average of 4 days after cervical stabilization procedure. They found seven suspected tracheostomy site infections in patients who underwent anterior stabilization with only one patient developing infection with the same organism at both the tracheostomy site and the anterior stabilization site. This cross-infection was associated with no evidence of deeper infection or subsequent nonunion, and it was managed with antibiotics. No patient required further surgical intervention. The authors concluded that early tracheostomy after spinal stabilization is associated with a low risk of infection even after the anterior approach.

During posterior approach to the cervical spine, stripping procedure can devascularize the musculotendinous tissue. Debridement of obviously devitalized areas has been proposed to decrease the risk of secondary contamination within the necrotic regions, but it is not commonly performed because of concerns of inadequate bony coverage and increased bleeding.

The incidence of surgical site infection following spinal surgery usually increases with the addition of instrumentation. Obviously, infections associated with surgical implants are generally more difficult to manage, because they require a longer period of antibiotic therapy and repeated surgical procedures.

13.2.3 Classification

Wound infections are generally classified as superficial and deep.

A superficial infection is located superficial to the deep fascia. Classical features include pain, tenderness, and signs of the infection (swelling, erythema, fluctuation, drainage, and fever). Superficial wound infection must be managed aggressively, because of the risk of extension below the deep fascia.

Deep infections are, by definition, located below the deep fascia. The wound may have completely normal features, and the patient may complain of progressive neck pain and fever.

Osteomyelitis, an infective process accompanied by bone destruction, is not a necessary component of a deep wound infection, particularly when managed early. Osteomyelitis can occur as the consequence of direct intraoperative contamination, by a deep wound infection, or hematogenous or lymphatic route.

Discitis is an infection of the disc space, which can develop whenever the disc is violated, as in discectomy, discometry, discography, interbody fusion procedures, and minimally invasive disc surgery (percutaneous nucleotomy, chemonucleolysis, and microdiscectomy).

The intervertebral disc is the largest avascular structure of the human body. It receives the nutrient supply by diffusion through the endplates and the blood vessels in the annulus fibrosus. Pathogens are introduced by direct inoculation at the time of penetration, although infection can also develop following spread from a contiguous focus. Staphylococci (*S. aureus* and coagulase-negative *Staphylococci*) are the most common pathogens responsible for infections. Aerobic gram-negative bacilli and *Propionibacterium* spp. account for most of the remainder.

In recent decades, increasing popularity of imaging and surgical procedures violating the intervertebral space was the main factor contributing to the rise in the incidence of iatrogenic discitis. Also, magnetic resonance imaging scanning is currently a valuable tool in the diagnosis of iatrogenic discitis, and is significantly more sensitive than radiography and computed tomography scanning, which were used in the past. The risk of disc space infection (overall incidence rating from <1 to 5%) depends on the type of intervention, but is generally lower in patients undergoing simple discectomy (0–3%). Despite the low incidence of iatrogenic discitis, the incidence of long-term morbidity among the affected patients is high, and the percentage of patients unable to resume their normal work ranges from 55.4 to 87.5% [17].

The patient may present with chills, fever, axial or radicular pain, and night sweats. Epidural abscesses may complicate discitis. They are of special interest to spine surgeons because they often result in acute neurological deterioration and require a combination of surgical and conservative treatments.

Particular organisms can lead to necrotizing fascial infections. Necrotizing wound infections are extremely rare, but life-threatening. Kauffman et al. [9] described a case of synergistic rapidly progressive necrotizing gangrenous fasciitis after spinal surgery in a 39-year-old man. The infection was successfully managed with serial debridements, appropriate antibiotics, and hyperbaric wound oxygenation.

13.2.4 Diagnosis

A high index of suspicion is central to the diagnosis of cervical osteomyelitis. The clinical presentation and timing of postoperative cervical spinal infection is variable, depending on the infected structure.

13.2.4.1 Laboratory Findings

The white blood cell (WBC) count may be increased, but is generally aspecific. C-reactive protein (CRP) and erythrocyte sedimentation rate (ESR) are usually used to determine the presence of infection. However, they are normally increased postoperatively. Thelander et al. [21] prospectively measured CRP and ESR after four types of uncomplicated lumbar spinal surgeries. In all patients, preoperative normal CRP increased, with peak levels on the second day after microdiscectomy and anterior fusion, and at the third day after conventional discectomy and posterolateral interbody fusion, with normalization in 5–14 days. Peak levels were not related to bleeding, transfusion, operation time, administered drugs, age, or sex. ESR increased to peak levels about 5 days postoperatively, followed by a slow and irregular decrease, and often remained elevated at 21–42 days postoperatively. Unfortunately, such data are not available for patients undergoing cervical spinal surgery.

Takahashi et al. [19] prospectively measured the WBC count and WBC differential after spinal instrumentation surgery with or without surgical wound infection to investigate the usefulness of WBC differential for early diagnosis of surgical wound infection after spinal instrumented surgery. They proposed that lymphopenia representing immunodepression status indicates the increased susceptibility to infection, which may occur postoperatively. If lymphopenia is diagnosed as early as possible, surgical wound infection can be managed promptly without removing the instrumentation.

Plasma procalcitonin increases rapidly during bacterial infections, but remains low in viral infections and other inflammatory processes. We used it as a useful marker in the diagnosis of osteomyelitis.

The presence of bacteria at Gram stain or culture is diagnostic of infection. Wound exploration and debridement are mandatory, and tissue samples for cultures may be obtained intraoperatively.

13.2.4.2 Imaging

Imaging studies are often not specific enough to guide the choice of management.

Radiographs are normally ineffective to diagnose an acute postoperative infection, because wide bone loss is necessary before being detectable on radiographs. However, conventional radiographs may provide additional information, such as loosening of spinal alignment or hardware or graft position, reduction of the disc space, and segmental kyphosis.

Lucency around hardware, grafts, or within the vertebrae is characteristic of infection in patients with more delayed infections. The presence of air in the soft tissues may indicate a gas-forming fascial infection or an esophageal tear [6].

The postoperative findings revealed by computed tomography and magnetic resonance imaging (edema, seroma, and hematoma) are difficult, if not impossible, to differentiate from infection.

Magnetic resonance imaging has a key role in the diagnosis of epidural abscess, and is important in preoperative planning of decompression.

Contrast magnetic resonance imaging is the method of choice for a reliable diagnosis in clinically suspicious cases [10].

Computed tomography-guided biopsy may be of utility in the presence of a suspicious lesion or fluid collection.

Bone scan maintains a well-reserved place in the diagnosis of infection of the cervical spine. The ability to radiolabel inflammatory cells that migrate to the foci of infection was a significant milestone in the evolution of infection imaging. Labeled leukocyte imaging is a useful tool to diagnose osteomyelitis, allowing distinguishing infections from other cervical spinal pathologies.

13.2.5 Management

The management of postoperative cervical spinal infection represents one of the greatest challenges to the spine surgeon. These infections are often complex and difficult to manage, and result in acute neurological deterioration and require a combination of adequate conservative and operative management options.

13.2.5.1 Wound Infections

Wound complications involving large subcutaneous tissue represents a significant issue for the surgeon. The cornerstone of the management of cervical spine wound infection includes:

- Exploration and debridement
- Antibiotic therapy
- Proper nutrition and medical management
- Appropriate wound care

The management of wound infection must be performed without delay. Exploration and debridement are mandatory, with the removal of all the devitalized tissues. Samples for cultures must be obtained at surgery. Subcutaneous tissue must be abundantly irrigated and debrided. Some authors, in the case of intact deep fascia and absence of signs of septicemia, proposed to limit the debridement to the superficial planes, performing aspiration of the subfascial planes. According to Massie et al. [12], we preferred to perform a debridement down to the bone in every patient. Infected or loosened bone graft must be removed. A growing body of evidence seems to support that hardware may be left in place, unless it has failed [6].

The wound closure options include closure over drains in each layer, open packing with delayed closure, and open packing with healing by second intention [6]. The indication and technique depend on the type of infection, the features of the wound, and the patient's risk factors. In patients with lesion of the esophagus, the wound is left open and heals by secondary intention.

13.2.5.2 Discitis

Nonoperative management, including intravenous antibiotic therapy and external immobilization, at the early stages are appropriate in the absence of neurological signs or symptoms, instability, deformity, or spinal cord compression. Standard initial management of postoperative cervical discitis is bedrest, hard collar, and intravenous antibiotics.

Antibiotics are usually administered empirically, although some surgeons may opt to obtain tissue culture from a percutaneous biopsy [6]. In our clinical practice, we always attempt to perform a biopsy to determine the pathogen responsible for the disease and administer selective antibiotics.

Despite the intervertebral disc being an avascular structure, antibiotics are frequently successful in the management of cervical spinal infections. Surgical debridement is indicated in patients with neurological signs or symptoms, instability, deformity, or spinal cord compression.

13.2.5.3 Vertebral Osteomyelitis

The management of postoperative osteomyelitis follows standard principles of primary bone infection. The involved area is exposed and necrotic bone is removed until a healthy bleeding surface is exposed, with care to protect the neural elements. The wound is copiously irrigated to remove all loose pieces. Stability must be ascertained. Large defects must be reconstructed. Both allograft and autograft appear suitable for this purpose, even in the presence of active infection. In our clinical practice, we use both allograft and autograft, and avoid the use of cages, whose implantation is not indicated in the site of infection [6]. The use of instrumentation in cervical spine osteomyelitis remains debated because of the perceived risk of persistent infection related to any spinal hardware. In our settings, after performing a wide debridement of the infected structures, if internal fixation is required, we insert the screws in the noninfected adjacent vertebrae.

In particular, there is a lack of information available for the long-term follow-up of patients undergoing instrumentation in spinal osteomyelitis. Osteomyelitis generally requires a long course of postoperative antibiotic therapy, depending on the infecting pathogen. Installation of peripheral intravenous catheters may facilitate drug administration.

Core Messages. Take Home Messages

- Spinal infections have a highly variable outcome, with dramatic consequences in some patients. Mortality is estimated around 1–20%, depending on the infecting agent and the general health status of the patient.
- In the suspicion of cervical spine infection, prompt diagnosis and management are a must. Reconstructive surgery for cervical spinal infection has become more aggressive after the development of chemotherapeutic drugs. Radical surgical excision and antibiotic therapy are currently regarded as the cornerstone of the management of such infections. Internal fixation is frequently used to stabilize the operated segment. Chemotherapeutics provide ancillary support for excision procedure in the majority of the patients.
- Generally, osteomyelitis can be classified as acute, subacute, or chronic, depending on the

duration of the symptoms. Osteomyelitis can also be classified as pyogenic or nonpyogenic. The mechanism of infection can be classified as exogenous or hematogenous. Exogenous osteomyelitis can occur by direct infection (through surgical manipulation or trauma), or by local spread from contiguous infected local structures.

- Hematogenous osteomyelitis of the cervical spine can be the consequence of any condition determining bacteremia, including urinary, respiratory tract, and soft-tissue infections.
- Intrinsic risk factors for iatrogenic spinal infections include genetic disorders (i.e. Down's syndrome).
- Diabetes mellitus, inflammatory diseases, organ transplantation, HIV.
- Extrinsic risk factors for iatrogenic spinal infections include the increased invasiveness and length of the surgical procedures, the use of a single glove, the use of additional intraoperative equipment, a high number of personnel in the operating room.
- Double gloving, limiting traffic, and conversation in the operative room, handling tissues carefully, and periodically releasing self-retaining retractors to allow reperfusion of muscles are measures that decrease the incidence of intraoperative infections.
- Intraoperative fluoroscopy is used routinely in the operating room for many spinal procedures. The upper portions of the C-arm drape should not be considered to be sterile in these situations, and avoiding contact with these areas may probably decrease the risks of intraoperative contamination and possibly postoperative infections.
- Traffic in and out of the operative room should be kept to a minimum. Self-retaining retractors should be periodically removed or released, and the wound must be irrigated with saline solution.
- Transoral surgeries have been historically related to a greater incidence of infections, upto 66%. Despite the initial negative experiences, after the introduction of the operating microscope, operative magnification, and micro-instrumentation, the improvement of preoperative imaging with more definite localization of pathology, availability of antibiotics, and new devices and techniques to manage dural tears, the incidence of infections after transoral surgery currently rates between 0 and 3%, similar to anterolateral or posterior approaches.
- In the anterolateral approach, perforation of the esophagus may lead to life-threatening infections, because of the risk of sequelae from mediastinitis, purulent spondylitis, meningitis, or septicemia.
- During posterior approach to the cervical spine, stripping procedure can devascularize the musculotendinous tissue.
- Infections associated with surgical implants are generally more difficult to manage because they require a longer period of antibiotic therapy and repeated surgical procedures.
- A high index of suspicion is central to the diagnosis of cervical osteomyelitis. The clinical presentation and timing of postoperative cervical spinal infection is variable, depending on the infected structure.
- The WBC count may be increased, but is generally nonspecific. Hence, CRP and ESR are usually used to determine the presence of infection.
- Plasma procalcitonin increases rapidly during bacterial infections, but remains low in viral infections and other inflammatory processes. We use it as a useful marker in the diagnosis of osteomyelitis.
- The presence of bacteria at Gram stain or culture is diagnostic of infection. Wound exploration and debridement are mandatory, and tissue samples for cultures may be obtained intraoperatively.
- Imaging studies are often not specific enough to guide the choice of management.
- Contrast magnetic resonance imaging is the method of choice for a reliable diagnosis in clinically suspicious cases.
- Bone scan maintains a well-reserved place in the diagnosis of infection of the cervical spine. The ability to radiolabel inflammatory cells that migrate to the foci of infection was a significant milestone in the evolution of infection imaging. Labeled leukocyte imaging is a useful tool to diagnose osteomyelitis, allowing

distinguishing infections from other cervical spinal pathologies.

- Wound complications involving large subcutaneous tissue represents a significant issue for the surgeon. The cornerstone of the management of cervical spine wound infection includes exploration and debridement, antibiotic therapy, proper nutrition and medical management, and appropriate wound care.
- The management of wound infection must be performed without delay. Exploration and debridement are mandatory, with the removal of all the devitalized tissues. Samples for cultures must be obtained at surgery. Subcutaneous tissue must be abundantly irrigated and debrided.
- After performing a wide debridement of the infected structures, if internal fixation is required, we can insert the screws in the non-infected adjacent vertebrae.

References

1. Acosta FL Jr, Chin CT, Quinones-Hinojosa A et al (2004) Diagnosis and management of adult pyogenic osteomyelitis of the cervical spine. Neurosurg Focus 17:E2
2. Berney S, Opdam H, Bellomo R et al (2008) An assessment of early tracheostomy after anterior cervical stabilization in patients with acute cervical spine trauma. J Trauma 64:749–753
3. Biswas D, Bible JE, Whang PG et al (2008) Sterility of C-arm fluoroscopy during spinal surgery. Spine 33:1913–1917
4. Brown EM, Pople IK, de Louvois J et al (2004) Spine update: prevention of postoperative infection in patients undergoing spinal surgery. Spine 29:938–945
5. Caird MS, Wills BP, Dormans JP (2006) Down syndrome in children: the role of the orthopaedic surgeon. J Am Acad Orthop Surg 14:610–619
6. Clarck CR (2005) The cervical spine, 4th edn. Lippincott Williams &Wilkins, Philadelphia
7. Kaibara T, Hurlbert RJ, Sutherland GR (2001) Intraoperative magnetic resonance imaging-augmented transoral resection of axial disease. Neurosurg Focus 10:E4
8. Karadimas EJ, Bunger C, Lindblad BE et al (2008) Spondylodiscitis. A retrospective study of 163 patients. Acta Orthop 79:650–659
9. Kauffman CP, Bono CM, Vessa PP et al (2000) Postoperative synergistic gangrene after spinal fusion. Spine 25: 1729–1732
10. Liebergall M, Chaimsky G, Lowe J et al (1991) Pyogenic vertebral osteomyelitis with paralysis. Prognosis and treatment. Clin Orthop Relat Res (269):142–150
11. Luck JV Jr, Logan LR, Benson DR et al (1996) Human immunodeficiency virus infection: complications and outcome of orthopaedic surgery. J Am Acad Orthop Surg 4:297–304
12. Massie JB, Heller JG, Abitbol JJ et al (1992) Postoperative posterior spinal wound infections. Clin Orthop Relat Res (284):99–108
13. Menezes AH (2008) Surgical approaches: postoperative care and complications "transoral-transpalatopharyngeal approach to the craniocervical junction". Childs Nerv Syst 24: 1187–1193
14. Mik G, Gholve PA, Scher DM et al (2008) Down syndrome: orthopedic issues. Curr Opin Pediatr 20:30–36
15. Orlando ER, Caroli E, Ferrante L (2003) Management of the cervical esophagus and hypofarinx perforations complicating anterior cervical spine surgery. Spine 28: E290–E295
16. Petsatodis G, Symeonidis PD, Karataglis D et al (2007) Multifocal Proteus mirabilis osteomyelitis requiring bilateral amputation in an HIV-positive patient. J Bone Joint Surg Br 89:249–251
17. Rohde V, Meyer B, Schaller C et al (1998) Spondylodiscitis after lumbar discectomy. Incidence and a proposal for prophylaxis. Spine 23:615–620
18. Spitzer R, Rabinowich JY, Wybar KC (1961) A study of abnormalities of the skull, teeth and lenses in mongolism. J Can Med Assoc 84:567–572
19. Takahashi J, Shono Y, Hirabayashi H et al (2006) Usefulness of white blood cell differential for early diagnosis of surgical wound infection following spinal instrumentation surgery. Spine 31:1020–1025
20. Tanner J, Parkinson H (2006) Double gloving to reduce surgical cross-infection. Cochrane Database Syst Rev (3): CD003087
21. Thelander U, Larsson S (1992) Quantitation of C-reactive protein levels and erythrocyte sedimentation rate after spinal surgery. Spine 17:400–404
22. Wimmer C, Gluch H, Franzreb M et al (1998) Predisposing factors for infection in spine surgery: a survey of 850 spinal procedures. J Spinal Disord 11:124–128
23. Winslow C, Bode RK, Felton D et al (2002) Impact of respiratory complications on length of stay and hospital costs in acute cervical spine injury. Chest 121:1548–1554

Pitfalls Related to Inflammatory Disorders 14

Alberto Di Martino, Luca Denaro, Umile Giuseppe Longo, and Vincenzo Denaro

Contents

A. Di Martino (✉)
Department of Trauma and Orthopaedic Surgery, University Campus Biomedico of Rome, Via Alvaro del Portillo 200, 00128 Trigoria, Rome, Italy
e-mail: a.dimartino@unicampus.it

14.1 General Considerations

Surgery for spinal inflammatory disorders represents a measure to manage progressive conditions nonresponding to conservative treatment. Surgery in these often fragile patients has to deal with their associated systemic illnesses, including low bone density, poor renal and metabolic function, secondary diabetes from corticosteroid treatment, secondary immunodeficiency from the use of immunosuppressant drugs, and poor respiratory function. The treatment of these conditions requires highly specialized centers providing integrated care, with dedicated anesthesiologists, rheumatologists, and surgeons. Surgery is necessary in a minority of patients, and most surgeons will never perform this surgery, which is difficult, risky, and often life-threatening.

Analysis of complications of surgery in inflammatory disorders of the cervical spine will deal with patients affected by rheumatoid arthritis (RA) and ankylosing spondylitis (AS), which are the most common inflammatory diseases affecting this spinal segment. RA normally affects the hypermobile segments. Therefore, the cervical spine is the most common involved spinal segment in patients with RA, because of its hypermobility.

14.2 Pitfalls Related to Patients with Rheumatoid Arthritis

Involvement of the cervical spine in RA reaches up to 85% of patients with moderate to severe disease [1], although only a small proportion of these patients will be symptomatic. Symptoms can range from mild discomfort at the occipito-cervical level to severe occipital pain, and neurologically from mild intermittent weakness to

L. Denaro et al. (eds.), *Pitfalls in Cervical Spine Surgery*,
DOI: 10.1007/978-3-540-85019-9_14, © Springer-Verlag Berlin Heidelberg 2010

sudden quadriparesis. Cervical spine involvement can be atlanto-axial (early and more frequent) or subaxial (late), but both may co-exist. Surgery is indicated if there is progressive neurological deterioration or intractable pain.

If left untreated, AR cervical spine involvement with neurological deficits carries a poor prognosis, with up to 50% of patients dying in 6 months [2, 3]. Several years ago, sudden unexplained deaths in these patients were attributed to strokes or heart attacks; more recently, it has been demonstrated that over half of the reported "sudden deaths" in patients with RA were actually associated with instability of the cervical spine and spinal-cord compression [4]. CT, and then MRI scans, showed that brain stem and upper cervical-cord compression of RA were more common than previously estimated, and disability was due to mechanical spinal-cord compression, leading to progressive myelopathy [5]. The databases collected by Corbett et al. [6] and Kauppi et al. [7] outlined the natural history of this complication: cervical myelopathy rarely appears in the first decade after the onset of the disease, because the etiology is represented by repeated minor spinal-cord injuries over time [8]. Once established, however, neurological deterioration can be rapid, with half of those patients who develop myelopathy dying within a year and most patients dying within 7 years [9].

It is important to remark that often the patients attribute the diminution of their functional status to impaired function of the limbs from the local evolution of the rheumatic disease, and therefore, the diagnosis of myelopathy is usually performed late, following compression of the spinal cord from instability.

In a recent observational study on survival between operated and nonoperated patients, it was demonstrated that once patients meet the criteria to undergo surgery (i.e., neurological compromise or intractable pain), they will undergo a decrease in overall survival, despite appropriate surgery being performed [8]. Moreover, in neurologically compromised patients, surgery is associated with substantial risks [10], with postoperative morbidity and mortality being related to the degree of pre-existing neurological impairment [2]. Despite these reports, surgery is often performed too late and associated with a high rate of complications, so that surgery in a quadriparetic patient is associated with a mortality rate up to 30% [11]. Therefore, more attention is presently focused toward early treatment before irreversible neurological damage occurs [12].

For this reason, patients with RA should be managed by a multidisciplinary team, which has access to full-trained cervical spine surgeons, experienced in managing problems and complications of surgery in patients with RA, as the highest complication rate occurs following surgeries performed by inexperienced surgeons [13]. In fact, since the realization of specialized centers and the use of new drugs, surgical outcome has progressively improved, with 66–89% of symptomatic patients who improve after surgery, and a decreased rate of associated surgical complications [10, 14, 15]. Moreover, as in joint surgery, medical teams have realized that surgery should be performed to prevent deformity and neurological symptoms and to treat specific neck pain, leading to more elective preventative operations in patients who are relatively well in general status [14, 16, 17]. It is important to remember that prophylactic surgery is performed on patients with poor general conditions for the disease, often with osteoporosis, acquired immunodeficiency, metabolic, respiratory, and kidney disorders. Therefore, judicious evaluation of every single patient is required to decide the correct indication for surgery. In fact, surgery in these patients can present several complications, and therefore the decision to operate should depend on the initial neurological damages. As stated earlier, RA predominantly affects hypermobile joints (especially, diarthrosis and synovial joints) with involvement of the capsuloligamentous structures stabilizing the joint. In addition, in the cervical spine, the most mobile joints (in order: the joints of the upper cervical spine, the posterior articulations, and the intervertebral disk) are most commonly involved in the disease.

This is the reason why vertical subluxation (basilar invagination), atlanto-axial subluxation, atlanto-axial rotatory subluxations, occipito-cervical scoliosis, subaxial ankylosis or subluxations, pannus formation, and spinal-cord compression should be carefully checked out when planning surgical interventions. MRI in this clinical setting could show the true extent of subluxation and cord compression and allows for adequate preoperative study: MRI allows the study of the rheumatoid pannus as well as the vertical translocation and significantly adds information over conventional flexion–extension radiographs. In these cases, a judicious clinical evaluation of the patient, imaging (dynamic radiographs and MRI), and electrophysiological studies allow the orthopedist to monitor the evolution of the disease. The transverse ligament in RA is at first involved by the inflammatory process arising from the synovial articulation with the dens and leads to segmental instability with more than 4–5 mm anterior displacement in forward head motion [18]. Pannus decreases once early segmental surgical stabilization is performed [19], suggesting that its formation is mainly related to segmental instability [20].

In a histological analysis of surgical specimens harvested from 33 chronic rheumatoid patients during transoral decompression, O'Brien et al. [8] identified two different histological types, a chronic active rheumatoid synovium that represents an earlier stage of the chronic disease and an end-stage type of synovium that represents the response of the joint to instability, with the synovium reduced to a fibrotic tissue. The latter stage is associated with advanced upper cervical spine disease and osseous destruction with myelopathy due to subluxation, erosion of the dens, and vertical translocation, which reduce the space available for the spinal cord.

14.2.1 Considerations for Fixation and Fusion

Decompression, stabilization, and fusion of the rheumatoid cervical spine are technically demanding. Fixation may take many forms and comprehend screws, hooks, and sublaminar wires, which can be attached to either plates or rods.

Even after a successful surgery, careful follow-up is required. RA slowly progresses and continues to affect the untreated cervical segments [21]. In fact, the ligamentous laxity due to the primary disease and the increased segmental motion adjacent to any fused segment can promote adjacent-level degeneration. This phenomenon more commonly occurs in the subaxial spine after long lever arm occipito-cervical stabilizations [22], above all when some kind of pre-existing adjacent disk degeneration is present [17, 23]. This result is not surprising because fusion of the craniocervical junction results in considerable loss of motion, which is then transferred to the adjacent disk level and results in accelerated degeneration and subaxial subluxations [24–26]. Zygmunt et al. reported the rate of adjacent subaxial subluxation in 163 patients undergoing occipito-cervical fusion for RA, with 4% (7/163) of patients requiring further surgery [26]. In the study of Kraus, 36% (9/24) of enrolled patients required further surgery for subaxial subluxation after occipito-cervical fusion in 2–3 years [25].

Conversely, adjacent segment degeneration is more rarely encountered when stabilizations are limited to C1–C2 segment, which is often possible when fusion is performed early in the course of the disease [25, 27]. Preservation of the occipito-atlantal and subaxial movement, in fact, decreases the abnormal mechanical loadings and protects the subaxial cervical spine from increased mechanical stresses.

Recently, anatomo-clinical correlations have been performed with the aim to standardize surgery, because as cited earlier, different clinical and radiological pictures are related to different kinds of pannus and cervical spine involvement.

14.2.2 Anterior Approaches

At the cranio-cervical junction, anterior procedures are performed via a transoral route, which can be extended to exposure up to the clivus, C1 and C2 [28–33].

Nonetheless, as stated before, the management of rheumatoid instability at the upper cervical spine can require combined anterior and posterior procedures or be managed by posterior approach alone, provided that resolution of the pannus often occurs when posterior immobilization is performed [1, 24, 34]. In patients with a fixed kyphotic deformity and brain-stem compression due to impingement of anterior bony structures on the spinal cord, however, transoral decompression allows to directly decompress the neural structures [35]. In selected cases, a limited anterior decompression could be obtained by performing a partial odontoidectomy without complete resection of the ring of C1. This attitude would keep stability, allow for anterior decompression, and prevent further interventions, but it is feasible in only few patients [36]. Basilar invagination of the dens into the foramen magnum is, in fact, often found in this patient population and requires full transoral decompression by complete resection of the anterior arch of C1 and, occasionally, also the resection of the inferior margin of the clivus to expose the invaginated dens to be removed. Once osseous resection is performed by the anterior route, fixation is required: anterior stabilization with instrumentation can be achieved using bone grafting for segmental reconstruction plus anterior C1–C2 plate screws systems up to the clivus [37].

Table 14.1 Complications of transoral decompression in patients with RA

Complication	Consequences	Tips/tricks
Brain-stem and spinal-cord injury	Severe neurological deficits, with CSF leaks, respiratory paralysis, and death	Adequate learning curve before performing surgery
Vertebral artery injury	Uncontrollable bleeding and potential neurological deficits	Preoperative study of VA position Risk increased in Cl- rotation/ subluxation leading to midline position of the VA
Soft palate dehiscence and infection	Resuture required	Adequate antibiotic prophylaxis
General complications	Pneumonia and emboli, respiratory distress, and even death	General complication risk increased because of fragile patients
Plate/screws or graft mobilization	Dysphagia and relapse of deformity	Revision surgery required Always perform combined anterior plus posterior fixation

In selected specialized centers, using the transoral procedure is not associated with a significant increase in morbidity and is related to a relatively low incidence of direct surgical complications, which eventually can be catastrophic (Table 14.1). Casey et al. [38] reported that in experienced hands, the transoral approach is a reasonably safe procedure. The learning curve is fundamental. Crockard et al. [29] presented the results of surgery for RA at the upper cervical spine in 23 patients and reported the experience with the transoral approach in 17 patients. The most serious complication was an incidental bleeding from a displaced vertebral artery (VA) during odontoid removal. One of the potential reasons for VA injury in that case was believed the Cl rotation and subluxation, leading the vessel to stay in the midline anteriorly. Despite attempted hemostasis, the decompression had to be abandoned, and eventually, neurological deterioration progressed. Another complication in the same series was resuturing of the soft palate in two patients. A summary of the management and overall outcome of the 23 patients revealed two patients with minimal neck pain and paresthesia, one of which eventually developed progressive myelopathy and required reoperation. Another patient was not eligible for repeat surgery and two refused despite progressive neurological deterioration. One patient died after surgery of progressive respiratory failure. At follow-up, two patients deteriorated: one at 3 years because of subsequent C6–C7 subluxation, while the other was the above-mentioned patient with profuse bleeding from the VA, who became quadriparetic. Using skull traction was associated with pulmonary emboli in two patients and pneumonia in three. All other patients who had transoral surgery or anterior subaxial surgery reported cessation of their neck pain, and 15 out of the 17 patients improved. There were no perioperative deaths.

Anterior approaches to the subaxial spine in RA are the same as for any cervical spondylosis and are more extensively described in another section (Chap. 10). A major cause of complication often encountered in these patients is severe osteoporosis, and the stability of plate–screw systems (particularly when the screws are convergent) should be carefully double-checked intraoperatively: in case, an additional posterior stabilization and/or solid external immobilization should be added to promote fusion and prevent implant mobilization or instrumentation failure. To maximize the chance of instrumentation fixation, the use of diverging screws and high–thread, high-diameter screws is helpful. Using converging screws, in fact, can be related to vertebral fracture and loss of fixation. When performing anterior reconstruction in the subaxial spine, it is important to maintain the vertebral endplate for weight bearing and better use tricortical iliac crest bone graft, either allograft or autograft. Hard cortical spacers or cages should not be used because of subsidence and high risk of mobilization or missed bony integration. In our experience, surgery is effective in the treatment of symptomatic subaxial subluxation in patients with RA, via either an anterior or posterior approach. Surgery consists of anterior stabilization and fusion with bone grafting in most cases; this allows for segmental stabilization and neurological recovery in most cases. Alternatively, patients can be managed by performing a posterior fixation. Laminectomy is only rarely required for neurological decompression. Combined anterior and posterior approaches can be performed in case of fixed kyphotic segmental deformity: the anterior approach using tricortical iliac crest bone graft and plating allows restoration of cervical lordosis and decreases the risk of instrumentation failure [39].

14.2.3 Complications of Occipito-Cervical Decompression and Fusion Procedures

Every procedure aimed at suppression of the movement at the occipito-cervical hinge leads inevitably to a serious disability for the patient, because of the suppression of rotation and flexion–extension movements of the head over the neck. Apart from patients with RA, this technique is commonly used in the treatment of invasive tumors, severe instabilities (primary, secondary, or iatrogeneic), atlanto-axial instabilities without integrity of the posterior ring of C1, and congenital cranio-cervical diseases such as invagination of the dens and assimilation of the atlas to the occiput [40, 41]. This procedure can be associated with foramen magnum enlargement and sometimes with the removal of the posterior arch of the atlas when required.

Several techniques have been described to achieve an occipito-cervical stabilization. Since the first report of occipito-cervical stabilization performed by Foerster in 1927 [42], surgeons have employed several fixation methods in the occipito-cervical region, including bone graft, wires, rods, plates, screws, and poly(methyl methacrylate) (PMMA). When autologous bone graft alone is used, stability is achieved after the integration of the bone graft, and solid fusion occurs. To achieve fusion, the constant use of bracings and external fixation such as Halo cast, Halo jackets, or Minerva casts is fundamental, provided that collars do not allow for adequate immobilization and expose the patient to an increased risk of nonunion (see Chap. 19). Bone grafts in this technique should bridge between the occiput and the rostral cervical vertebrae and are anchored tightly by the use of screws on both the cervical lateral masses and occipital bone (Fig. 14.1). Bone graft is classically harvested from the posterior iliac crest, whose curved shape anatomically contours to the occipito-cervical hinge. Provided that fusion procedures require bone graft on both sides, the whole piece of bone graft harvested from the iliac crest can be split into two halves, thus obtaining both a cortical and a trabecular aspect for each piece. After adequate preparation of the graft bed with exposure of the trabecular bone after decortication of the occiput and the rostral cervical vertebrae, the bone graft is posed on its sponge side for better osteo-integration. Once the bone graft is posed on site, it is tightened with the screws at the occiput and lateral masses of the cervical spine [43].

Screw insertion at the occiput is performed at less than 15 mm laterally from the external occipital protuberance, and the screws are usually fixed in a bicortical fashion (better with screws of 3.6–4.5 mm diameter), with screw length requiring the tip of the screw to stop on the inner cortex of the occiput: the definitive length of the screw should take into account the width of the bone graft plus the occiput. Screws at the occiput can be gently tapped using a high-speed drill to decrease the risk of meningeal lesions: more recent self-tapping screws allow for easy insertion through the external cortex. In case of cerebrospinal fluid leakage, the hole can be filled with spongostan and fibrin glue before inserting the screw. Laterally, the bone graft is extended up to the lateral masses of C2, C3, or even up to C4 [44].

Results of occipito-cervical surgery improved dramatically once dedicated posterior instrumentation was designed, which ensures adequate stabilization. Newer instrumentation systems together with proper bone-grafting techniques are crucial in this surgery, provide immediate stability, and promote osteointegration and fusion.

The design of contoured plates and screws systems allows for primary stability in this problematic region: this big result arose from the efforts of Roy–Camille and, more recently, Grobb [45, 46]. Roy–Camille plates are "L" shaped and are designed to allow safe anchoring of the screw to the occiput and the lateral masses of the lower cervical spine. Minimum width for screw insertion at the occiput is 6–8 mm. Grob designed the "Y" plates, with stable fixation over the occiput performed with a single central plate anchored to the outer cortex (where the width is bigger and allows for more solid anchoring). Screw insertion at this level is safe and can only be complicated by meningeal lesion in few cases. The two distal diverging branches are moldable and can be secured to the lateral masses posteriorly. Other instrumentation systems available in commerce allow for anchoring to the skull with hooks, which are connected to the longitudinal bars and secured distally with screws at the lateral

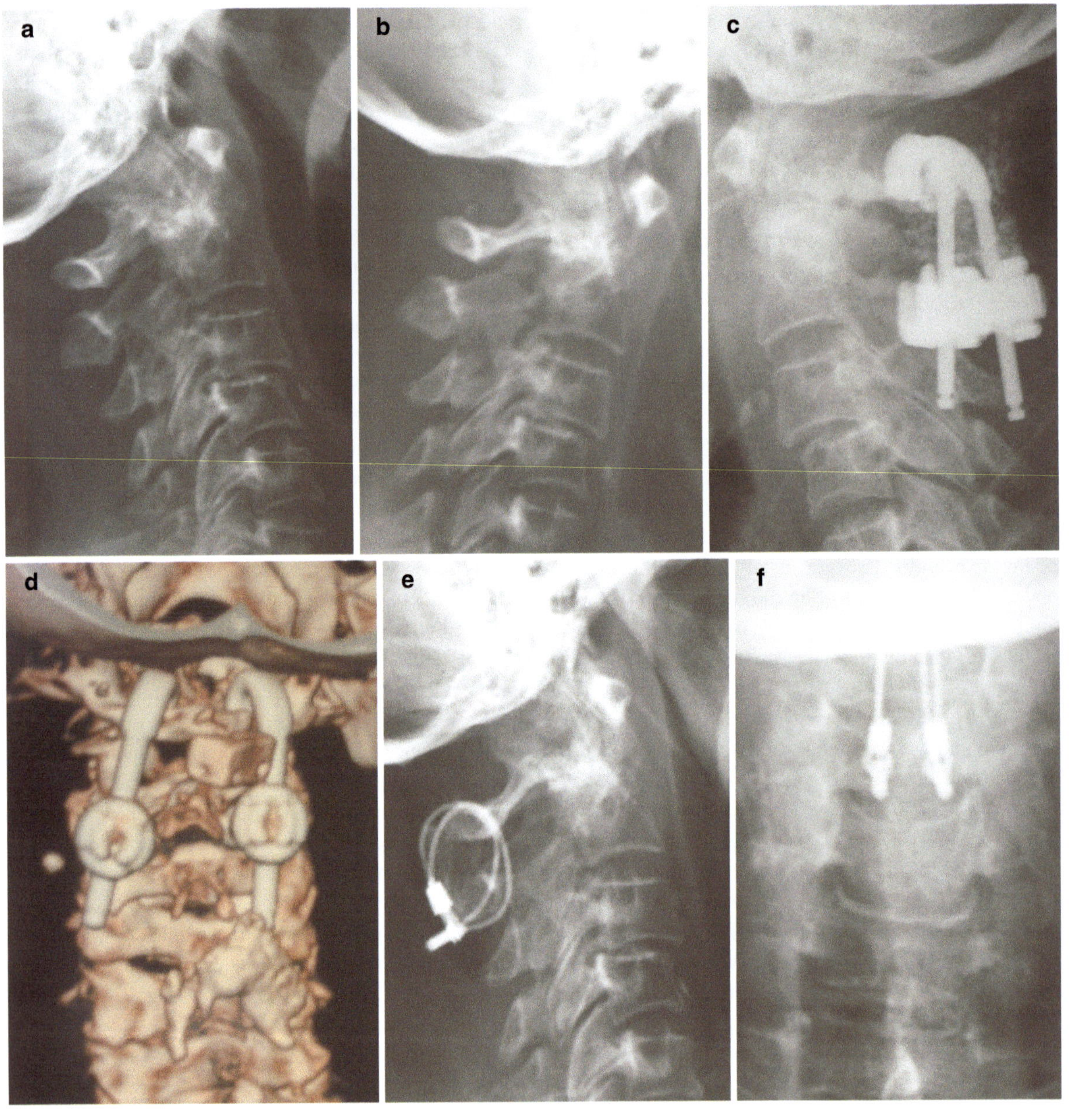

Fig. 14.1 (**a**, **b**) Lateral dynamic radiographs of a patient with RA with atlanto-axial instability and myelopathy under corticosteroid management. The dislocation of the arch of the atlas in comparison with the axis is superior to 5 mm. (**c**) Postoperative radiograph and (**d**) CT scan showing the C1–C2 stabilization with hooks and rods and hydroxyapatite graft, with successive mobilization and deep infection. Postoperative lateral (**e**) and antero-posterior (**f**) radiographs after revision surgery with wide debridement, showing the arthrodesis performed with Songer cables and autoplastic iliac bone graft

masses and/or laminar hooks at the subaxial spine. Length of fixation depends on subaxial involvement.

Recently, newer bar-polyaxial screws systems or plate–screws systems became available for this surgery. These systems keep a fixed angle between the occiput and the cervical spine to allow the patient for a normal visual field. In fact, patients candidate to occipito-cervical fusion require a preoperative adjustment of the sagittal orientation before fixation. This tip allows avoiding abnormal segmental kyphosis or lordosis, provided that the occipito-cervical angle should not be far from 110° [27, 47].

Matsunaga et al. [48] reported a 10-year follow-up of a cohort of 16 patients with RA with myelopathy, who underwent occipito-cervical instrumented fusion with a rectangular rod. Patients had irreducible atlanto-axial dislocation, and 11 also had vertical dislocation of the axis. Surgery had an effect mainly on the occipital pain, which resolved or decreased in all cases. Neurological function also improved with surgery, with myelopathy improving in 75% (12/16) patients with respect to the preoperative neurological condition. Despite the survival rate at 10 years after surgery being 38%, mortality was related mainly to the primary disease and patient's age at surgery. Fusion instead was achieved in all cases. Subaxial subluxation developed in 31% of patients after surgery but was asymptomatic in all but one patient.

In a mixed cohort of 58 patients candidate to occipito-cervical fusion and affected by several diseases (ranging from tumor to inflammatory conditions), fusion was attempted in 51 of the 58 patients, while 7 underwent decompression and stabilization alone due to advanced tumor disease [49]. Fusion was achieved in 48 out of the 51 patients (94%). Of the three nonfused patients, two underwent instrumentation failure and required reoperation, while the other developed asymptomatic nonunion. Complications occurred in 30% of patients. Early complications occurred in 15% of patients and included cervical wound infections (5%), bone graft site infection (5%), and medical complications (5%). Medical complications were most commonly pneumonia. There was one death (1.7%) due to a cardiac event. Adjacent-level degeneration was noted in four patients (7%): two of them required extension of their fusion to include lower levels, whereas others were managed conservatively. Other studies reported similar complication rates with this procedure [50].

Surgical complications in occipito-cervical fixation and fusion (Table 14.2):

Meningeal, Neural, and nerve root lesions
Vascular injuries
Instrumentation failure

14.2.3.1 Complications to Meninges, Spinal Cord, and Nerve Roots

Meningeal, spinal cord, and bulbar lesions can occur either during decompression maneuvers at the occiput or during widening of the foramen magnum and opening of the tectory membrane. Meningeal lesions then would require repair with dural grafts or pieces of Liodura. Liquoral leak can occur even after procedures of screw insertion and hook anchorage to the skull. In most cases, the CSF leak can be stopped with fibrin glue and small pieces of spongostan, followed by screw insertion or hook blockage. If these measures are not effective, opening a bony breech and direct lesion repair is required and/or the application of a lumbar drain. An important issue is the reciprocal position of the head with respect to the cervical spine. When odontoid protrusion or other cranio-cervical malformations occur, the aim of this surgery is to keep approximately the same reciprocal position of head and neck before surgery. In

Table 14.2 Complications of occipito-cervical decompression and fusion

Complication	Consequences	Tips/tricks
Meningeal, neural, and nerve root lesions	Meningeal and bulbar lesions during decompression maneuvers Liquoral fistulae also during screw insertion and hook anchorage	Repair meningeal lesions with dural grafts or Liodura Use fibrin glue and small pieces of spongostan plus screw insertion or hook blockage to stop CSF leak
Vertebral artery lesions	Hemorrhage Loss of visual field Need for ligation Neurological deficits	Dissection at the atlasextending <1.5 cm from midline (1.0 cm in children) Risk increased in patients with congenital malformations or dens invaginations
Instrumentation failure	Mobilization of instrumentation Loss of correction Kyphosis Swan neck deformity Neurological deficits	Proper bone grafting technique to increase solid fusion Rigid neck external support postoperatively
Vicious fusion position	Loss of visual field Dysphagia	Adjustment of the sagittal orientation before fusion and instrumentation Keep occipito-cervical angle not far from 110°

fact, any attempt of deformity reduction would change the reciprocal relationship between bony and neural structures, thus provoking irreversible spinal-cord lesions, extending up to encephalic trunk. Postoperative infections occurring at this level can also be associated to serious life-threatening conditions such as meningitis or encephalitis. Infections can be severe, provided it decreases immune response in this patient population.

14.2.3.2 Vascular Lesions

Vascular lesions consist in most cases in lesions to the vertebral artery, mainly in its portion out of the bony spine, where the artery exits the foramen lateral to the apophysis of C2 and turns upward and medially to lay on the posterior arch of the atlas running from lateral to medial [11, 51]. When a laminectomy at this level is performed, the artery is encountered and is easy to injure, also in its intratechal portion, where it turns more lateral to concur to the circle of Willis. When dissecting the posterior arch of the atlas, a dissection extending more than 1.5 cm from the midline (1.0 cm in children) increases the risk of vertebral artery injury. This anatomical picture is far more complicated in patients affected by congenital malformations with segmental stenosis, such as in the forms of assimilation of the atlas to the occiput, and much more risky in patients with dens invaginations associated with occiput-C1 and C1–C2 arthritis such as in patients with RA[43].

14.2.3.3 Mobilization of Instrumentation

Mobilization of the instrumentation in occipito-cervical stabilizations and fusions occurs because of long lever arms with high torsional forces applied by the head over the cervical spine. The only, often underestimated, way to achieve good, long-term results is in any case to put much attention, once instrumentation is performed, in preparing a proper grafting bed with abundant bone to increase the chances of a solid fusion. As an adjunct, a rigid neck external support (better Halo jacket) should be kept enough time to achieve fusion. Despite modern advances in technology, cranio-cervical fixation represents a demanding surgery for most spinal surgeons. Screw malpositioning at the occipito-cervical segment is associated with a risk of lesion to the main neurovascular structures, such as bulb and spinal cord, nerve roots, and vertebral artery. In the subaxial spine, screws are secured to the lateral masses; complications are secondary to the exit of the tip of the screw from the external cortex during burring, screw malpositioning, and use of too long screws. This risk increases when bicortical anchoring is purchased [52, 53]. Other complications associated with the implant of screws in the lateral masses are screw pull-out, foraminal iatrogeneic stenosis, facet violation, screw breakage, and overload adjacent to the segmental fusion [47]. In case of occipito-cervical fixation failure because of the progression of subaxial disease below the fixed segment, inferior extension of the fixation is required.

Hardware mobilization can have catastrophic consequences. Recently, the first report of mediastinal migration of the distal aspect of a posterior occipito-thoracic screw–rod construct (C0–T2) in a patient with severe RA was described [54]. In this patient, 1-year postoperative radiographs demonstrated asymptomatic screw loosening at C7, T1, and T2. Eighteen months after surgery, the patient developed acute airway obstruction due to cricoarytenoid arthritis for which an emergency tracheotomy was performed, which required neck hyperextension. This was followed by bilateral hand weakness, dysphagia, upper thoracic pain, and lateral tilt of the head and neck. In this patient, forced hypextension during tracheotomy provoked a fracture-subluxation of T1/2 and T2/3 with the bilateral C7, T1, and T2 screws migrating in the mediastinum, causing tracheal and esophageal compression. The patient required removal of the instrumentation and revision of instrumentation plus prolonged halo fixation.

14.2.4 Posterior Fixation at C1–C7 in Patients with RA

The posterior approach allows rapid access to wide exposures to obtain safe bony fixation points for hooks, screws, and metal wires [22, 26, 41, 47, 50, 53, 55–61]. For these reasons, posterior approaches are the mainstay for stabilization of the rheumatoid cervical spine, also in case of severe osteoporosis. The posterior approach also allows for segmental decompression when required [62, 63]; in any case, posterior decompression without stabilization should not be performed in patients with RA, because it leads to segmental kyphosis and eventual worsening of the neurologic deficit.

When C1–C2 fusion is required, after careful and gentle reduction, fixation can be performed using bone graft and wiring techniques or using transarticular screws [26]. In the casuistic of Ito, transarticular screw fixation has been performed to achieve C1–C2 fixation in patients with RA. The technique was associated with posterior bone grafting and the metal or polyethylene wires. The author reported lower fusions of the posterior graft in patients with RA (77.4%) compared with patients without RA (100%), and the use of polyethylene wires had a lower posterior graft union rate (75.9%) when compared with metal wires (100%), confirming results available in literature [64].

Alternatively, in case of atlanto-axial subluxation, pedicle screws in C2 and lateral mass screws at C1 allow stable segmental fixation [65]. Instrumentation in these patients can be extended if subaxial cervical spine involvement occurs [37, 38]; when instrumentation must be carried in the subaxial spine, lateral mass screws can be used, despite failure of subaxial fixation often been encountered in patients with RA. Pedicle screws can be used in (C7) T1 and T2 to maximize the pullout strength at the caudal end of a long construct. Nonunions are reported in 20–30% of patients. This low fusion rate has led some authors [31, 59] to suggest that perhaps instrumentation without fusion is not an option provided that stabilization is the primary goal in these low demand patients, but we consider a fusion attempt worthy for long-term results in this patient population.

14.3 Pitfalls Related to Patients with Ankylosing Spondylitis

AS affects the cervical spine in 30% of patients and leads to a progressive anterior protraction of the head; cervical spine involvement is more typical in the female population [66, 67]. Appropriate conservative management allows most patients to continue a normal life.

The initial evaluation of a patient with AS and a suspected cervical deformity are focused on identifying the primary area needing correction, which could also be at the hips or the thoracolumbar spine. Examination includes assessment of the patient standing upright with extended hips; accessory evaluation should check for patients' position in both seated and supine positions. Patients with a primary cervical deformity exhibit persistent cervical flexion, despite lying flat; conversely, hip or thoracic/lumbar deformities tend to correct in the sitting or supine positions, respectively. If multiple areas require surgery, usually the less complicated surgery should be performed first (i.e., hip flexion deformities should be corrected first). Surgery for cervical flexion deformity is reserved only for patients who have continued sagittal-plane deformity, despite appropriate surgical balancing of the other segments.

The cervical flexion deformity is measured by the chin–brow to vertical angle (CBA) method, which is an angle measured between the chin–brow line and the vertical line with the patient standing with the hips and knees extended. In the healthy patient, the CBA is about 0°, but in patients with severe AS, cervical deformities can arise up to 90°. Angle measure is necessary to assess the degree of correction required: after surgery, a CBA of 10° will allow the patient to work at a desk or to see forward while walking.

Computed tomography and MRI are essential to find the bony points of fixation for instrumentation and to study the spinal cord to spinal canal relationship. It is important to remember that some patients can present concurrent atlanto-axial instability, which represents a potential risk of neurologic injury during both intubation maneuvers and surgery. As an adjunct, patients with severe cervical flexion deformity may suffer nutritional imbalance for swallowing difficulties, and perioperative tube feeding or parenteral nutrition may be necessary.

14.3.1 Treatment of Cervical Flexion Deformity in AS

Patients who present with only painful arthropathy and mild cervical kyphosis may initially undergo conservative management. The initial stages of cervical kyphosis may be responsive to behavior modification, such as sleeping without a pillow under the head.

Indications for cervical osteotomy depend on the grade and extension of the deformity, the age and general conditions of the patient, and by the will of the patient to accept the risks connected to such complex procedure. Contraindications are mainly related to the general status of the patient.

Urist first described the use of cervical extension osteotomy for correction of a chin-to-chest deformity in a patient with AS [40]. This procedure was modified from the Smith–Petersen procedure of lumbar osteotomy for flexion deformities [68]: the technique described by Urist and later modified by Simmons involved removing a posterior wedge of bone from C7 with subsequent gradual extension of the head and neck to "close" the osteotomy defect and achieve sagittal correction [40, 69].

14.3.1.1 Surgical Technique of Cervical Extension Osteotomy

Because of its relatively high risk of neurovascular complications, cervical osteotomy still remains one of the most challenging procedures in spinal surgery and is associated to a high rate of complications (Table 14.3). This technique can be performed in a sitting position on a dental chair with local anesthesia or in a prone position under fiber-optic-guided general anesthesia and electrophysiological intraoperative continuous monitoring by evoked potentials, to monitor spinal cord function. Endotracheal intubation guarantees emergency airway access and allows the surgeon to perform the procedure in the prone position, facilitating the use of instrumentation and reducing the risk of air embolism. This latter, conversely, is more commonly associated with the sitting position: the low-pressure venous system at the base of the neck produces a negative pressure during inspiration that can "aspirate rather than bleed." To monitor this condition, a Doppler monitor is routinely fixed to the patient's chest before surgery and allows for detection of any air embolisms when sitting position is used during surgery.

General anesthesia, however, impairs the ability to monitor neurological function, particularly immediately after the corrective extension maneuver performed intraoperatively: spinal cord injury in this setting is secondary to an acute translational injury or to an impingement of the spinal cord with the bony structures while closing the osteotomy wedge. Some authors [70] use the intra-operative wake-up test to assess the neurological function after spinal deformity correction, but there is a "critical time window" for deficit reversal that may be spent while waiting for the patient to recover from anesthesia.

In the original technique by Urist or Simmons, surgery is performed on the awake patient in sitting position on a dental chair. In the operating room, a halo ring is fixed to the patient's head and placed on traction of approximately 10 lb in direct line with the neck [40, 69].

After midline surgical exposure, a fluoroscopic level confirmation is mandatory: the surgeon can often use the C6 spinous process (which is the last bifid) as

Table 14.3 Complications of cervical spine surgery in patients with AS

	Complication	Consequences	Tips/tricks
Deformity cervical extension osteotomy	Acute subluxation during cervical extension maneuver Spinal-cord lesion and C8-palsy Nonunion Air embolism	Spinal cord injury Severe neurological deficits Motor and sensory disturbances Resurgery required Cardiac arrest and death	Intraoperative electrophysiological monitoring Careful halo handling of the head during extension maneuver Surgery with the awake collaborating patient allows for prompt treatment Completely unroof of nerve root Adequate bone grafting or instrumentation Postoperative immobilization (halo jacket) Occurs in sitting position
			Use of continuous Doppler intraoperative monitoring
Fractures	Aortic or tracheal rupture Usually unstable lesions General complications and death	Life-threatening complications High risk of postoperative deformity and instrumentation failure Pneumonia respiratory failure, postoperative wound infections,anddeep venous thrombosis	Check for these complications Often combined anterior and posterior approached Neck fixation in the supposed preoperative alignment to avoid further spinal cord injury High rates of complications related to general health status

a landmark. The preferred level for osteotomy is at the C7–T1 vertebrae, because the spinal canal is wider and the C8 root has a nice mobility in this area. Moreover, eventual compromise of the C8 nerve root is associated with an acceptable level of disability. Another important issue is the reciprocal position of the vertebral artery in respect to the spine at this level: it courses anteriorly to the transverse process of C7 to enter the C6 foramen, so at this level is safe from manipulations during the osteotomy maneuver. The area of bone removal consists of the complete C7 lamina plus the inferior edge of C6 and the superior laminar edge of T1. Once bony resection is performed, wide exposure of the dural sac and spinal cord is obtained. The emerging C8 nerve root is identified, followed laterally in the nerve root canal, and protected with a probe. In the sitting position, the awake patient will be able to collaborate and refer any sensory or motor disturbance while manipulating the nerve roots and spinal cord. The bony roof of the nerve root canal is removed laterally in a way that at the end of surgery, the two lateral resections will be symmetrical (to avoid coronal imbalance), and the C7 and T1 lateral masses will be in contact posteriorly after cervical extension. Pedicles are undercut to obtain a new root canal for the C8 nerve root.

Once decompression is obtained, the surgeon extends the neck of the patient by levering on the halo ring, up to contact between the adjacent lateral masses. With closure of the osteotomy, a circumferential instability is obtained, and the surgeon should carefully monitor that acute subluxation does not occur while extending the neck [71]. Once reduction is obtained, the halo ring is connected to the jacket. At surgeons' preference, a long instrumented fusion with lateral mass and thoracic pedicle screws can be performed. It is helpful to place the deep sutures before the osteoclasis, as these are somewhat difficult to insert following closure of the osteotomy. Proper bone-grafting technique is mandatory in all cases. Postoperative immobilization is guaranteed by the application of a halo vest/jacket to allow consolidation of the bone graft. Even in patients where instrumentation was used, the use of a Halo vest in the postoperative period is suggested to increase the chance of bony fusion [61]. After surgery, the patient is referred to the intensive care unit.

With the introduction of spinal instrumentation in this surgery, several techniques and newer implants are used to prevent acute instrumentation translation during extension maneuver. Shimizu et al. [72] reported the use of sublaminar wires and a prebent Hartshill rectangular loop rod for controlled correction during extension osteotomy. Once the prebent rod is attached with wires at the thoracic levels, cervical wires are gradually tightened to the rod while checking for sagittal and coronal balance.

Mehdian et al. [73] have described the use of a provisional malleable rod connected to posterior cervical and thoracic screws to prevent acute instrumentation mobilization during extension. When the desired correction is achieved, the thoracic screws are tightened to one provisional rod, and the other is replaced by a titanium rod bent to match the corrected angle. After final tightening of the titanium rod to the screws, the same procedure is performed on the contralateral rod.

14.3.1.2 Complications of Cervical Extension Osteotomy

The complication rate in these patients is very high [70] and comprehends neurological deficits (ranging from transient root palsy up to tetraparesis), nonunion requiring resurgery, and subluxation at the cervicothoracic hinge. Nonetheless, in well-selected patients, clinical results can dramatically improve the quality of life, because angle deformity correction can reach more than 50° [74]. In a recent analysis of all series with at least ten patients with AS who underwent cervical extension osteotomy, it has been found that 5 of 183 (2.7%) patients had significant spinal-cord injury, which included one case of paraparesis, one case of hemiparesis, and three cases of tetraparesis [71]. In the overall population, six patients (3.3%) died within 3 months from surgery. Minor neurological complications were also observed, mainly consisting in self-resolving palsy at the C8 nerve root (35 patients, 19%): in such cases, patients immobilized in halo vest without internal fixation underwent gentle distraction of the halo to relieve foraminal compression of the C8 nerve root. Other complications included transient postoperative dysphagia that generally resolved within few weeks. Nonunion was a rare complication and was probably due to delayed subluxation at the osteotomy site. Simmons et al. reported six nonunions occurring in 131 patients, and McMaster found two cases of nonunion in

15 patients. In both series, the patients with nonunions had no instrumentation at first surgery [75].

14.3.2 Cervical Spine Fractures in AS

Spinal fractures are often described in AS, because of the high rate of osteoporosis in this population; in fact, patients with AS present a fourfold risk of fracture in their lifetime when compared with the healthy population [76]. The ankylosed spine is brittle and rigid: the combinations of these factors results in unstable fractures prone to translation even after minimal traumas [77, 78]. Neurological deficits are commonly observed in these patients [78] and do not always resolve with surgery. Moreover, even neurologically intact patients have a high risk of secondary displacement with neurological deficits.

A patient with AS developing painful progressive flexion deformity even after minor trauma should be considered as having a cervical-spine fracture until proven otherwise.

Unrecognized fractures in this patient population proceed to gradual erosion and can eventually heal in vicious position, leading to a painless fixed neck flexion deformity that requires osteotomy. Fractures are usually located at the cervico-thoracic junction, ranging from C6 to T2. The patient is usually aware of the difference in head position and may tend to hold the head with the hands.

In the systematic review by Westerveld et al., a delay in diagnosis of cervical spine fracture (>24 h) was found in 17.1% (59/345) of patients [79]. Interestingly, in 31 out of the 59 patients (52.5%), diagnosis delay was due to the doctor underestimating the trauma and in 28 out of 59 (47.6%) in a delay of the patient to seek medical attention.

Clinically, fractures can lead to immediate spinal-cord injury, directly consequent to the trauma itself and fragment displacement, or late neurological deficit during patient manipulation or transfer to another hospital. Commonly, patients with ankylosed spines present with an unexpected straight neck that was flexed before trauma. As an initial measure, the emergency team should ask the patient and relatives which was the previous segmental alignment, and a halo should be fixed after gentle traction according to the supposed alignment before trauma. Application of a halo vest should be performed even before radiological studies are undertaken to prevent further displacement or neurological deficits. Multislice spiral CT scan is the best method to study the involved segment.

Surgery in these patients can have catastrophic complications and should be performed with the awake collaborating patient to monitor neurological function and prevent further major spinal-cord injury: determinants of new neurological deficits can be related to intubation maneuvers and preoperative patient positioning. Patient can be safely operated in the sitting position under local anesthesia as already reported for cervical extension osteotomy.

In the past, techniques for stabilization of the fractured AS cervical spines were similar to those we extensively used to stabilize the cervical spine with metastasis in patients with poor prognosis: with this technique, by the use percutaneous Steinman pins, methylmethacrylate and metal wirings, immediate stabilization is achieved [43, 80, 81].

More recently, open reduction and internal fixation with rods and screws systems followed by immobilization in halo jacket is the standard treatment. Because of the osteoporotic bone and the long lever of arm at the instrumentation site, long fixation is required, but instrumentation failure occurs. This is one of the reasons supporting circumferential fusion at the fracture site.

The other area subjected to traumas in patients affected by AS is the occipito-cervical hinge. In fact, erosive fractures through the posterior arch of C1 and C1–C2 subluxations can present as painless flexion deformities with or without neurological symptoms. Cause of this deformity is destructive arthritis at the atlanto-occipital joints. In this case, the lateral radiographs show a relatively normal lordosis, suggesting the site of disease being the upper cervical spine. Treatment consists of stabilization with halo vest and subsequently atlanto-axial fusion for C1–C2 subluxation, or occipito-cervical fusion in case of occipito-cervical instability.

Some patients affected by AS develop a typical aseptic spondylodiscitis. This clinical picture is often related to trauma and seems the consequence of a stress fracture of the endplate or of the articular processes [69]. Differential diagnosis is with infective spondylodiscitis. Treatment is conservative but nonunion. If it develops, surgery consisting in anterior discectomy and fusion or, better, circumferential instrumented fusion is required.

14.3.2.1 Complications of Surgery for Cervical Spine Fractures in AS

Fractures in the cervical spine in patients with AS can be lethal or can result in severe spinal-cord lesions, leading to quadriplegia [36, 82]. In a recent review on complications related to spine fractures in patients with AS, aortic dissection and tracheal rupture were reported in the setting of trauma and led to death in four out of seven reported cases. Lesions of the aorta could be due to aortitis, direct trauma associated with the fracture mechanism, and the shearing forces applied to the aorta firmly adherent to the calcified anterior longitudinal ligament. Some kind of neurological deficit at the time of trauma has been found in up to 67.2% of patients (232/345). In the study, after treatment, 48/345 patients (13.9%) developed delayed neurological deficits. Patients treated with surgery reported no change in neurological function in 59.4% of cases (111/187 patients). Fifty-one out of 187 patients (27.3%) showed some improvement in neurological function postoperatively, and 28/187 (26.7%) improved further at follow-up. A total 17.7% of patients (61/345) deceased within 3 months of injury. The most frequent cause of death was pneumonia and/or respiratory failure, occurring in the postoperative period and at follow-up [79]. Moreover, patients who underwent surgery developed a wide range of complications, comprehending postoperative wound infections, deep venous thrombosis, and respiratory failure [83–97].

Core Messages

- Most spinal surgeons will never perform surgery in patients affected by RA or SA at the cervical spine, provided that this surgery is difficult, risky, and often life-threatening.
- Decompression and deformity correction followed by instrumented fusion at the inflammatory cervical spine are technically demanding, and these surgeries should be carried out by experienced surgeons only.
- Patients with RA are medically and physically frail, and systemic illnesses such as lower bone density, poor renal and metabolic function, secondary diabetes from corticosteroid treatment, and poor respiratory function are common and lead to frequent intra-operative complications and postoperative instrumentation failures.
- In patients with AS, surgery can be considered in either severe deformity or in the trauma setting. Surgery in these patients is related to a high risk of spinal-cord lesion, postsurgical deformity, and even death.
- Because of the osteoporotic bone encountered in inflammatory diseases and the long lever of arm at the instrumentation site, long fixations in these patients are quite common and circumferential fusion can be required.

References

1. Bland JH, Eddy WM (1968) Hemiplegia and rheumatoid hemiarthritis. Arthritis Rheum 11:72–79
2. Boden SD, Dodge LD, Bohlman HH, Rechtine GR (1993) Rheumatoid arthritis of the cervical spine. A long term analysis with predictors of paralysis and recovery. J Bone Joint Surg 75A:1282–1297
3. Mark JS, Sharp J (1981) Rheumatoid cervical myelopathy. Q J Med 199:307–319
4. Plotz GM, Schutz U, Grob D (1998) Occipitocervical fusion in chronic polyarthritis. Z Rheumatol 57:147–158
5. Henderson FC, Geddes JF, Crockard HA (1993) Neuropathology of the brainstem and spinal cord in end stage rheumatoid arthritis: implications for treatment. Ann Rheum Dis 52:629–637
6. Corbett M, Dalton S, Young A, Silman A, Shipley M (1993) Factors predicting death, survival and functional outcome in a prospective study of early rheumatoid disease over fifteen years. Br J Rheumatol 32:717–723
7. Neva MH, Myllykangas-Luosujarvi R, Kautiainen H, Kauppi M (2001) Mortality associated with cervical spine disorders: a population-based study of 1666 patients with rheumatoid arthritis who died in Finland in 1989. Rheumatology 40:123–127
8. O'Brien MF, Casey AT, Crockard A, Pringle J, Stevens JM (2002) Histology of the craniocervical junction in chronic rheumatoid arthritis: a clinicopathologic analysis of 33 operative cases. Spine 27(20):2245–2254
9. Casey AT, Crockard HA, Bland JM, Stevens J, Moskovich R, Ransford A (1996) Predictors of outcome in the quadriparetic nonambulatory myelopathic patient with rheumatoid arthritis: a prospective study of 55 surgically treated Ranawat class IIIb patients. J Neurosurg 85:574–581
10. Casey AT, Crockard HA (1995) In the rheumatoid patient: surgery to the cervical spine. Br J Rheumatol 34:1079–1086
11. Brislin BT, Hilibrand AS, Taylor BA (2002) Complications of anterior and posterior cervical instrumentation. In:

Vaccaro AR, Betz RR, Zeidman SM (eds) Principles and practice of spine surgery. C.V. Mosby, St. Louis
12. Casey AT, Crockard HA, Bland JM et al (1996) Surgery on the rheumatoid cervical spine for the non-ambulant myelopathic patient - too much too late? Lancet 347:1004–1007
13. Christensson D, Saveland H, Rydholm U (2000) Cervical spine surgery in rheumatoid arthritis. A Swedish nationwide registration of 83 patients. Scand J Rheumatol 29:314–319
14. Hamilton JD, Gordon MM, McInnes IB et al (2000) Improved medical and surgical management of cervical spine disease in patients with rheumatoid arthritis over 10 years. Ann Rheum Dis 59:434–438
15. Redlund-Johnell I (1985) Cervical dislocations in rheumatoid arthritis. Lakartidningen 82:4510–4512
16. Casey ATH, Crockard HA, Pringle J, O'Brien MF, Stevens JM (2002) Rheumatoid arthritis of the cervical spine: current techniques for management. Orthop Clin North Am 33:291–309
17. Santavirta S, Konttinen YT, Sanelin J et al (1990) Operations for the unstable cervical spine in rheumatoid arthritis: sixteen cases of subaxial subluxation. Acta Orthop Scand 61:106–110
18. Eulderink F, Meijers KAE (1976) Pathology of the cervical spine in rheumatoid arthritis: a controlled study of 44 spines. J Pathol 120:91–108
19. Larsson EM, Holtas S, Zygmut S (1989) Pre- and postoperative MR imaging of the craniocervical junction in rheumatoid arthritis. Am J Rheumatol 152:561–566
20. Halla JT, Jr Hardin JG (1990) The spectrum of atlanto-axial facet joint involvement in rheumatoid arthritis. Arthritis Rheum 33:325–329
21. Krieg JC, Clark CR, Goetz DD (1993) Cervical spine arthrodesis in rheumatoid arthritis: a long-term follow-up. Yale J Biol Med 66:257–262
22. Olerud C, Larsson BE, Rodriguez M (1997) Subaxial cervical spine subluxation in rheumatoid arthritis: a retrospective analysis of 16 operated patients after 1–5 years. Acta Orthop Scand 68:109–115
23. Santavirta S, Konttinen YT, Laasonen E et al (1991) Ten-year results of operations for rheumatoid cervical spine disorders. J Bone Joint Surg 73:116–120
24. Agarwal AK, Peppelman WC, Kraus DR et al (1992) Recurrence of cervical spine instability in rheumatoid arthritis following previous fusion: can disease progression be prevented by early surgery? J Rheumatol 19:1364–1370
25. Kraus DR, Peppelman WC, Agarwaal AK et al (1991) Incidence of subaxial subluxation in patients with generalized rheumatoid arthritis who have had previous occipital cervical fusions. Spine 16(Suppl10): 486–489
26. Zygmunt SC, Christensson D, Saveland H et al (1995) Occipito-cervical fixation in rheumatoid arthritis – an analysis of surgical risk factors in 163 patients. Acta Neurochir (Wien) 135:25–31
27. Matsunaga S, Onishi T, Sakou T (2001) Significance of occipitoaxial angle in subaxial lesion after occipitocervical fusion. Spine 26:161–165
28. Crockard HA, Calder I, Ransford AO (1990) One-stage transoral decompression and posterior fixation in rheumatoid atlanto-axial subluxation. J Bone Joint Surg Br 72B:682–685
29. Crockard HA, Essigman WK, Stevens JM et al (1985) Surgical treatment of cervical cord compression in rheumatoid arthritis. Ann Rheum Dis 44:809–816
30. Crockard HA, Pozo JL, Ransford AO et al (1986) Transoral decompression and posterior fusion for rheumatoid atlanto-axial subluxation. J Bone Joint Surg Br 68B:350–356
31. Crockard HA (1995) Spine update: surgical management of cervical rheumatoid problems. Spine 20(23):2584–2590
32. Crockard HA (1985) The transoral approach to the base of the brain and upper cervical cord. Ann R Coll Surg Engl 67:321–325
33. Crockard HA (1995) Transoral surgery: some lessons learned. Br J Neurosurg 9:283–293
34. Grob D, Wursch R, Grauer W et al (1997) Atlantoaxial fusion and retrodental pannus in rheumatoid arthritis. Spine 22(14):1580–1583
35. O'Brien MF (1998) The craniocervical junction: anterior problems and surgical solutions. In: Devlin VJ (ed) Anterior spinal column surgery: spine: state of the art review. Hanley & Belfus, Philadelphia, pp 529–570
36. Dickman CA, Locantro J, Fessler RG (1992) The influence of transoral odontoid resection on stability of the craniovertebral junction. J Neurosurg 77(4):525–530
37. Kandziora F, Mittlmeier T, Kerschbaumer F (1999) Stage-related surgery for cervical spine instability in rheumatoid arthritis. Eur Spine J 8:371–381
38. Casey ATH, Crockard HA, Stevens J (1997) Vertical translocation. Part II. Outcomes after surgical treatment of rheumatoid cervical myelopathy. J Neurosurg 87:863–869
39. Denaro V (1992) Artrite reumatoide a localizzazione cervicale bassa (C3–C7). Giornale Italiano di Ortopedia e Traumatologia. Estratti dal LXXVII congresso della SIOT. 131–136
40. Urist MR (1958) Osteotomy of the cervical spine. J Bone Joint Surg Am 40:833–843
41. Vale FL, Oliver M, Cahill DW (1999) Rigid occipitocervical fusion. J Neurosurg 91(Suppl 2):144–150
42. Vanden Berghe A, Ackerman C, Veys E et al (1991) Occipitocervical fusion in rheumatoid arthritis. Acta Orthop Belg 57(Suppl 1):94–98
43. Denaro E (1991) Stenosis of the cervical spine causes, diagnosis and treatment. Springer, Berlin
44. Roy-Camille R, Mazel CH, Saillant G (1987) Treatment of cervical spine injuries by a posterior osteosynthesis with plate and screws. In: Kehr P, Weidner A (eds) cervical spine I. Springer, Berlin
45. An HS (1995) Internal fixation of the cervical spine: current indications and techniques. J Am Acad Orthop Surg 3: 194–206
46. Wertheim SB (1987) Occipitocervical fusion: indications, techniques, and long term results in thirteen patients. J Bone Joint Surg Am 69:833–836
47. Mc Cullen GM, Garfin SR (2000) Spine update: cervical spine internal fixation using screw and screw-plate constructs. Spine 25:643–652
48. Matsunaga S, Ijiri K, Koga H (2000) Results of a longer than 10-year follow-up of patients with rheumatoid arthritis treated by occipitocervical fusion. Spine 25(14):1749–1753
49. Deutsch H, Haid RW, Rodts GE, Mummaneni PV (2005) Occipitocervical fixation: long-term results. Spine 30(5):530–535
50. Heidecke V, Rainov NG, Burkert W (1998) Occipito-cervical fusion with the cervical Cotrel-Dubousset rod system. Acta Neurochir (Wien) 140(9):969–976
51. An HS, Cooper M (1998) Cervical spine instrumentation. In: An HS (ed) Principles and techniques of spine surgery. Williams & Wilkins, Philadelphia, pp 65–73

52. Ebraheim NA, Rupp RE, Savolaine ER, Brown JA (1995) Posterior plating of the cervical spine. J Spinal Disord 8:111–115
53. Grob D, Dvorak J, Panjabi MM et al (1994) The role of plate and screw fixation in occipitocervical fusion in rheumatoid arthritis. Spine 19:2545–2551
54. Joseph V, Al Jahwari AS, Rampersaud YR (2008) Mediastinal migration of distal occipito-thoracic instrumentation. Eur Spine J 17(Suppl 2):S257–S262
55. Edwend M, Ducker TB (1993) Rheumatoid C1–2 spinal instability. J Spinal Disord 6:535–536
56. Eyres KS, Gray DH, Robertson P (1998) Posterior surgical treatment for the rheumatoid cervical spine. Br J Rheumatol 37:756–759
57. Fehring TK, Brooks AL (1987) Upper cervical instability in rheumatoid arthritis. Clin Orthop 221:137–148
58. Grob D, Dvorak J, Panjabi M et al (1991) Posterior occipitocervical fusion: a preliminary report of a new technique. Spine 16(Suppl 3):S17–S24
59. Millbrink J, Nyman R (1990) Posterior stabilization of the cervical spine in rheumatoid arthritis: clinical results and magnetic resonance imaging correlation. J Spinal Disord 3:308–315
60. Shen FH, Samartzis D, Jenis LG, An HS (2004) Rheumatoid arthritis: evaluation and surgical management of the cervical spine. Spine J 4:689–700
61. Szpalski M, Gunzburg R (2002) What are the advances for surgical therapy of inflammatory diseases of the spine? Best Pract Res Clin Rheumatol 16(1):141–154
62. Christensson D, Saveland H, Zygmunt S et al (1999) Cervical laminectomy without fusion in patients with rheumatoid arthritis. J Neurosurg 90(Suppl 4):186–190
63. Stambough JL, Balderston RA, Grey S (1990) Technique for occipito-cervical fusion in osteopenic patients. J Spinal Disord 3:404–407
64. Ito H, Neo M, Fujibayashi S, Miyata M, Yoshitomi H, Nakamura T (2008) Atlantoaxial transarticular screw fixation with posterior wiring using polyethylene cable. Spine 33(15):1655–1661
65. Harms J, Melcher RP (2001) Posterior C1-C2 fusion with polyaxial screw and rod fixation. Spine 26:2467–2471
66. Calin A, Elswood J (1988) The relationship between pelvic, spinal and hip involvement in ankylosing spondylitis–one disease process or several? Br J Rheumatol 27(5):393–395
67. Calin A (1985) Ankylosing spondylitis. In: Kelley WN (ed) Textbook of rheumatology. WB Saunders, Philadelphia, pp 993–1006
68. Smith-Petersen MN, Larson CB, Aufranc OE (1945) Osteotomy of the spine for correction of flexion deformity in rheumatoid arthritis. J Bone Joint Surg Am 27:1–11
69. Simmons ED, DiStefano RJ, Zheng Y, Simmons EH (2006) Thirty-six years experience of cervical extension osteotomy in ankylosing spondylitis. Spine 31(26): 006–3012
70. McMaster MJ (1997) Osteotomy of the cervical spine in ankylosing spondylitis. J Bone Joint Surg Br 79(2): 197–203
71. Hoh DJ, Khoueir P, Wang MY (2008) Management of cervical deformity in ankylosing spondylitis. Neurosurg Focus 24(1):E9
72. Shimizu K, Matsushita M, Fujibayashi S, Toguchida J, Ido K, Nakamura T (1996) Correction of kyphotic deformity of the cervical spine in ankylosing spondylitis using general anesthesia and internal fixation. J Spinal Disord 9:540–543
73. Mehdian SM, Freeman BJ, Licina P (1999) Cervical osteotomy for ankylosing spondylitis: an innovative variation on an existing technique. Eur Spine J 8:505–509
74. McAfee PC, Cassidy JR, Davis RF et al (1991) Fusion of the occiput to the upper cervical spine: a review of 37 cases. Spine 16(Suppl 10):S490–S494
75. Sansur CA, Fu KG, jr Oskouian RJ, Jagannathan J, Kuntz C IV, Shaffrey CI (2008) Surgical management of global sagittal deformity in ankylosing spondylitis. Neurosurg Focus 24(1):E8
76. Graham AW, Swank ML, Kinard RE et al (1996) Posterior cervical arthrodesis and stabilization with a lateral mass plate. Spine 21:323–329
77. Hunter T, Dubo H (1978) Spinal fractures complicating ankylosing spondylitis. Ann Intern Med 88(4):546–549
78. Olerud C, Frost A, Bring J (1996) Spinal fractures in patients with ankylosing spondylitis. Eur Spine J 5(1):51–55
79. Westerveld LA, Verlaan JJ, Oner FC (2009). Spinal fractures in patients with ankylosing spinal disorders: a systematic review of the literature on treatment, neurological status and complications. Eur Spine J 18(2):145–156
80. Denaro V, Gulino G, Papapietro N, Denaro L (1998) Treatment of metastasis of the cervical spine. Chir Organi Mov 83:127–137
81. Denaro V (1988) Treatment of metastases and systemic tumors of the cervical spine. Neuro Orthopedics 6:101–110
82. Amamilo SC (1989) Fractures of the cervical spine in patients with ankylosing spondylitis. Orthop Rev 18(3): 339–344
83. Bland JH (1974) Rheumatoid arthritis of the cervical spine. J Rheumatol 1:319–341
84. Casey ATH, Crockard HA, Geddes JF, Stevens J (1997) Vertical translocation: the enigma of the disappearing atlantodens interval in patients with myelopathy and rheumatoid arthritis. Part I. Clinical, radiological, and neuropathological features. J Neurosurg 87:856–862
85. Crockard HA, Johnston F (1993) Development of transoral approaches to lesions of the skull base and craniocervical junction. Neurosurgery Q 3:61–82
86. Eleraky MA, Masferrer R, Sonntag VK (1998) Posterior atlantoaxial facet screw fixation in rheumatoid arthritis. J Neurosurg 89:8–12
87. El-Khoury GY, Wener MH, Menezes AH, Dolan KD, Kathol MEH (1980) Cranial settling in rheumatoid arthritis. Radiology 137:637–642
88. Finkelstein JA, Chapman JR, Mirza S (1999) Occult vertebral fractures in ankylosing spondylitis. Spinal Cord 37(6):444–447
89. Graham B, Van Peteghem PK (1989) Fractures of the spine in ankylosing spondylitis. Diagnosis, treatment, and complications. Spine 14(8):803–807
90. Huang RC, Girardi FP, Poynton AR et al (2003) Treatment of multilevel cervical spondylotic myeloradiculopathy with posterior decompression and fusion with lateral mass plate fixation and local bone graft. J Spinal Disord Tech 16: 123–129
91. Magerl F, Seemann PS (1985) Stable posterior fusion of the atlas and axis by transarticular screw fixation. In: Kehr P, Weidner A (eds) Cervical spine. Springer, New York, pp 322–327
92. Matsunaga S, Sakou T, Sunahara N et al (1997) Biomechanical analysis of buckling alignment of the cervical spine:

predictive value for subaxial subluxation after occipitocervical fusion. Spine 22:765–771

93. Moskovich R, Crockard HA, Shott S et al (2000) Occipitocervical stabilization for myelopathy in patients with rheumatoid arthritis. J Bone Joint Surg Am 82A: 349–365
94. Paus AC, Steen H, Røislien J, Mowinckel P, Teigland J (2008) High mortality rate in rheumatoid arthritis with subluxation of the cervical spine: a cohort study of operated and nonoperated patients. Spine 33(21):2278–2283
95. Ronkainen A, Niskanen M, Auvinen A, Aalto J, Luosujarvi R (2006) Cervical spine surgery in patients with rheumatoid arthritis: longterm mortality and its determinants. J Rheumatol 33:517–522
96. Stanley D, Laing RJ, Forster DM et al (1994) Posterior decompression and fusion in rheumatoid disease of the cervical spine: redressing the balance. J Spinal Disord 7: 439–443
97. Szpalski M, Gunzburg R (2002) Surgical therapy and spinal inflammatory disease. Best Practice Res Clin Rheum 16(1):141–154

Section V

Complications related to neural diseases

15 Spinal Cord Neoplasms

Luca Denaro and Domenico D'Avella

Contents

L. Denaro (✉)
Department of Neuroscience, University of Padua,
Via Giustiniani 5, 35128 Padua, Italy
e-mail: lucadenaro@hotmail.com

15.1 Primary and Metastatic Intradural Cervical Spine Tumors

Spinal cord neoplasms are an uncommon cause of back pain, radicular pain, or sensorymotor deficits. Primary tumors that involve the spinal cord or nerve roots may arise from glial cells located within the parenchyma of the cord, Schwann cells of the nerve roots, or meningeal cells covering the cord. Metastatic spinal cord tumor can result from dissemination of a primary systemic cancer or, more rarely, from drop metastasis of primary intracranial lesions. According to the literature, spinal tumors are divided on the basis of their location into three major groups: intradural intramedullary, intradural extramedullary, and extradural tumors. Intradural tumors are contained in the thecal sac and they can originate within the spinal cord tissue, classified as intramedullary, or adjacent but extrinsic to the cord, classified as extramedullary lesions.

15.2 Intradural Intramedullary Neoplasms

Intradural intramedullary spinal cord tumors (IMSCTs) are neoplasms that arise within the substance of the spinal cord invading or displacing the cord tissue depending on their histological nature. IMSCTs account for 3% of all central nervous system tumors and for approximately 25% of spinal neoplasms. Astrocytomas, ependymomas, and hemangioblastomas are the most common subtypes, accounting for 45, 35, and 10%, respectively. Other tumor types include lipomas, dermoids, teratomas, neuroblastomas, schwannomas, oligodendrogliomas, PNETs, and metastases [1–3]. The

L. Denaro et al. (eds.), *Pitfalls in Cervical Spine Surgery*,
DOI: 10.1007/978-3-540-85019-9_15, © Springer-Verlag Berlin Heidelberg 2010

clinical presentation is variable and insidious. Symptoms begin several months before diagnosis with an evolution that depends on the histological characteristic of the tumor. A malignant lesion becomes clearly symptomatic within 10 months while a myelopathy due to a slow growing tumor can be clear even after years. Acute neurological defects are correlated to intratumor hemorrhage, a typical event of ependymomas. Neck pain is the most common manifestation of these lesions followed by upper extremity paraesthesia, sensory loss, progressive unilateral or bilateral spasticity, and weakness. Bowel, bladder, or sexual dysfunctions are symptoms of advanced disease. Spinal MR with injection of gadolinium is the gold standard for the diagnosis and preoperative evaluation of IMSCTs; a precise localization and the presence of cysts or syrinx are achieved while the signal intensity can suggest the nature of the lesions. Surgery is a fundamental step of the therapeutic strategy of these lesions. The first surgical objective is to obtain a precise diagnosis remembering that interpretation of a biopsy fragment can be inaccurate. Different histological tumors have different capacity to infiltrate the spinal cord tissue. The presence of a plane between the tumor and the spinal cord is the principal condition to achieve a gross total resection of the lesions preserving the preoperative neurologic function.

15.2.1 Astrocytomas

Spinal astrocytomas account for approximately 3% of central nervous system astrocytomas and 6% of all spinal cord tumors. They are most prevalent in the first three decades of life; 60% of them occur in the cervical and cervico-thoracic segments [4, 5]. Cystic lesions rostral or caudal to the tumor mass may represent either tumor cysts or benign reactive syrinx. Histologically, spinal cord astrocytomas, according to the Kernohan grading scheme, are classified as low-grade and high-grade lesions. Low-grade astrocytomas are more frequent, accounting for 70–80% in adults and 90–80% in children [6, 7]. To reach and remove the tumor, a myelotomy should be performed along the midline extending over the entire length of the solid portion and the cysts. Astrocytomas are eccentrically located within the cord and typically infiltrate the surrounding tissue owing to an asymmetric expansion and distortion of the cord that make the identification of the dorsal median sulcus difficult. The sulcus can be localized as the midline between the two dorsal root entry zones or as the line formed by the veins emerging from the dorsal raphe [8]. Typically, it is very difficult, if not impossible, to recognize a cleavage plane between an astrocytoma and the surrounding nervous tissue, and a complete resection of the tumor can be achieved only with unacceptable risks of deficits. In such instances, subtotal resection, preserving neurological function, is indicated to obtain the histological diagnosis, to decompress the cord and to reduce the mass in preparation of adjunctive therapy. However, in some cases, low-grade lesions can have a dissection plane, and a macroscopic gross total resection can be achieved with a good clinical result. Commonly, in the immediate postoperative period, a neurological deterioration from the preoperative baseline is seen even when resection is limited to grossly apparent tumor. Preoperative neurological function is the best prognostic indicator for functional outcome [3, 7, 9].

15.2.2 Ependymomas

Intramedullary ependymomas are the most common spinal cord tumors in adults representing 35% of all central nervous system ependymomas and approximately 60% of all intramedullary tumors in adults. Originating from the ependymal rests in the central canal, ependymomas usually have a central location. The tumor does not disrupt the symmetry of the cord displacing the cortical spinal tracts anteriorly and laterally allowing the localization of the midline easier [8]. Like astrocytomas, ependymomas are un-encapsulated neoplasms, but differently, especially low-grade lesions, do not infiltrate the spinal cord tissue but pushed aside it maintaining a good cleavage plane. This characteristic often allows a complete tumor excision and a good long-term prognosis. Different subtypes of histologic variety have been recognized graded 1–4, grade 4 being the most malignant. In 65% of cases, the lesion is associated with syrinx or cysts particularly when the tumor is located in cervical spinal cord [9–12]. Vascularization is very variable with vessels coming prevalently from the anterior spinal artery that may be attached to the tumor and at risk of damages during surgery. The noninfiltrative behavior often allows a complete tumor excision and a good long-term prognosis. Gross total resection is the treatment of choice and intraoperative biopsy has the role to encourage the surgeon to look for the cleavage plane or vice versa to be less aggressive in case of a histologically malignant tumor. Surgical strategy should be adjusted on the peculiarity of each lesion. Small tumor can be removed in block once the cleavage plane is identified while a large tumor should be reduced before a plane is found to limit the risks to damage the surrounded tissue. Even if ependymomas do not have an infiltrative growth, they have origin from the spinal cord and there is a point where the neoplasm blends with the normal tissue [9–12].

15.2.3 Hemangioblastomas

Hemangioblastomas represent 2–5% of primary intramedullary spinal cord neoplasm. They are benign, sharply circumscribed but not encapsulated, highly vascular tumors that are usually located in the dorsal aspect of the cord. They are typically composed of a cystic lesion associated with a mural nodule enhancing on MR, commonly located on the dorsal or dorsolateral surface of the spinal cord, immediately apparent on the surface with a collection of vessels that feed and drain it. The neoplasm does not infiltrate the cord preserving a clear plane of dissection with the nervous tissue and can be completely resected. To isolate the tumor cleavage plane between the tumor and the cord, it is advisable to start dissection at the level of the associated cyst avoiding to enter the lesion until the vascular supply is interrupted totally; to facilitate the dissection limiting manipulation and damage to the surrounding nervous tissue, the lesion can be progressively shrunk by bipolar coagulation of the surface. Because of the high vascularization, it is imperative to coagulate superficial feeding arteries first and during dissection the arteries exposed preserving venous outflow until the end of the resection. This is to avoid swelling of the tumor and a possible blood loss that may be difficult to control [3, 8]. One-third of the cases of hemangioblastomas are related with the von Hippel–Lindau disease. When a hemangioblastoma is encountered, patients should be investigated for von Hippel–Lindau disease because of the possibility to have multiple lesions along the neuraxis and because of the risks to develop new tumors during lifetime [13, 14].

15.2.4 Intramedullary Spinal Cord Metastases

Intramedullary spinal cord metastases account for 1–8% of all intramedullary spinal cord tumors and affect 0.1–0.4% of all cancer patients; 24% of them localized in the cervical cord tract [15]. They can be often clinically silent and be recognized only at autopsy [16]. Any metastatic tumor can theoretically spread to the spinal cord. The most common primary sources include broncogenic cancer, small cell lung cancer, breast cancer, melanoma, lymphoma, colon adenocarcinoma, and renal cell carcinoma [15, 17]. The presence of intramedullary spinal cord metastases is correlated with brain or leptomeningeal localizations and is an indicator of advanced systemic involvement. Metastases are vascular lesions that maintain a cleavage plane with the adjacent tissues. Surgical technique is similar to removal of primary spinal cord neoplasm. If surgery is planned, administration of radiation treatment should be done after the surgery to avoid scarring and obscuration of tissue planes. Surgery is indicated only in case of large tumors because an intra-operating localization of small lesions with a major risk of neurological deficits may be difficult [15]. To limit postoperative complications, planning surgery is mandatory to evaluate patient's general conditions, immunosuppression from primary disease, or therapy and nutritional state. Poor wound healing, higher infection rates, and higher postoperative morbidity are reported [18]. Furthermore, surgical risks must be weighed against expectancy and quality of life. Radical resection can offer a better quality of life to these patients who, however, have a mean survival of 1 year.

15.3 Intradural Extramedullary Neoplasms

Intradural extramedullary tumors (EMSCTs) account approximately for 70% of intradural spinal cord tumors in adults. The most common derive from meningial cells (meningiomas), which constitute about 85% of all EMSCTs and from sheath cells of the spinal nerve roots (nerve sheath tumors (NSTs) as shwannomas and neurofibromas). Rare are other tumor types as lipomas, paragangliomas, hemangiopericytomas, epidermoid, and dermoid cysts. Generally, EMSCTs are slow-growing tumors that cause pain and symptoms of spinal cord compression as other nonneoplastic conditions. Local or radicular pain is the most common symptom that evolves into myelopathy as the lesion enlarges enough to compress the cord. Myelopathy has a slow evolution similar to those of intramedullary and extradural tumors or nonneoplastic conditions as spondylotic myelopathy. Radicular pain can be the consequence of direct root compression or direct involvement by NSTs. Local pain is more typical of dural irritation from meningiomas. Nocturnal pain is a potential spinal cord tumor sign. MR is the radiological procedure of choice to identify and localize the lesion, to suggest the histological nature, and to define the involvement of the spinal cord and the other structures such as roots, vertebral body, or vertebral artery.

15.3.1 Meningiomas

Meningiomas account for 25% of all primary intraspinal neoplasms and 12% of all meningiomas [19]; most commonly, they occur in the thoracic spine (80%); cervical tumors are less common (17%) and lumbar are rare (3%) [20]. They arise from arachnoid villi cells embedded in the dura at the nerve root sleeve and, in fact, they are more frequently lateral or ventrolateral [3]. Meningiomas are well circumscribed and slow-growing lesions with no tendency to infiltrate surrounding tissue and gross total resection is achieved in 90% of patients [21]. Malignant subtypes are very rare. Almost in all cervical cases, a posterior approach is sufficient to reach and remove a meningioma. Because of the slow growth pattern, the tumor usually reaches a relatively significant size before being symptomatic and, in the main time displaces the cord providing a quite safe access to the anterior and anterolateral portion of the spinal canal. Total surgical resection of the tumor and its base of implant is the primary strategy of treatment. After a correct identification of the level, a laminectomy is performed and the dura is opened. The tumor is internally debulked using microsurgical technique or ultrasonic aspirator and the arachnoid plane is identified. The lesion in then removed from its dural attachment and where possible the base of the implant is resected or coagulated using bipolar cauterization. A water-tight suture is then performed using a dural graft if needed [22].

15.3.2 Nerve Sheath Tumors

NSTs are schwannomas and neurofibromas that account for 26% of spinal tumors [23], 25% of intradural tumors in adults with a peak of incidence in the fourth through the sixth decade. Schwannomas arise from the Schwann cells of dorsal nerve roots and neurofibromas from mesenchymal cells. NSTs are mainly benign lesions with a favorable prognosis. The malignant peripheral NST is a rare entity characterized by an aggressive course and a poor prognosis. These tumors can occur sporadically or they can be associated with neurofibromatosis 1 or 2. These tumors may extend with the nerve root through the neural foramen or may be purely extradural. Transdural growth is common in cervical spine NSTs because the intradural root segment is short [24, 25]. NST tumors are relatively avascular, globoid, and without calcification. The involved root appears distended in a fusiform shape with no apparent plane of dissection between the tumor and the nerve. Surgical excision is the treatment of choice preserving the involved nerve or at list limiting the sacrifice of the only root of origin. Resection of the nerve root is usually not associated with significant motor or sensory deficit. If the tumor is attached to the spinal cord or to vital structures in the cervical region, subtotal resection is an option [2].

15.4 Surgical Technique and Complication Avoidance

Patient selection is at the base of a correct and safe surgical treatment. The diagnosis of an intramedullary mass lesion is not an indication for surgery by itself. The surgeon has to consider the general condition and the neurological state of the patient in contrast to the expectations and the risks of neurologic deterioration as a result of an operation. The goal of surgery on a cervical IMSCT, besides achieving the histological diagnosis, is to stop or slow neurologic deterioration and possibly to improve motor and sensory function; preservation, rather than restoration, of neurologic function, is the reasonable expectation after intramedullary tumor resection. Patients who are only minimally symptomatic receive the greatest benefit, and are at the least risk of surgery for intramedullary tumors [26, 27]. The cervical region of the cord is the most dangerous site for surgical intervention because of the important autonomic functions (maintenance of respiration and blood pressure) that may become compromised. In particular, if the tumor involves the brain stem, respiratory impairment can require prolonged intubation. Before surgery, if the patient presents an important motor deficit in lower limbs, a Doppler study of the deep venous system is performed to exclude a deep venous thrombosis. All patients go to surgery wearing anti-embolism compression stockings and, in the postoperative period, thromboprophylaxis with low molecular weight heparin is given until they are ambulatory. Intraoperative neurophysiologic monitoring is recommended to detect surgically induced lesions of the cord even if the true efficacy remains unclear. Collaboration among surgeon, neuro-physiologist, and anesthetist is essential to obtain good results. For example, halogenated volatile anesthetics modify sensory evoked potentials, and they should be avoided [28]. The preservation of sensory evoked potentials encourages proceeding, but the loss of them is of little value. Motor-evoked potentials (MEPs) are more closely correlated with postoperative motor function; a >50% decrease in MEP amplitude is a warning sign that the surgeon should stop and wait until restoration of normal signals [29, 30]. In this time, to help improvement and limit the risk of ischemia, abundant irrigation of the surgical field and administration of papaverin is recommended. Cervical IMSCT are generally approached in a prone position with the head placed in a three-pin headholder. Care should be taken in positioning the pins to avoid damages to the venous sinus, epidural hematomas or skull fractures, and in freeing the thorax and abdomen from pressure to minimize venous hypertension and bleeding during surgery. A midline incision is used and the laminae are exposed. Before laminectomy, an accurate intraoperative check of the vertebral level is mandatory. In adult patients, to minimize the risk of postoperative kyphosis, laminectomy is performed preserving the lateral masses, while in pediatric population, in which postoperative deformity is more probable, laminotomy with laminoplasty reconstruction is a better choice. When it is possible, sparing the midline intervertebral ligament reduces the risk of ligamentous instability [28, 31]. A careful hemostasis is recommended at any step of surgery. Even a small bleeding coming from skin incision, muscles, or bone is to be controlled before dura opening and the surgical field must be kept very clean during microsurgical dissection. Once the dura is exposed, before opening it, ultrasound is used to confirm the location of the mass lesion minimizing the dural opening. Under operative microscope, using a micro scalpel, a midline incision is made and the dura is opened by just pulling the edges with micro-forceps. This limits the danger to damage the arachnoid or the dorsal aspect of the spinal cord. After dural retention sutures are placed, dissection and opening of arachnoid is made and sutures are placed to apply a gentle traction on it. Spinal cord splitting is preferably performed along the midline throw of the posterior median sulcus, but if the tumor is located in the surface or reaches it, myelotomy is not necessary. Because of the deformation of the cord, the location of the midline can be very difficult. To localize it, help can be offered by the vessels that converge toward the midline or calculating the midway between the left and right dorsal roots [3, 28]. The vertically running vessels are dissected and mobilized laterally and never coagulated. The spinal cord splitting, using a fine blade or micro-scissor along the midline, allows one to separate the posterior columns, to reach the tumor minimizing the risk of lesions to the surrounding nervous tissue [32]. The myelotomy should be extended to expose the superior and inferior poles of the tumor. Pial traction suturing improves the exposure and reduces the severity of repeated trauma resulting from dissection [28]. After exposing the tumor, a biopsy is taken to adjust the surgical strategy. Debulking of the tumor before searching for a cleavage plane allows for a simpler dissection and limits traction on the spinal cord. In case of nonvascular tumor, reduction of the mass volume is achieved by ultrasonic surgical aspirator with an inside-out technique. The surgeon must be aware that the aspirator does not distinguish between tumor and spinal cord: it is better to regulate suction and vibratory force at the lowest level [28]. If the mass is highly vascular, tumor reduction is obtained using a microsurgical technique in a piecemeal fashion. After decompression, retracting the tumor into the obtained cavity, a cleavage plane between tumor and normal tissue can be identified and a gross total resection can be achieved. In case of infiltrating lesions, the resection should be stopped as soon as the dissection plane becomes indistinguishable or until a modification in the evoked potentials are detected. Great attention has to be paid to preserve the vascularity of the spinal cord remembering that the anterior spinal artery may be dislocated by the mass, and easily injured during dissection [8]. Patients suffering unilateral symptoms due to unilateral or eccentrically located tumors experience the worst neurological postoperative scenario. In these patients, the location of the tumor predisposes the normal hemicord to increased risk of surgical injury during resection or manipulation of the normal tissue; centrally located tumors are usually technically easier to resect and are associated with less risks of injury to adjacent tissue [30]. After the tumor resection is completed, a careful hemostasis of the surgical bed is done to avoid a postoperative intraspinal hematoma that can be a disastrous complication. The myelotomy and the pial layer are not sutured while a meticulous water-tight closure of the dura using a nonabsorbable suture must be performed to prevent cerebrospinal fluid leak. If necessary, in case of a swollen cord or for the presence of residual tumor, a patch should be used avoiding any tension on the cord.

EMSCTs are predominantly histologically benign slow-growing lesions that typically displace the cord saving a good plane of dissection with the cord. These biological characteristics allow a complete surgical excision that is the optimum treatment [33]. The posterior midline approaches permit one to reach the mass even if it has a ventral origin because the cord is displaced laterally. If necessary, to facilitate the mobilization of the cord, one or more dentate ligaments can be cut. Generally, a clear cleavage plane between the arachnoid and the tumor is found. Large tumors should be debulked internally limiting the manipulation of the adjacent tissue in a piecemeal fashion or with the aid of ultrasonic surgical aspirator, while small tumors can be excised en bloc. To limit recurrence of meningiomas, its dural attachment has to be resected or coagulated. Complete resection of meningioma with the involved dura, followed by a patch graft, is the better solution but an alternative strategy, especially in cases of anterolateral implant, is coagulation of the area of tumor implant. Another strategy that can lower the risk of cerebrospinal fluid leakage is separation of the inner and outer dural layers, resection of the inner layer, where the tumor is implanted, preserving the outer layer that is sutured [31, 34]. Anterior, en plaque, recurrent meningiomas with arachnoid scarring and calcifications do not respect tissue planes. Adhesions cause cord tethering and it is difficult to distinguish between scar, meningioma, and spinal cord; poor functional outcomes are reported in these patients as a result of the additional manipulations required to dissect the tumor [22]. The risk to damage the anterior spinal artery should be always kept in mind, especially in the cases of tumor growing close to radicomedullary artery [35]. NSTs typically originate on the dorsally sensory roots and it is generally possible to spare motor functions. The dorsal rootlets entering the tumor are necessarily sacrificed: from C2 to C4 they can be sectioned safely with no major sensitive deficit. To limit postoperative painful neuralgia, the nerve root should be sectioned proximal to the ganglion [36]. Lesions extending in a "dumbell" fashion into the foramen require extensive exposure. The intradural portion is resected as a first step to minimize spinal cord manipulation. Despite the use of modern sterile techniques, wound complications occur during surgery, and cause significant morbidity [35]. Complications related to dehiscence, infection, and cerebrospinal fluid leak are much more common in patients who have undergone prior surgery or radiation therapy [5, 26]. These complications rarely resolve with conservative therapy, and early re-operation is imperative to avoid exacerbation [25]. In case of CSF fistula, before revision surgery, the use of a lumbar drainage can be curative. Patients operated on to remove a metastasis may be subjected to immunosuppression from the underlying disease or treatments and may have poor nutritional status increasing the risk of wound sepsis, would healing, and general postoperative complications [18].

Core Messages

Primary and metastatic intradural cervical spine tumors

- Spinal cord neoplasms are divided into intradural intramedullary, intradural extramedullary, and extradural tumors. The clinical presentation is variable and insidious.
- Neck pain is the most common manifestation of these lesions followed by upper extremity paraesthesia, sensory loss, progressive unilateral or bilateral spasticity, and weakness.
- Nocturnal pain is a potential spinal cord tumor sign.
- Spinal MR with injection of gadolinium is the gold standard for the diagnosis and preoperative evaluation: a precise localization and the presence of cysts or syrinx are achieved while the signal intensity can suggest the nature of the lesions.
- IMSCTs are neoplasms that arise within the substance of the spinal cord invading or displacing the cord tissue depending on their histological nature.
- Surgery is a fundamental step of the therapeutic strategy of these lesions. Patient selection is at the base of a correct and safe surgical treatment.

- The diagnosis of an intramedullary mass lesion is not an indication for surgery by itself. The goal of surgery on a cervical IMSCT is to stop or slow neurologic deterioration and possibly to improve motor and sensory function; preservation, rather than restoration, of neurologic function, is the reasonable expectation after intramedullary tumor resection.
- Patients who are only minimally symptomatic receive the greatest benefit, and are at the least risk of surgery for intramedullary tumors.
- Intraoperative neurophysiologic monitoring is recommended to detect surgically induced lesions of the cord even if the true efficacy remains unclear.
- The presence of a plane between the tumor and the spinal cord is the principal condition to achieve a gross total resection of the lesions preserving the preoperative neurologic function.
- Typically, it is very difficult, if not impossible, to recognize a cleavage plane between an astrocytoma and the surrounding nervous tissue, and a complete resection of the tumor can be achieved only with unacceptable risks of deficits. In such instances, subtotal resection is indicated to decompress the cord and to reduce the mass in preparation of adjunctive therapy.
- Cystic lesions rostral or caudal to the tumor mass may represent either tumor cysts or benign reactive syrinx.
- To reach and remove the tumor, a myelotomy should be performed along the midline extending over the entire length of the solid portion and the cysts. The sulcus can be localized as the midline between the two dorsal root entry zones or as the line formed by the veins emerging from the dorsal raphe.
- Vascularization is very variable with vessels coming prevalently from the anterior spinal artery that may be attached to the tumor and at risk of damages during surgery.
- Commonly, in the immediate postoperative period, a neurological deterioration from the preoperative baseline is seen even when resection is limited to grossly apparent tumor. Preoperative neurological function is the best prognostic indicator for functional outcome.

References

1. Colosimo C, Cerase A, Denaro L, Maira G, Greco R (2003) Magnetic resonance imaging of intramedullary spinal cord schwannomas. Report of two cases and review of the literature. J Neurosurg Spine 99(1 Suppl):114–117
2. Traul DE, Shaffrey ME, Schiff D (2007) (2007) Part I spinal-cord neoplasms: intradural neoplasms. Lancet Oncol 8(1):35–45
3. Zeidman SM (2004) Intradural intramedullary and extramedullary tumors. In: Clark CR (ed) The cervical spine, 4th edn. The Cervical Spine Research Society Editorial Committee. Lippincott Williams & Wilkins, Philadelphia, pp789–804
4. Bourgouin PM, Lesage J, Fontaine S, Konan A, Roy D, Bard C, Del Carpio O'Donovan R (1998) A pattern approach to the differential diagnosis of intramedullary spinal cord lesions on MR imaging. AJR Am J Roentgenol 170:1645–1649
5. McCormick PC, Stein BM (1990) Intramedullary tumors in adults. Neurosurg Clin N Am 1:609–630
6. Bouffet E, Pierre-Kahn A, Marchal JC, Jouvet A, Kalifa C, Choux M, Dhellemmes P, Guérin J, Tremoulet M, Mottolese C (1998) Prognostic factors in pediatric spinal cord astrocytoma. Cancer 83:2391–2399
7. Epstein FJ, Farmer J-P, Freed D (1993) Adult intramedullary spinal cord ependymomas: the result of surgery in 38 patientes. J Neurosurg 79:204–209
8. Jallo GL, Kothbauer KF, Epstein FJ (2001) Intrinsic spinal cord tumor resection. Neurosurgery 49(5):1124–1128
9. Samii M, Klekamp J (1994) Surgical results of 100 intramedullary tumors in relation to accompanying syringomyelia. Neurosurgery 35:865–873
10. Helseth A, Mork SJ (1989) primary intraspinal neoplasms in Norway 1955–1986. A population-based surgery of 467 patients. J Neurosurg 71:842–845
11. Mork SJ, Loken AC (1988) Ependymoma: a follow up study of 101 cases. Cancer 40:907–915
12. Schwartz T, Parsa AT, McCormick PC (2005) Intramedullary ependimomas. In: Berger MS, Prados MD (eds) Textbook of neuron-oncology. Elsevier, Amsterdam, pp 497–500
13 Lonser LR, Oldfield EH (2005) Spinal cord hemangioblastomas, Chapter 68. In: Berger MS, Prados MD (eds) Textbook of neuron-oncology. Elsevier, Amsterdam, pp 506–510
14. Lonser RR, Wait SD, Butman JA, Vortmeyer AO, Walther MM, Governale LS, Oldfield EH (2003) Surgical management of lumbosacral nerve root hemangioblastomas in von Hippel-Lindau disease. J Neurosurg (Spine) 99:64–69
15. Chi JH, Parsa AT (2005) Intrinsic metastatic spinal cord tumors, Chapter 12. In: Berger MS, Prados MD (eds) Textbook of neuron-oncology. Elsevier, Amsterdam
16. Schiff D, O'Neill BP (1996) Intramedullary spinal cord metastases:clinical features and treatment outcome. Neurology 47:906–912
17. Potti A, Abdel-Raheem M, Levitt R, Schell DA, Mehdi SA (2001) Intramedullary spinal cord matastases and non-small cell lung carcinoma:clinical patterns, diagnosis and therapeutic considerations. Lung Cancer 31:319–323
18. Wise JJ, Fischgrund JS, Herkowitz HN, Montgomery D, Kurz LT (1999) Complication, survival rates, and risk factors of surgery for metastatic disease of the spine. Spine 24(18)1943–1951
19. Rubinstein LJ (1972) Tumors of the central nervous system. Atlas of Tumor Pathology. Armed Forces Institute of Pathology, Washington, DC

20. Ciappetta D, Domenicucci M, Raco A (1988) Spinal meningiomas: prognosis and recovery factors in 22 cases with severe motor deficits. Acta Neurol Scand 77:27–30
21. Solero CL, Fornari M, Giombini S et al (1989) Spinal meningiomas: review of 174 operated dases. Neurosurgery 25: 153–160
22. Gottfried ON, Gluf W, Quinones-Hinojosa A, Kan P, Schmidt MH (2003) Spinal miningiomas: surgical management and outcome. Neurosurg Focus 14(6):2–8
23. Waldron J, Weinstein PR (2005) Nerve sheath tumor of the spine, Chapter 63. In: Berger MS, Prados MD (eds) Textbook of neuron-oncology. Elsevier, Amsterdam, pp 485–488
24. Schwartz TH, McCormick PC (2003) Spinal Cord tumors in adults. In: Winn HR (ed) Youmans neurological surgery. Saunders, Philadelphia, pp 4817–4834
25. Seppälä MT, Haltia MJ, Sankila RJ, Jääskeläinen JE, Heiskanen O (1995) long term outcome after removal of spinal schwannoma: a clinicopathological study of 187 cases. J Neurosurg 83:621–636
26. Cooper PR (1985) Outcome after operative treatment of tntramedullary spinal cord tumours in adults: intermrdiate and long-term results in 51 patients. Recent experience in 29 patients. J Neurosurg 63:492–499
27. Epstein FJ, Farmer JP, Freed D (1992) Adult intramedullary astrocytomas of the spinal cord. J Neurosurg 77:355–359
28. Botchi J (2002) Intrinsic spinal cord tumor resection. Neurosurgery 50(5):1059–1063
29. Costantini S, Miller DC, Allen JC, Rorke LB, Freed D, Epstein FJ (2000) Radical excision of intramedullary spinal cord tumors: surgical morbidity and long term follow upevaluation in 164 children and young adults. J Neurosurg 93(suppl 2):183–193
30. McGirt MJ, Chaichana KL, Atiba A, Attenello F, Yao KC, Jallo GI (2008) Resection of intramedullary spinal cord tumors in children: assessment of long-term motor and sensory deficits. J Neurosurg Pediatrics 1:63–67
31. Misra SN, Morgan HW (2003) Avoidance of structural pitfalls in spinal meningioma resection. Neurosurg focus 14(6):9–15
32. Maira G, Amante P, DenaroL MA, Colosimo C (2001) Surgical treatment of cervical intramedullary spinal cord tumors. Neurol Res 23:835–842
33. Klekamp J, Samii W (1999) Surgical results for spinal meningiomas. Surg Neurol 52(6):552–562
34. Saito T, Arizono T, Maeda T, Terada K, Iwamoto Y (2001) A novel technique for surgical resection of spinal meningioma. Spine 26(16):1805–1808
35. Roux FX, Nataf F, Pinaudeau M, Borne G, Devaux B, Meder JF (1996) Intraspinal meningiomas, review of 54 cases with discussion of poor prognosis factors and modern therapeutic management. Surg Neurol 46:458–464
36. Hajjar MV, Smith DA, Schmidek HH (2000) Surgical management of tumors of the nerve sheath involving the spine. In: Schmidek HH (ed) Operative neurosurgical techniques. WB Saunders, Philadelphia, pp 1843–1854

Syringomyelia

16

Luca Denaro and Domenico D'Avella

Contents

L. Denaro (✉)
Department of Neuroscience, University of Padua,
Via Giustiniani 5, 35128 Padua, Italy
e-mail: lucadenaro@hotmail.com

16.1 Syringomyelia and the Chiari Malformations

Syringomyelia is a chronic and progressive condition caused by a longitudinal fluid-filled cavity within the spinal cord. The term includes hydromyelia, which is referred to a dilatation of the central canal by cerebrospinal fluid usually in communication with the fourth ventricle [1]. This condition is the consequence of an impaired cerebrospinal fluid dynamics due to an obstruction of the spinal subarachnoid space. Different are the causes: acquired as trauma, infections, inflammations that cause arachnoid scars obstructing the spinal subarachnoid space below the foramen magnum (primary syringomyelia), or congenital anomalies, as the Chiari I malformations and other conditions associated with a small posterior fossa, that obstruct the subarachnoid space at the level of the foramen magnum (secondary syringomyelya) [2].

16.2 Pathogenesis and Development Theories

Chiari malformation is a hindbrain herniation without associated mass lesions. Hans Chiari [3], in 1891, classified the hindbrain herniation through the foramen magnum in three types: type I characterized by the herniation of cerebellar tonsils below the foramen magnum with no spinal cord anomalies; type II is the herniation of the cerebellar vermis, the forth ventricle and part of medulla and pons are associated with lumbar myelomeningoceles and hydrocephalus; type III is the herniation of the posterior fossa content in a cervical–occipital meningocele.

L. Denaro et al. (eds.), *Pitfalls in Cervical Spine Surgery*,
DOI: 10.1007/978-3-540-85019-9_16, © Springer-Verlag Berlin Heidelberg 2010

The mechanism at the base of syringomyelia formation has been studied extensively by Oldfield and colleagues [2, 4, 5], who described the descended tonsils as acting as pistons against the somewhat isolated spinal fluid compartment beneath the tonsils, thereby driving fluid from the subarachnoid space into the cord parenchyma. There are no studies about the pathophysiology of syringomyelia not associated with Chiari I, but Batzdorf assumes that when pulsatile CSF encounters scar tissue, cyst membrane, or tumor, it fulfills the role of the "piston" [2].

16.3 Symptomatology

Batzdorf [6] subdivided the symptoms of syringomyelia in symptoms referable to syringomyelic cavity and the associated symptoms related to the hindbrain descend (Chiari syndrome). Syringomyelic cysts are often asymmetric and consequently neurological deficits can involve, in different ways, the two sides of the spine. Anterior horn cells destruction is responsible for upper extremity weakness and atrophy, loss of temperature sensation results from spinothalamic tract lesions, while corticospinal tract lesions are responsible for spasticity. Dysesthetic pain and loss of sweating, often in the area of sensory loss, result from the lesion of the intermediolateral columns [6]. Symptoms related to Chiari syndrome are due to the impaired cerebrospinal fluid dynamics responsible for headache, typically at the base of the skull or upper neck, brought on by situations associated with a Valsalva maneuver rarely accompanied by transient visual obscuration. The involvement of brain stem and lower cranial nerve are responsible of ocular symptoms, as double vision or nystagmus, dizziness, vertigo. Aspiration, impaired coughing and swallowing, and alteration of the voice are due to the involvement of the lower cranial nerve [6].

16.4 Diagnosis and Evaluation

MR allow accurate identification and characterization of the syringomyelic cavity. In T1-weighted images, the syrinx cavity appear hypointense in contrast with the spinal tissue. T1-weighted images are useful to study the morphology and extension. Sagittal images show the rostral and caudal extension of the cavity and septations if present. Axial images detect eccentricity of the lesion and the size of the cord. In T2-weighted images, the cavity appear hyperintense in the absence of flow whereas as a contrary, in the presence of a CSF movement, it can be seen as areas of signal void. Detecting the presence of a hindbrain descend is essential in the diagnostic procedures to plan therapeutic strategy. At present, the cerebellar tonsils descending below the foramen magnum up to 3 mm is considered normal, between 3 and 5 is borderline, and greater than 5 mm is pathological. Pointed or wedge-shaped tonsils are considered pathological [6, 7]. In some cases when the syrinx cavity has no explanations on the MR, a myelography with water-soluble contrast medium can be used in association with a CT scan. In patients who are diagnosed with syringomyelia with no signs of posterior fossa anomalies or negative history for causative event as trauma or infections, it is mandatory to perform a MR scan with contrast injection, to exclude the presence of a tumor.

16.5 Surgical Treatment and Complications Avoidance

Surgical treatment of syrinx aim to prevent the progression of myelopathy and to improve symptoms. Syrinx formations are related to a spinal fluid circulation disturbance; therefore, the goal of therapy is to eliminate the causes of impaired circulation. If this is not possible or in case of a failure, other methods such as syrinx shunting have to be considered. In some cases, different procedures are performed in the same patient.

All patients go to surgery wearing antiembolism compression stockings and, in the postoperative period, if they are not ambulatory soon, thromboprophylaxis with low-molecular-weight heparin is given. Surgical related complications are of general type as wound infections, meningitis, cerebrospinal fluid leak, and venous thrombosis, and specific for each treatment. Laminectomy preserving the lateral masses in adult patients and laminotomy in pediatric patients prevent the postoperative delayed spinal deformity and instability. Intraoperative level confirmations are recommended.

16.5.1 Primary Syringomyelia: Decompression of Subarachnoid Space

In primary syringomyelia, the obstruction is due to the scar tissue located along the spinal cord. Batzdorf and Williams [8, 9] proposed the resection of the scar tissue and the expansion of the subarachnoid space. This technique provides a more physiologic solution avoiding an incision into the spinal cord and the introduction of a foreign body. Careful preoperative studies are necessary to localize the exact level of the scar. A wide laminectomy, with respect of the facet joints is performed on the identified level of obstruction and extended, rostrally and caudally, to create enough space to insert a dural graft. A mid line dural incision is made using a micro scalpel. To open the dura leaving the arachnoid intact, it is possible, after a short incision, to open it only pulling the edges of the dura using microforceps. After dural retention sutures are placed, resection of the scar is performed extending to each side of the spinal cord. The area of scar resection is bridged and closed using a dural graft of autologous fascia lata or bovine pericardium or other biological membranes. The risk of scar tissue adhesion may be reduced by using an inner layer of Gortex dura graft substitute and dural tenting sutures. In pseudomeningocele patients, recurrence and failure of the procedure are the major problems reported [8]. Batzdorf concluded that this technique is most applicable in patients with very focal areas of scarring or an arachnoid band, while it is not indicated in cases of arachnoid scarring that extends over several spinal segments. [8]. Klekamp reported a 83% stabilization or reduction in size of syrinx in 35 patients operated on for focal arachnoid scarring, but in only 17% of patients in whom extensive scarring had been demonstrated [10]. Similar conclusions are reported by Lee, in a small series of seven patients in whom he observed a clinical improvement in four cases for localized scar tissue [11]. Furthermore, he underlined that the most important point in clinical improvement is the reversal of the pathological mechanism of CSF alteration rather than the size decrease of the syrinx. Particular case is syringomyelia associated with an uncorrected posttraumatic spinal deformity. In these patients, the displaced bone fragments compress the spinal cord and cause an obstruction of CSF circulation resulting in syrinx formation. Epidural decompressive surgery may result in the reduction of the syrinx and neurological improvement [12].

16.5.2 Shunting Procedures for Syringomyelia

Historically, drainage procedures were the first to be used to treat syringomyelia, draining the fluid from the cysts into the subarachnoid space or into other body cavities. [8]. Shunting of the syrinx to the subarachnoid, pleural, or peritoneal space is still accepted to treat patients with syringomyelia, in which arachnoid scarr extends over several spinal segments, when the resection of scar tissue failed or in case of recurrent scar tissue formation in the postoperative time [13]. On the basis of RM findings, the level where the cavity is wider is identified and a two-level laminectomy is performed preserving the facet joint. The dura is incised along the midline or, in case of an hemilaminectomy, in the center of the exposed area [14]. Special care is necessary not to damage the arachnoid that is than incised and tended to the dural edges. Meticulous hemostasis is recommended, because blood in the subarachnoid space may cause meningeal irritation, arachnoiditis, and shunt fail. To open the syrinx, a 2–3 mm myeloyomy is made utilizing a microscalpel. Multiple options have been used: midline myelotomy, myelotomy through the thinnest portion of the syrinx, postero-lateral myelotomy, or dorsal root entry zone myelotomy [15]. Syringomyelic cavities are often not simple, confluent fluid spaces. Rather, they may be quite complex, with separate channels that may or may not communicate with each other. In case of septated syringes, attempts should be made to place the tube in the largest cavity . The catheter is sutured to the pia mater at the myelotomy site, a pad of fascia can be placed around the entry site of the tube as a further insurance against siphonage of spinal CSF, which might enter the syrinx at this site and be drained. The dura and the arachnoid are sutured maintaining the integrity of the subarachnoid space. The caudal end of the catheter is placed either in the ventral subarachnoid space, anterior to the dentate ligament or a subcutaneous tunnel is created to reach the thorax or abdomen. In these cases of syringoperitoneal or syringopleural shunt, some authors recommend the use of a one-way low pressure or programmable valve to avoid overdrainage phenomena as transient positional headhaches [16, 6]. If the distal end is placed in the subarachnoid space, no valve should be used because the majority of syringomyelia patients have a normal overall cerebrospinal fluid pressure. Follow ing surgery, the syrinx rarely disappears, but the patients may show good clinical improvement. In patients with no clinical improvement and persistent syrinx, the cause is generally related to technical consideration. Shunting of the syrinx to the subarachnoid space, pleura, or peritoneum carries the risk of significant morbidity: spinal cord injury at myelotomy site or due to the insertion of the catheter, hemorrhage, shunt dysfunction, disconnection, or infection [5, 17, 18]. The most common complication related to shunting is malfunction of the shunt, which may occur by dislodgment of the proximal or distal ends, development of local arachnoiditis obliterating the distal catheter, incomplete penetration of syrinx septation, or infections [19, 20]. Failure of a shunt to function may occur because of simple shunt disconnection, separation at the site of a connector, inappropriate placement of the distal tip of the cyst-to-subarachnoid shunt into the subdural rather than the subarachnoid space or placement of the distal tip into a partially scarred subarachnoid space. One problem that can complicate the technique is the excessive efficiency of the system. This can produce energetic flattening of the cord imposing an immediate stress on the cord. Another complication is the syrinx collapse around the tube blocking it, or the evenience of glial tissue that grows in it closing the hole of the catheter (Fig. 16.1). The syrinx will then reform leaving the drain immured in the wall of the cavity [21]. In some patients who have ongoing or progressive neurological symptoms, with an adequate drainage of the cyst, a tethering cord could be the cause. Cord tethering occurs at the site of spinal injury in patients affected by posttraumatic syringomyelia but the role of the shunt tube as an anchoring mechanism of the dorsal spinal cord has been recognized in particular in the most mobile cervical spine [21–23]. After laminectomy, the development of postoperative deformity, in children for shunt insertion, recurrent pleural effusion, and distal shunt migration in the pleural space has been reported [9, 14].

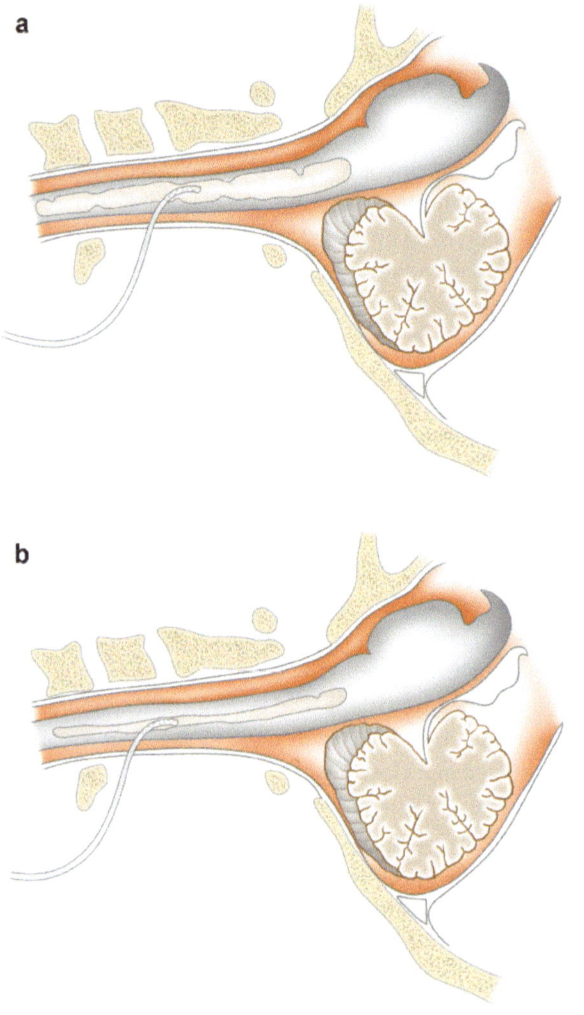

Fig. 16.1 (**a**) Positioning of the tube into the syrinx (**b**) The syrinx may collapse around the tube blocking it

16.5.3 Syringomyelia and Chiari Malformation: Posterior Fossa Decompression

The current trend regarding the surgical treatment of syringomyelia associated with Chiari 1 malformations is to try to restore the normal flow of CSF at the foramen magnum as the first step. Drainage of the syringx is advocated as an adjuvant only if the first surgery fails [24]. Posterior fossa decompression may involve complications from anesthesia, craniectomy, opening of the dura and arachnoid, intradural intra-arachnoid exploration, dural closure, hematoma, and infection. As in all patients harboring a cervical cord or medullary compression due to any causes, excessive neck motion should be avoided during intubation and positioning. The neural elements are already compressed by the cerebella tonsils or the syrinx. Marked flexion of the neck during surgery may cause postoperative neurological deficit or respiratory problems [25]. Intubation in the awake patient or monitoring of evoked potentials, are preferable. It is important to avoid hypotension to protect an already compromised spinal cord. The small size of the posterior fossa in these patients may make for protrusion or ptosis of the cerebellum through the craniectomy. The posterior fossa craniectomy should not be large to prevent postoperative cerebellar ptosis. An opening of the occipital bone no larger than 3 cm in width and 2.5 cm far from the edge of the foramen magnum maintains the support of the cerebellum; furthermore, extension farther laterally risks injury to the vertebral artery. C1 laminectomy can be a necessity to achieve decompression of the descended tonsilla (Fig. 16.2). The size of the decompression dose not matter; what matters is the adequacy of the decompression in the zone where craniospinal pressure dissociation is engendered. When bleeding from the venous plexus is encountered, it is treated by packing with Surgicel or Gelfoam [26]. The dura is opened in a Y-shaped fashion, being careful enough to keep the arachnoid intact (Fig. 16.3). The occipital sinus is either coagulated or clipped. The dural opening should be carried inferior to the tonsils. The arachnoid is separated from the dura. The author's current treatment, in the first instance, is to maintain the arachnoid intact and to cover it with a dural graft. Theoretically, if only the dura is opened, potential complications related to CSF leakage are

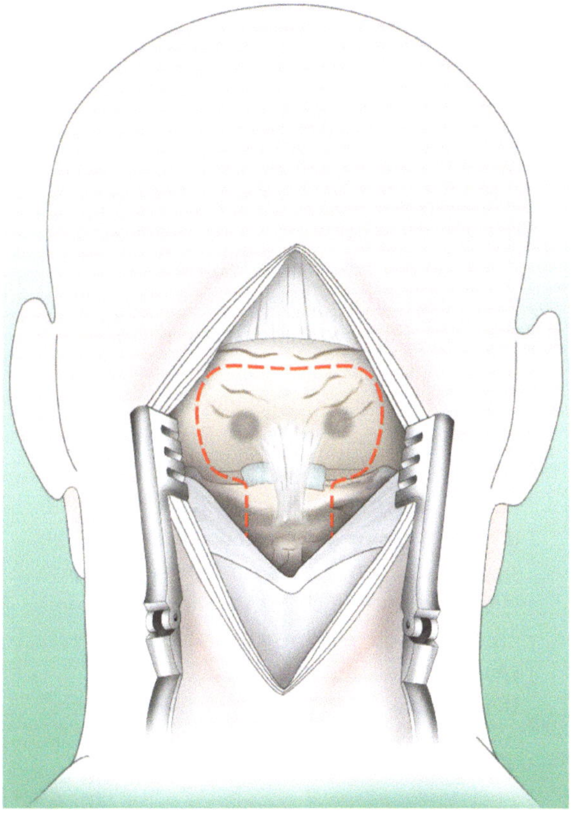

Fig. 16.2 Craniectomy should be no larger than 3 cm in width and 2.5 cm far from the edge of the foramen magnum. In same cases, C1 laminectomy can be necessary to achieve decompression of the descended tonsilla

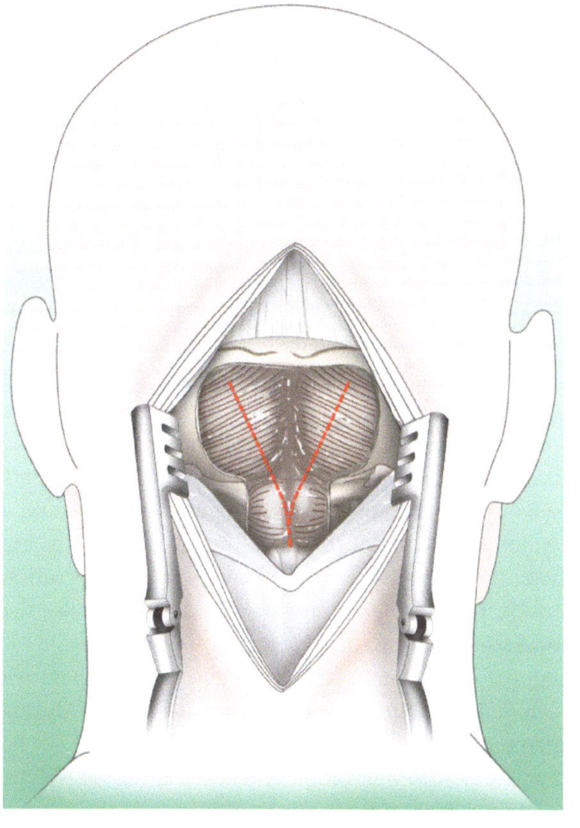

Fig. 16.3 The dura is opened in a Y-shaped fashion, being careful to keep the arachnoid intact

avoided. In case of a pinpoint opening seal, control with bipolar coagulation or fibrin glue is recommended. The dura is then patched with a watertight closure to prevent postoperative complications of pseudomeningocele, CSF leak, or meningitis. The tightness of the dural closure is tested with a Valsalva maneuver. Isu [17] proposed to remove only the outer layer of dura. They found this technique to be effective in the reduction of the size of the syrinx on postoperative MRI [17]. If intradural exploration in needed, for example, when the tonsils appear as they did before first operation, the presence of fibrosis increases the risks. In these patients, a reoperation and an attack on the tonsils is necessary. The surgery may be more difficult if a graft has been inserted owing to the fibrosis involving the arachnoid and the pia over the tonsils and the medulla with an increased risk of both, vascular and medullary damage. If it is necessary to perform an intra-arachnoid exploration, even if the tonsils can be separated easily, vascular damages are possible. Any sizable artery should be spared and the posterior inferior cerebellar artery should be respected. There may be small strands with vessels that appear to run from the medulla to the cerebellum. The rule is not to cauterize anything that could possibly be supplying the medulla. Damage to the medulla can be severe. Even a covering of tissue that appears extremely thin should not be myelotomized or excised [27]. Chiari malformation is often accompanied by hydrocephalus. Batzdorf [27, 28] notes a minor degree of hydrocephalus can be ignored, although vigilance in the postoperative period is necessary. Major hydrocephalus has to be treated.

All patients are given prophylactic antibiotics. In the postoperative period, deterioration can be observed. In addition to hydrocephalus that should be treated, other complications can be seen. Patients who do not breathe well after operation constitute a major problem. Mortality following surgery is not unknown. Patients are maintained under observation in the intensive care unit for the day following the operation. Vasospasm of a major blood vessel supplying the cerebellum can be the cause of postoperative cerebellar ataxic symptoms. Persistence of dysesthetic pain after syringomyelia therapy should not be confused with neurological deterioration. This type of pain is very resistant to treatment and may remain troublesome for patients who are otherwise doing well [24, 29–31].

Core Messages

Syringomyelia and the Chiari Malformations

- Surgical treatment of syrinx aim to prevent the progression of myelopathy and to improve symptoms.
- Syrinx formations is related to a spinal fluid circulation disturbance; therefore, the goal of therapy is to eliminate the causes of impaired circulation. If this is not possible or in case of a failure, other methods as syrinx shunting are to be considered.
- In primary syringomyelia, the resection of the scar tissue and the expansion of the subarachnoid space is the therapy of choice.
- The area of scar resection is bridged and closed using a dural graft of autologous fascia lata or bovine pericardium or other biological membranes.
- Shunting of the syrinx to the subarachnoid, pleural, or peritoneal space is still accepted to treat patients with syringomyelia, in which arachnoid scarr extends over several spinal segments, when the resection of scar tissue failed or in the case of recurrent scar tissue formation in the postoperative time.
- Meticulous hemostasis is recommended, because blood in the subarachnoid space may cause meningeal irritation, arachnoiditis, and shunt fail.
- The current trend regarding the surgical treatment of syringomyelia associated with Chiari 1 malformations is to try to restore the normal flow of CSF at the foramen magnum as the first step.
- Drainage of the syringx is advocated as an adjuvant only if the first surgery fails. The posterior fossa craniectomy should not be large to prevent postoperative cerebellar ptosis. The size of the decompression dose not matter; what matters is the adequacy of the decompression in the zone where craniospinal pressure dissociation is engendered.
- If intradural exploration is needed, the presence of fibrosis increases risks.
- Any sizable artery should be spared and the posterior–inferior cerebellar artery should be respected. The rule is not to cauterize anything that could possibly be supplying the medulla.

References

1. Wisoff JH, Epstein F (1989) Management of hydromyelia. Neurosurgery 25:562–571
2. Batzdorf U (2005) Primary spinal syringomyelia. J Neurosurg Spine 3:429–435
3. Chiari H (1987) Concerning alterations in the cerebellum resulting from cerebral hydrocephalus. Pediatric Neurosci 13:3–8
4. Heiss JD, Patronas N, DeVroom HL (1999) Elucidating the pathophysiology of syringomyelia. J Neurosurg 91:553–562
5. Oldfield EH, Murasko K, Shawker TH et al (1994) Pathopysiology of syringomyelia associated with Chiari I malformation of the cerebellar tonsils. Implications for diagnosis and treatment. J Neurosurg 80:3–15
6. Batzdorf U (2000) Microsurgery of syringomyelia and syringomyelia cord syndrome. In: Schmidek HH, Sweet WH (eds) Operative neurosurgical techniques. Saunders, Philadelphia, pp 1946–1954
7. Schnk M, Ruggeri P (1997) Imaging of syringomyelia and the Chiari malformation. In: Anson JA, Benzel EC, Awad A (eds) Syringomyelia and the Chiari malformations. Neurosurgical topics. The American Association of Neurological Surgeons, Park Ridge, pp 41–56
8. Batzdorf U (2000) Primary spinal syringomyelia: a personal perspective. Neurosurg Focus 8: Article 7
9. Vernet O, Farmer JP, Montes JL (1996) Comparison of syringopleural and syringosubarachnoid shunting in the treatment of syringomyelia in children. J Neurosurg 84: 624–628
10. Klekamp J, Batzdorf U, Samii M et al (1997) Treatment of syringomyelia associated with arachnoid scarring caused by arachnoiditis or trauma. J Neurosurg 86:233–240
11. Lee JH, Chung CK, Kim HJ (2002) Decompression of the spinal subarachnoid space as a solution for syringomyelia without Chiari malformation. Spinal Cord 40:501–506
12. Holly LT, Johnson JP, Masciopinto JE et al (2000) Treatment of posttraumatic syringomyelia with extradural decompressive surgery. Neurosurg Focus 8: article 8
13. Iwasaki Y, Koianagi I, Hida K (1999) Syringo-subarachnoid shunt for syringomyelia using partial hemilaminectomy. Br J Neurosurg 13:41–45
14. Colak A, Boran BO, Kutlay M et al (2005) A modified technique for syringo-subarachnoid shunt for treatment of syringomyelia. J Clin Neurosci 12:677–679
15. Rhoton AL (1976) Microsurgery of Arnold Chiari malformation in adults with and without hydromyelia. J Neurosurg 45:473–483
16. Lesion F, Petit H, Thomas CEIII et al (1986) Use of syringoperitoneal shunt in the treatment of syringomyelia. Surg Neurol 25:131–136
17. Isu T, Sasaki H, Takamura H et al (1993) Foramen magnum decompression with removal of the outer layer of the dura as treatment for syringomyelia occurring with Chiari I malformation. Neurosurgery 33:845–850
18. Schlesinger EB (1992) Letter to the editor. Surg Neurol 38(161–163):10
19. Hida K, IwasakiY IH et al (1994) Posttraumatic syringomyelia: its characteristic magnetic resonance imaging findings and surgical management. Neurosurgery 35:886–891
20. Kern MB, Anson JA et al (1997) Shunting procedures for syringomyelia in Chiari malformations. Syringomyelia and the Chiari malformations. Neurosurgical topics. The American Association of Neurological Surgeons, Park Ridge, pp 151–157
21. Batzdorf U, Klekamp J, Johnson JP (1998) A critical appraisal of syrinx cavity shunting procedures. J Neurosurg 89:382–388
22. Sgouros S, Williams B (1995) A critical appraisal of drainage in syringomyelia. J Neurosurg 82:1–10
23. Steinmetz A, Aschoff A, Kunze S (1993) Complications. Evaluation of surgical treatment. The iatrogenic tethering of the cord. Acta Neurochir 123:219–220
24. Batzdorf U (1997) Complications and deterioration following surgery. In: Anson JA, Benzel EC, Awad A (eds) Syringomyelia and the Chiari malformations. Neurosurgical topics. The American Association of Neurological Surgeons, Park Ridge, pp 159–165
25. Mullan S, Raimondi AJ (1962) Respiratory hazards of the surgical treatment of the Arnold-Chiari malformation. Neurosurgery 19:675–678
26. Duddy MJ, Williams B (1991) Hindbrain migration after decompression for hindbrain hernia: a quantitative assessment using MRI. Br J Neurosurg 5:141–152
27. Williams B (1997) Management schemes for syringomyelia: surgical indications and nonsurgical management. In: Anson JA, Benzel EC, Awad A (eds) Syringomyelia and the Chiari malformations. Neurosurgical Topics. The American Association of Neurological Surgeons, Park Ridge, pp 125–143
28. Batzdorf U (1991) Syringomyelia related to abnormalities at the level of the craniovertebral junction. In: Badzdorf U (ed) Syringomyelia: current concepts in diagnosis and treatment. Baltimore, Williams & Wilkins, pp 163–182
29. Dyste GN, Menezes AH, VanGilder JC (1989) Symptomatic Chiari malformations. An analysis of presentation, management and log-term outcome. J Neurosurg 71:159–168
30. Batzdorf U (1993) Chiari malformation and syringomyelia. In: Apuzzo MJL (ed) Brain surgery: complication avoidance and management. Churchill Livigstone, New York
31. Lam S, Batzdorf U, Bergsneider M (2008) Thecal shunt placement for treatment of obstructive primary syringomyelia. J Neurosurg Spine 9:581–588

Section VI

Miscellanea

Complications Related to Graft

17

Umile Giuseppe Longo, Luca Denaro, Nicola Maffulli, and Vincenzo Denaro

Contents

U. G. Longo (✉)
Department of Orthopaedic and Trauma Surgery,
Campus Biomedico University, Via Alvaro del Portillo,
200, 00128 Rome, Italy
e-mail: g.longo@unicampus.it

L. Denaro et al. (eds.), *Pitfalls in Cervical Spine Surgery*,
DOI: 10.1007/978-3-540-85019-9_17, © Springer-Verlag Berlin Heidelberg 2010

17.1 Introduction

Arthrodesis of the spine is a commonly employed procedure for several cervical spinal pathologies, including deformity, instability, trauma, and degenerative diseases [1–5]. Failure of fusion is always a therapeutic challenge. Bone graft is used in cervical spine surgery to achieve several goals: to enhance bone healing reducing the risk of nonunion [6], to reconstruct bony defects, to restore the load-bearing capacity of the cervical spine, and, when adequately shaped, to restore the physiological lordosis of the cervical spine [7, 8].

Integration of the graft depends on multiple factors. The presence of any detrimental condition may diminish the osteogenic potential of the fusion site, and contribute to the development of a nonunion. Numerous systemic risk factors may inhibit bone formation, including use of tobacco or other drugs, advanced age of the patient, and metabolic comorbidities (i.e., diabetes or osteoporosis) [9] (see Chap. 1). Structural instability, improper preparation of the host bone, and poor vascularity are other factors that may contribute to unsuccessful arthrodesis of the spine [5].

The three primary types of bone graft materials used are autografts (graft from the patient's own bone), allografts (graft from bone harvested from other subjects), and synthetic bone graft substitutes (bone graft materials and synthetic substitutes) [10]. An ideal bone graft will have osteogenic, osteoconductive, and osteoinductive properties, increasing the regenerative capacity of the host bone and load-bearing capacity (Table 17.1). Graft osteogenesis is the transplant of osteogenic precursor cells, able to form new bone, that may originate from a graft or host bed [11]. Osteoinduction is the property of the graft by which pluripotential mesenchymal cells are recruited from a surrounding host tissue to differentiate into osteoblasts [12]. Osteoconduction refers to a process in which the three-dimensional structure of a substance is conducive for the ongrowth and/or ingrowth of newly formed bone [13].

17.2 Autograft

Autograft bone is biologically superior to allograft for multiple reasons, being at the same time osteoconductive, osteoinductive, and osteogenic. It houses cells, minerals, connective tissue, and proteins able to facilitate new bone growth [14]. Because autograft bone is identical to its host, there is no incompatibility of the major histocompatibility complex seen in allogeneic transplants. This lack of immunogenicity seen with the use of autografts facilitates graft incorporation. Another advantage to the use of autograft is the lack of disease transmission, a major potential complication of allogeneic transplants [14]. Autologous bone also is available in various contours, it is generally available, and it is not necessary to store it before transplantation.

Despite these advantages, the incidence of donor site morbidity has led to the evaluation of alternatives to autograft use. Blood loss, nerve damage, infection, cosmetic deformity, and chronic pain are some of the complications that can arise from harvesting of autograft bone [15, 16]. Although autograft (i.e., iliac crest autograft) remains the gold standard for fusion, the quantity of autograft bone available is limited in a given patient, its procurement results in more extensive surgical trauma, necessitates a separate operative incision, and it has been associated with significant donor site morbidity [3, 13]. Age of the patient, previous surgery or bone harvesting in the area, and donor site pathologic features are factors contributing to insufficient availability of autograft.

Grafts may be constituted of purely cancellous bone, purely cortical bone, or a mixture of cortical and cancellous bones. Pure cancellous grafts consist of bone marrow cells, bone matrix proteins, and mineral for scaffolding. They have the highest fusion rates [14], and are frequently used in posterior spinal fusions. In anterior column reconstruction procedures, they carry only 60% of the compressive strength of tricortical grafts, and they cannot withstand the compressive forces required in anterior reconstructive spinal surgery [14, 17]. On the other hand, pure cortical grafts can be used to this aim, but they have decreased osteogenic capacity because they contain less cellular components and, as a consequence, lower fusion rates than cancellous bone [14, 17]. For this reason, in patients in whom strong structural support is needed, pure cortical grafts are commonly supplemented with an internal autogenous cancellous filler [14, 17]. Grafts containing a combination of autologous cancellous and allogeneic cortical bone are popular in anterior spinal reconstructive procedures because they can withstand high anterior compressive forces while retaining osteogenic potential. The composition of the graft, its ability to

Table 17.1 Properties of the most common employed grafts

	Osteogenic	Osteoinductive	Osteoconductive
Cancellous autograft	Yes	Yes	Yes
Cancellous allograft	No	No	Yes
Bone marrow aspirate	No	Yes	No
Platelet-rich plasma	No	Yes	No
Demineralized bone matrix	No	Yes	Yes
Bone morphogenetic proteins	Yes	Yes	No
Ceramics	No	No	Yes

stimulate the healing process, graft positioning, and graft stability once transplanted are important factors in graft incorporation [18]. Because few donor osteocytes survive transplantation, proper decortication of the host site is needed to provide adequate transference of mesenchymal osteoprogenitor cells [14].

General complications of all bone graft materials at the recipient site include osseous nonunion, delayed union, graft fracture, graft extrusion, and infection (see above).

17.3 Allografts

Allograft bone is an attractive alternative to autogenous bone, as it avoids donor site morbidity, is relatively abundant, and can be used off the shelf. Allograft bone is not considered to be osteogenic, because the donor cells are eradicated during tissue processing [13]. However, through its osteoconductive properties, allograft bone is used as a biologic scaffolding to facilitate the production of new bone by the host. The rate of fusion can be improved by adding growth factors obtained from autologous platelet gel or other osteoinductive materials. More recently, we used autologous bone marrow cell concentrates enriched with platelet-rich fibrin on corticocancellous bone allograft for posterolateral multilevel cervical fusion [19]. Allografts are prepared either by freezing or lyophilization (i.e., freeze-drying) to decrease their antigenicity and allow storage for long periods [20]. Disadvantages of the use of allografts include the possibility of disease transmission (although it should be acknowledged that this risk has become negligible because of tissue processing and sterilization procedures), the costs of a bone bank, host immune response, and inconsistent graft incorporation [5].

Miyazaki et al. [21] evaluated the levels of evidence of the studies containing original data on bone substitutes for cervical spinal fusion to elucidate their effect and to establish clinical guidance. They concluded that among many alternatives, there seems to be strong evidence only for osteoinductive proteins (rhBMP-2 and OP-1) to show that they can be used as bone enhancers and substitutes for any kind of spinal fusion. Detailed description of these studies is reported in Table 17.2.

17.3.1 Studies Comparing Allografts vs. Autografts

Brown et al. [22] conducted a radiographic evaluation to compare 53 patients who had 76 cervical interspaces grafted with frozen, bone marrow-free cadaver bone to 45 patients who received 63 iliac crest autografts for anterior cervical spine fusion. The roentgenograms were evaluated on the basis of achieving union, delayed union, nonunion, and the presence of graft collapse and extrusion. No significant difference was noted in the union rate, with allografts (94%) or with autografts (97%). In 21 patients, a higher rate of graft collapse was noted with allografts when compared with autografts in multilevel fusions. No difference in collapse rate was noted between allografts and autografts in 32 patients with single-level fusions. Insertion of frozen bone allografts into intervertebral spaces of the cervical spine did not produce adverse reactions.

Young et al. [23] conducted a retrospective comparison of patients undergoing cervical anterior spinal fusion through the Smith–Robinson technique, for both one- and two-level fusions, using cadaveric fibular allografts (23 patients) or autologous iliac crest grafts (25 patients). Evidence of radiographic fusion was achieved in 92% of the patients undergoing fusion

Table 17.2 Levels of evidence of the studies containing original data on bone substitutes for cervical spinal fusion

Author(years)	Type of study	Graft	Numbers of patients (vertebral levels)	Procedure	Plates	Postoperative immobilization	Nonunion	Statistical significance of results	Level of evidence
Brown et al. [21]	Retrospective study	Frozen iliac allografts	53	Smith–Robinson1 level (32)	No	6–8weeks	1	NS	III
				Smith–Robinson 2 levels (19)	No	6–8weeks	4	NS	
		Iliac crest autografts	45	Smith–Robinson 1 level (29)	No	6–8weeks	0	NS	
				Smith–Robinson 2–3 levels (16)	No	6–8weeks	2	NS	
Young et al. [23]	Retrospective study	Cadaveric fibular allografts	23	Smith–Robinson 1 level	No	Philadelphia Collar 6 weeks	2	NS	III
		Iliac crest autografts	25	Smith–Robinson 1 level	No	Philadelphia Collar 6 weeks	3	NS	
Savolainen et al. [24]	Retrospective study	Heterologous artificial bone graft (UnilabSurgibone | Unilab Inc. USA)	101	Smith–Robinson	No	Not reported	2	NS	III
		Iliac crest autografts	149	Smith–Robinson	No	Not reported	3	NS	
Zhang et al. [25]	Retrospective study	Allografts	20	Smith–Robinson	No	Not reported	10	S	IV
		Autografts	58	Smith–Robinson	No	Not reported	9	S	
Zdeblick et al. [26]	Retrospective study	Frozen iliac allografts	27	1 level (19)	No	Rigid collar for 6 weeks, then soft collar for 2 weeks	1	NS	III
				2-levels (8)	No	Rigid collar for 6 weeks, followed by soft collar for 2 weeks	5	$p=0.03$	
		Iliac crest autografts	60	1 level (41)	No	Rigid collar for 6 weeks, followed by soft collar for 2 weeks	2	NS	
				2–3 levels (19)	No	Rigid collar for 6 weeks, followed by soft collar for 2 weeks	3	$p=0.03$	

Bishop et al. [27]	Prospective study	Tricortical iliac crest allografts (49 patients)	32	Single-level	No	Philadelphia collar for 8 weeks	4	$p=0.004$	II
			17	Multilevel	No	Philadelphia collar for 8 weeks	4	$p=0.005$	
		Tricortical iliac crest autografts (83 patients)	60	Single-level	No	Philadelphia collar for 8 weeks	2	$p=0.004$	
			23	Multilevel	No	Philadelphia collar for 8 weeks	0	$p=0.005$	
Thalgott et al. [30]	Retrospective study	Coralline hydroxyapatite (Pro Osteon 200)	26	Smith–Robinson 1 level (14)	AO cervical spine locking plate	Philadelphia collar for 12 weeks	0		III
				Smith–Robinson Multilevel (12)	AO cervical spine locking plate	Philadelphia collar for 12 weeks	0		
An et al. [31]	Prospective study	Freeze-dried allograft augmented with demineralized bone matrix	39	Smith–Robinson 1 level (19)	No	Philadelphia collar for 6 weeks	9	NS	I
				Smith–Robinson 2–3 levels (20)	No	Philadelphia collar for 6 weeks	9	NS	
		Iliac crest autografts (38)	38	Smith–Robinson 1 level (19)	No	Philadelphia collar for 6 weeks	5	NS	
				Smith–Robinson 2–3 levels (19)	No	Philadelphia collar for 6 weeks	6	NS	
Baskin et al. [32]	Prospective pilot trial	INFUSE™ bone graft (rhBMP-2 applied to absorbable collagen sponge	18	Smith–Robinson 1 level (10)	ATLANTIS™ anterior cervical plate	Not reported	0	NS	I
				Smith–Robinson 2 levels (8)	ATLANTIS™ anterior cervical plate	Not reported	0	NS	
		Iliac crest autograft placed inside the CORNERSTONESR™ fibular allograft	15	Smith–Robinson 1 level (8)	ATLANTIS™ anterior cervical plate	Not reported	0	NS	
				Smith–Robinson 2 levels (7)	ATLANTIS™ anterior cervical plate	Not reported	0	NS	

using cadaveric fibular allografts, and in 88% of the patients undergoing fusion using autologous iliac crest grafts, without statistically significant differences. The mean duration of hospital stay was less in the allograft group (5.4 vs. 7.25 days). In addition, postoperative pain was less in the allograft group because the allograft group did not have pain from the donor site.

Savolainen et al. [24], in a retrospective comparison of 250 patients undergoing anterior cervical surgery with iliac crest (149 patients) and artificial bone grafts (101 patients), found that a stable fusion was achieved in 98% of patients in both groups and there was no significant difference in the clinical outcome. Donor site complications (severe pain and hematoma) were seen in one-sixth of the patients with autologous bone grafts.

Zhang et al. [25] conducted a retrospective analysis of patients with cervical spondylotic myelopathy managed by anterior fusion. Autografts were used in 83 patients and allografts in 38 patients. The rate of autograft fusion was 81.6%, and for allografts the rate was 50%.

Zdeblick et al. [26] performed a retrospective analysis of a consecutive series of 87 patients undergoing Smith–Robinson anterior cervical fusion. Freeze-dried tricortical iliac crest bone was used in 27 patients, and tricortical autograft bone was used in 60 patients. Radiographs showed delayed union at 3 months in 13% of patients with autograft and in 37% of patients with freeze-dried allograft. At 1 year, radiography showed nonunion in 8% of patients with autograft and in 22% of patients with allograft. One-level procedures had a delayed union rate of 7% for autograft and 21% for allograft. Nonunion in one-level procedures was 5% for both autograft and allograft. For two-level procedures, the nonunion rate was 17% for autograft and 63% for allograft. Graft collapse was more commonly seen with freeze-dried allograft (30%) than with autograft (5%).

Bishop et al. [27] conducted a prospective study in 132 patients requiring interbody fusion without instrumentation following anterior cervical discectomy to compare the efficacy of tricortical iliac crest allograft vs. autograft fusion substrates. Autograft tricortical iliac crest bone was found to be superior to allograft bone as an interbody fusion substrate after both single- and multiple-level anterior cervical decompression procedures with respect to maintenance of cervical interspace height, interspace angulation, and radiographic and clinical fusion success rates. Cigarette consumption had a significant adverse effect on successful anterior cervical interbody fusion for both autograft and allograft substrates.

17.4 Bone Graft Substitutes

Bone graft substitutes, alternatives to allografts and autografts, are frequently used in cervical spine surgery [11, 12, 28, 29]. They have primarily osteoconductive properties. Currently used bone graft substitutes are subdivided into three primary groups: demineralized bone matrix, ceramics, and composite grafts. Clinical studies on bone graft substitutes are still in their infancy. It remains a great challenge to design an ideal bone graft that emulates nature's own structures or functions. Because of the distinct biological conditions and biomechanical forces that are specific to the anterior spinal column and the posterior elements, it is very likely that the efficacy of each bone graft material for generating successful fusion will also be dependent on the particular clinical application for which it is being used (i.e., interbody fusion vs. posterolateral fusion).

17.4.1 Ceramics

Thalgott et al. [30] conducted a nonrandomized, retrospective human study of 26 patients requiring anterior cervical discectomy and reconstruction to determine the efficacy of coralline hydroxyapatite as a bone replacement in conjunction with rigid plate fixation. They found no evidence of plate breakage, screw breakage, resorption of the implant, or pseudoarthrosis. Two patterns of incorporation were identified. The implant incorporated totally in 100% of the disk spaces. Average hospital stay was 1.6 days, and the average decrease in pain was 75.8%.

17.4.2 Demineralized Bone Matrices

An et al. [31] analyzed the fusion results of an allograft-demineralized bone matrix composite (39 patients) vs. autograft (38 patients) in a prospective series of patients undergoing anterior cervical fusion surgery for cervical disk disease. They found nonunion in 46.2% of patients (33.3% of levels) in the allograft-demineralized bone matrix group when compared with 26.3% (22% of levels) in the autograft group. For patients undergoing two-level fusions, 37.5% of allograft-demineralized bone matrix failed, compared with 23.5% of autografts. For single-level fusions, 47.4% of allograft patients developed a pseudoarthrosis, compared with 26.3% in the autograft group. Graft collapse of ≥3 mm was noted in 11% of the autograft group vs. 19% in the allograft-demineralized bone matrix group ($p=0.32$). Graft collapse of ≥2 mm occurred in 24.4% of autograft patients compared with 39.7% of the allograft-demineralized bone matrix group ($p=0.09$). Smokers had an increased rate of pseudoarthrosis (47.1%) when compared with non-smokers (27.9%, $p=0.13$). Then, the authors concluded that the allograft-demineralized bone matrix construct gives a higher rate of graft collapse and pseudoarthrosis when compared with autograft although the differences were not statistically significant.

17.4.3 Osteoinductive Growth Factors

Baskin et al. [32] conducted a prospective pilot trial on 33 patients with degenerative cervical disk disease to compare a fibular allograft (CORNERSTONE-SR Allograft Ring) with an rhBMP-2-laden collagen carrier inside the graft along with an ATLANTIS anterior cervical plate vs. a fibular allograft with cancellous iliac crest autograft placed inside it, along with an ATLANTIS anterior cervical plate. All the patients evaluated had solid fusions 6, 12, and 24 months after surgery. There were no device-related adverse events.

Shields et al. [33] retrospectively reviewed 151 patients undergoing anterior cervical fusion using recombinant human bone morphogenetic protein (rhBMP)-2 with an absorbable collagen sponge (INFUSE; Medtronic Sofamor Danek, Minneapolis, MN). A total of 35 (23.2%) patients had complications after the use of high-dose INFUSE in the cervical spine. There were 15 patients diagnosed with hematoma, including 11 on postoperative day 4 or 5, of whom eight were surgically evacuated. Thirteen individuals had either a prolonged hospital stay (> 48 h) or hospital readmission because of swallowing/breathing difficulties or dramatic swelling without hematoma.

Vaidya et al. [34] conducted a retrospective study in 46 consecutive patients undergoing anterior spinal fusion and instrumentation following discectomy. Twenty-two patients treated with rhBMP-2 and PEEK cages were compared with 24 patients in whom allograft spacers and demineralized bone matrix was used. Dysphagia was a common complication and it was significantly more frequent and more severe in patients in whom rhBMP-2 was used. Postoperative swelling anterior to the vertebral body on lateral cervical spine X-ray was significantly larger in the rhBMP-2 group when measured from 1 to 6 weeks after which it was similar.

17.5 Donor Site Complications

Autogenous grafts remain the gold standard for bone grafts. The iliac crest, the tibia, and the fibula are the common donor sites of bone grafts in cervical spine surgery, with the iliac crest being the commonest source. The ability to harvest autologous bone is a well-established skill in the surgical armamentarium of the orthopedic surgeon. As with any surgical procedure, these operations have their own set of complications. The surgeon must be aware of these potential problems in an effort to avoid them when possible. Potential disadvantages of autogenous grafting include infection, wound drainage, hematomas, reoperation, fracture, prolonged pain, sensory loss, and keloids [15, 35–37]. Autogenous bone grafting generally requires the patient to undergo a second skin incision, and there are the costs of long anesthetic time and hospital stay [8].

17.5.1 The Iliac Crest

The most common source of graft is the iliac crest. This site has the potential to provide cortical, cancellous, or both cortical and cancellous graft.

The bone stock of the ilium is thickest in two regions [38]: (1) the area extending from 2 to 3 cm posterior to the anterior superior iliac spine to a point 6–8 cm posteriorly along the iliac crest and (2) the postero-inferior portion (sacroiliac surface area) of the ilium.

In our experience, the ideal site of harvest is the portion of the crest between the two anterior thirds and

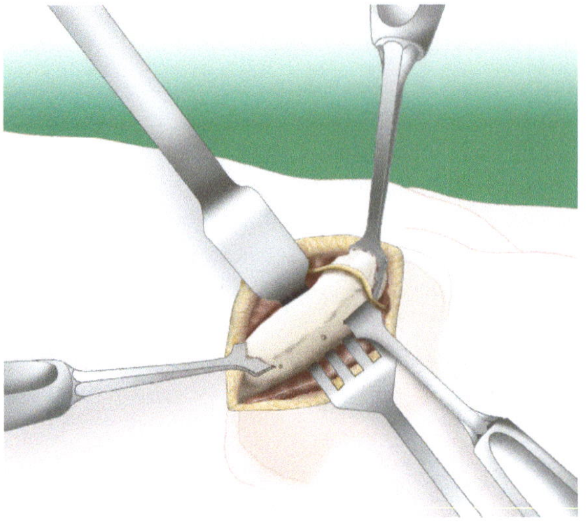

Fig. 17.1 When it is necessary to obtain a tricortical graft from the iliac crest following a corpectomy, the incision should be parallel to the iliac crest. The abdominal muscles and the gluteal muscles are detached on their respective sides. The iliac crest is exposed and full depth drill holes are used to delineate the margin of the resection. Chisels are placed proximally and distally, and are used as levers to hold and raise the graft, while a third scalpel is used to cut the graft in between the drill holes

the posterior third of the iliac wing, the latter being able to provide the greater amount of bone. It is important to begin harvesting of the graft from the front and work toward the back. The incision must start at least 5 cm from the anterior superior iliac spine. If the graft is harvested too anteriorly, the muscles may disrupt the bone at the anterior superior iliac spine. The major muscular pull will be from the tensors of the fascia lata and the sartorius muscle (Fig. 17.1). The choice of site will also depend on the position of the patient on the operating table (whether supine or prone) and on the type of graft required by the operative procedure [39]. The neurovascular structures adjacent to the ilium are the lateral femoral cutaneous, iliohypogastric, and ilioinguinal nerves anteriorly and the superior cluneal nerves and superior gluteal neurovascular bundle posteriorly. These structures are vulnerable to injury during bone graft harvesting [38].

Donor site complications after iliac bone graft harvesting and include chronic donor site pain [40–43], neurovascular injury [44–50], urethral injury [45], fracture of the iliac wing [51], hematoma [41, 42], infections [40], herniation of abdominal contents [52, 53], gait disturbance [40, 54], cosmetic deformity [40], sacroiliac joint instability [55], peritoneal perforation, hip subluxation, and tumor transplantation. The most relevant case series on donor site complications after iliac bone graft harvesting are reported in Table 17.3.

17.5.1.1 Donor Site Pain

Chronic pain (defined as persistent pain at least 3 months postoperatively) is the most common drawback of iliac bone graft harvesting [43] . It often interferes with early mobilization of the patient, and it may cause a longer stay in hospital and patient dissatisfaction [41, 42]. The incidence of chronic donor site in the most relevant studies is reported in Table 17.4.

Causes of donor site pain include both muscular or periosteal pain (because of the stripping of the abductors from the ilium), damage to the superior cluneal nerves [40, 43], and the weight bearing [40].

The incidence of donor site pain has been found to be higher in patients undergoing iliac bone graft harvesting for spine surgery than for those in whom the graft was harvested for no-spinal surgery [56].

It has been also proposed that an unsatisfactory outcome from spine fusion was associated with a significantly higher prevalence of donor site pain [43].

To overcome the problem of chronic donor site pain, the use of anesthetic regimens [57], a pneumatic gouge to harvest the bone [58], minimally invasive tools (limiting the degree of dissection and periosteal stripping) [59], vertical or oblique skin incisions to avoid cutting cutaneous nerves, incisions ≥3 cm dorsal to the anterior superior iliac spine, subperiosteal dissection with careful hemostasis, and a unicortical cancellous graft harvest technique has been proposed [60–62]. Data from the most relevant case series reporting on chronic donor site pain after iliac bone graft harvesting are reported in Table 17.4.

17.5.1.2 Nerve Injury

Nerve injury is one of the most commonly reported complications associated with iliac bone harvesting. The neural structures adjacent to the ilium are the ilioinguinal, iliohypogastric, lateral femoral cutaneous, sciatic, superior gluteal, femoral, and superior cluneal nerves. These neural structures are vulnerable to injury during bone graft harvesting [38]. Since the nerves exposed to major risk of damage are sensory, the characteristic symptoms include pain, numbness, burning, and itching in the distribution of the affected nerve. Damage to the nerves adjacent to the ilium, most likely results from direct transection or excessive traction. Specific peripheral nerve injuries are reported below.

The lateral cutaneous nerve of the thigh (also called the lateral femoral cutaneous nerve) is a cutaneous nerve that innervates the skin on the lateral part of the thigh. During anterior iliac bone graft harvesting, the lateral femoral cutaneous nerve may be damaged, causing meralgia paraesthetica (Bernhardt's syndrome), over the lateral aspect of the thigh (Table 17.5) [48, 50]. Although the lateral femoral cutaneous nerve usually emerges from the lateral border of the psoas major muscle and crosses the ilium toward the ASIS, its course is variable [63]. In some patients, it runs across the iliac crest 2 cm posterior to the ASIS and may be damaged at this site during exposure of the crest [63]. Occasionally, it crosses close to the iliacus muscle along the iliac crest and may be injured by ligation, diathermy, or retraction through the iliacus muscle.

Obviously, the risk of injuries to the lateral femoral cutaneous nerve will increase with increasing size of the harvested bone graft, because when large piece of the iliac bone is removed, the incision may be long and the iliacus muscle widely retracted [63]. The risk of nerve injury is also significantly higher in patients in whom graft is deeper than 30 mm is harvested [63]. Therefore, surgery in which grafts of large size are harvested carries a higher risk of injury to the lateral femoral cutaneous nerve. Patients should be informed and consented of the possibility of such injury, and surgeons should carefully consider the size of graft required before harvesting [63]. To preserve the nerve, Shamsaldin et al. [64] suggested to place skin incision at least 2 cm dorsal to the ASIS and to reduce dissection along the inner iliac wall performing gentle iliac muscle retraction.

Surgical decompression of the nerve or nerve ablation can be considered when patient's symptoms do not improve with occasional nerve blocks, analgesics, and desensitization. At surgery, the lateral femoral cutaneous nerve must be carefully evaluated for any cause of anatomic compression. Nerve section, when required, should be performed above the level of the inguinal ligament [65].

During posterior iliac bone graft harvesting, the superior cluneal nerves are more vulnerable to injury [66, 67]. The superior clunial nerves innervate the skin of the upper part of the buttocks. They are the terminal ends of the posterior rami of lumbar spinal nerves (L1, 2, 3). They constitute a group of three nerves, which pass vertically over the pelvic brim about 8 cm lateral to the posterior superior iliac spine [68].

Patients with injuries to the clunial nerves complain of posterior pelvic pain radiating into the buttocks, often worst by sitting. Local anesthetic injection to the proximal nerve is generally a sufficient measure to control pain. Sequential nerve blocks and desensitization should be considered when injections have failed to improve the patient's symptoms. In case of failure of nerve blocks and desensitization, exploration and neuroma resection can be required.

The ilioinguinal, iliohypogastric, superior gluteal, sciatic, and femoral nerves are also potentially at risk of injury.

The ilioinguinal nerve is a branch of the first lumbar nerve. It separates from the first lumbar nerve along with the larger iliohypogastric nerve. Its fibers are then distributed to the skin of the upper and medial part of the thigh. In males (anterior scrotal nerve), it provides sensation to the skin over the root of the penis and upper part of the scrotum; in females (anterior labial nerve), it provides sensation to the skin covering the mons pubis and labium majus.

Damages to the ilioinguinal nerve may occur when harvesting the inner cortex of the iliac crest, especially as a consequence of excessive medial retraction in this area when it descends from the spine along the iliacus muscle. Damage to the ilioinguinal nerve are very disabling for the patient, causing loss of sensibility to the pubic symphysis, base of penis and proximal scrotum or labia majora, and the anteromedial aspect of the thigh. Reduction of electrocauterization and iliac muscle retraction and avoidance of entrapment should prevent these injuries. Patients with symptoms nonresponsive to conservative treatment may be managed with segmental neurectomy [69].

The iliohypogastric nerve [40] is the superior branch of the anterior ramus of spinal nerve L1 after this nerve receives fibers from T12. Injury to this nerve may be the consequence of bone graft harvesting from the inner table of the anterior ilium, probably from vigorous retraction of the abdominal wall and iliacus muscles.

Table 17.3 Case series on donor site complications after iliac bone graft harvesting (NR: Not reported)

Study	Number of iliac bone graft harvesting	Wound dehiscence	Superficial infection	Deep infections	Hematoma	Fracture of the iliac wing	Vascular injury	Contour abnormalities of crest	Urethral injury	Nerve injuries: superior Cluneal nerve	Nerve injuries: lateral femoral cutaneous nerve	Painfulscar	Sacroiliac joint instability	Gait disturbance	Herniation of abdominal contents
Younger and Chapman [83]	217 pts	1	6	1	3	0	NR	NR	NR	3	0	6	0	NR	0
Laurie et al. [128]	60 pts	3	NR	NR	NR	0	NR	18	0	5	0	NR	NR	0	0
Keller and Triplett [129]	160 pts	3	NR	NR	NR	0	NR	NR	NR	NR	NR	NR	NR	NR	NR
Fernyhough et al. [68]	147 pts (151 iliac graft harvets)	NR	NR	NR	NR	NR	NR	NR	NR	NR	NR	NR	NR	NR	NR
Kreibich et al. [130]	58 pts (73 harvests)	NR	NR	NR	1	NR	NR	NR	NR	NR	NR	1	NR	NR	NR
Hu [51]	About 400 pts	NR	NR	NR	NR	14	NR	NR	NR	NR	NR	NR	NR	NR	NR
Hutchinson and Dall [131]	400 pts	NR	1	2	14	NR	NR	NR	NR	NR	NR	NR	NR	NR	NR
Savolainen et al. [24]	NR	NR	NR	NR	5	NR	NR	NR	NR	NR	NR	NR	NR	NR	NR
Banwart et al. [76]	180 pts (195 harvests)	1	1	NR	1	NR	NR	NR	NR	NR	0	4	0	0	0
Arrington et al. [81]	414 pts	NR	5	7	20 (16 minor and 4 deep)	2	Three superior gluteal artery. A retractor in the sciatic notch was used on each of three	NR	NR	3	3	NR	NR	NR	2
Colterjohn and Bednar 1997 [132]	57 pts	0	3	0	3	0	0	0	0	0	0	2	0	0	0
Beirne et al. [133]	137 pts (154 anterior iliac crest harvesting)	NR	5	NR	NR	NR	NR	17	NR	NR	1	5	NR	0	NR
Kalk et al. [134]	65 pts (68 harvest)	3	NR	NR	5	1	NR	NR	NR	2	2	NR	0	NR	NR
Goulet et al. [56]	191 pts	NR	3	1	NR	NR	NR	NR	NR	3 (numbness)	NR	NR	NR	11	NR
Hill et al. [135]	73	NR	NR	NR	NR	NR	NR	NR	NR	NR	NR	11	NR	NR	NR

Skaggs et al. [136]	214 children (223 posterior harvests)	NR	2	NR	NR	NR	Onesuperior glutealartery injury at the sciatic notch	NR	NR	1 (numbness)	NR	NR	1 sacroiliac penetration	NR	NR
Robertson and Wray 2001 [82]	106	0	0	1	0	0	0	NR	0	13 (numbness)	0	10	NR	NR	NR
Ahlmann et al. [137]	88 pts (108 harvests)														
	Anterior($n=66$)	NR	NR	NR	2	NR	NR	NR	NR	0	3 (numbness)	3	NR	NR	1
	Posterior($n=42$)	NR	NR	NR	0	NR	NR	NR	NR	1 (numbness)	NR	NR	NR	NR	0
Heary et al. [138]	105 pts (120 iliac crest, 87 anterior and 33 posterior)	0	2	0	NR	0	0	NR	0	0	0	0	0	0	0
Cricchio and Lundgren [139]	70 pts	NR	1	NR	9	1	NR	2	NR	1	9	NR	NR	1	NR
Mazock et al. [140]	33 pts (35 harvests)	NR	NR	NR	3	NR	NR	NR	NR	1 (neurosen-sory deficit)	NR	NR	NR	NR	NR
Silber et al. [141]	134 pts	3	10	NR	2	0	NR	NR	NR	21	0	7	NR	17	NR
Joshi and Kostakis [142]	98 pts	NR	3	1	3	5	NR	NR	NR	11 (numbness)	1	NR	NR	NR	NR
DeOrio and Farber [143]	180 pts	1	1	0	12	0	0	0	0	0	1	0	0	0	0
Kessler et al. [144]	118 pts (127) harvests														
	81 pts anterior iliac crest	NR	1	NR	7	0	NR	NR	NR	NR	1	1	NR	8	0
	46 pts posterior iliac crest	NR	0	NR	2	0	NR	NR	NR	NR	0	0	NR	1	0
Kager et al. [145]	71 pts	NR	3	NR	NR	NR	NR	NR	NR	NR	NR	NR	NR	NR	NR
Shamsaldin [64]	50 pts	NR	1	NR	1	0	NR	NR	NR	NR	5 pts anterolateral thigh numbness	NR	NR	NR	0
Pollock 2008 et al. [146]	24 pts trephine method	0	0	0	1	0	0	0	0		1meralgia parasthetica			12	0
	52 pts trephine method	0	4	0	1	0	0	0	0		1 Meralgia parasthetica				0

Table 17.4 Case series reporting on chronic donor site pain after iliac bone graft harvesting

		3 months(%)	6 months(%)	12 months(%)	≥24 months(%)
Laurie et al. [128]					10
Summers and Eisenstein [43]					25
Younger and Chapman [83]			2.5		
Fernyhough et al. [68]				29	
Kreibich et al. [130]					9
Savolainen et al. [24]					14
Banwart [76]					
Kalk [134]		19			
Colterjohn and Bednar [132]			53		
Goulet et al. [56]		16.5	37.9		18.3
Schnee et al. [42]		2.8			
Sawin et al. [41]		17			
Arrington et al. [81]					6
Hill [135]					20
Eufinger and Leppanen [147]				0	
Mirovsky [148]		43		43	39
Skaggs et al. [136]					24
Robertson and Wray [82]				12	
Ahlmann et al. [137]					2
Heary [138]					34
Cricchio [139]		26			11
David [149]					35
Sandor et al. [150]			0		
Silber et al. [141]					26.1
Joshi [142]			10		
DeOrio [143]			4.5		
Kessler et al. [144]	Anterior iliac crest				0
	Posterior iliac crest				0
Sasso et al. [151]		59	41	33	
Kager et al. [145]					10
Shamsaldin et al. [64]				6	
Delawi et al. [152]					40.9
Singh et al. [153]	Infusion of 96-mL normal saline solution at the donor site (10 pts)				7 pts of 10
	Infusion of 96 mL of 0.5% Marcain at the donor site (9 pts)				0 pts of 9

Sciatic nerve [40] may be damaged either in, or in proximity to, the sciatic notch. The individual branches of the sciatic nerve may not coalesce to form the sciatic nerve itself until 1–5 cm distal to the proximal border of the sciatic notch. Therefore, damage to the nerve at the notch may mimic a lumbosacral nerve root injury, rather than result in a complete sciatic nerve injury.

Damage to the superior gluteal nerve in the region of the sciatic notch may result in weakness of hip abduction nerve [40].

Femoral nerve [40] is rarely injured after iliac bone graft harvesting. Femoral neuropathy from subfascial hematoma after iliac bone harvesting has been also reported. The patient underwent surgical decompression of the hematoma to facilitate femoral nerve recovery [70]. To minimize the risk of injury to this nerve, careful dissection and retraction near the iliac fossa during harvesting of bone from the inner table of the anterior ilium has been also proposed [40]. The most relevant case reports on nerve injuries after iliac bone graft harvesting are reported in Table 17.5.

17.5.1.3 Vascular Injury

Vascular injury is a infrequent but severe complication after iliac bone grafting [46, 47, 49]. The superior gluteal artery is the largest branch of the internal iliac artery. It enters the gluteal region through the proximal portion of the sciatic notch and supplies the bulk of the gluteal muscle [40].

Damage to the superior gluteal artery have related to harvesting iliac bone too close to the greater sciatic notch, excessive muscle retraction or the placement of retractors into the sciatic notch. Bleeding resulting from these arterial injuries is difficult to control.

False aneurysm and arteriovenous fistula of the superior gluteal vessels after removal of bone grafts have also been reported [44, 45]. Exploration and ligation or embolization can be used to control the bleeding from a lacerated artery [46, 47].

Direct exposure and ligation of the superior gluteal artery can be facilitated by the release of the gluteal muscular origin and notch resection. When the artery cannot be exposed through this approach, an anterior or retroperitoneal surgical approach may be necessary to ligate the artery. In this case, an angiographic embolization method may be preferred to stop the bleeding.

When the superior gluteal artery retracts into a relatively inaccessible intrapelvic location, surgeon should not blindly use a hemostat or clip because of the risk of sciatic or superior gluteal nerve damage. In such instances, additional surgical exposure, including removal of the sciatic notch, can be required to expose the transected artery.

Damage to the superior gluteal artery can also manifest late as a gluteal artery aneurysm [44]. These complications necessitate hospitalization, blood transfusion, surgical ligation, or invasive radiological procedures for arterial embolization. Injury to the superior gluteal artery has been also reported as a cause of compartment syndrome of the buttock [71]. The most relevant case reports on vascular injury following iliac bone graft harvesting are reported in Table 17.6.

17.5.1.4 Fractures of the Ilium

Fracture of the ilium occurs more commonly when the anterior portions of the iliac crest is harvested. Most often, the fracture consists in avulsion of the anterior superior iliac spine [51] from the action of the sartorius and tensor fascia lata muscles. This complication can be avoided by harvesting bicortical or tricortical grafts from an area not closer than 3 cm to the anterior superior iliac spine. Conservative management is effective in the majority of the patients, and consists in a short period of rest followed by assisted ambulation until the fracture heals. Open reduction and internal fixation of the fracture may be required in selected patients [72].

Hu [51] reported in 14 patients with fractures at an iliac crest graft harvest site. All but one of these patients were female. The patients with anterior cervical fusions experienced avulsion fractures of the anterior superior iliac spine. One patient with a posterior occipital cervical fusion experienced bilateral posterior iliac wing fractures, and one with posterior atlantoaxial fusion resulted in a unilateral iliac wing fracture. All patients were managed conservatively with protection of weight bearing until resolution of pain. All patients had satisfactory results at final follow-up ranging from 6 months to 5 years. Three patients had residual mild pain that did not affect activities of daily living. The most relevant case reports on fractures following iliac bone graft harvesting are reported in Table 17.7.

17.5.1.5 Violation of the Sacroiliac Joint

Involvement of the sacroiliac joint is a potential complication after posterior iliac bone graft harvesting, and occurs from damage to the posterior sacroiliac

Table 17.5 Case reports on nerve injuries after iliac bone graft harvesting

Study	Patient	Index surgery	Symptoms	Diagnosis	Management	Intraoperative findings	Outcome
Weikel [50]	50-year-old woman	Dorsal augmentation of her nose with left iliac graft	Postoperatively pain over the lateral anterior thigh	Meralgia paraesthetica	Conservative: analgesics, local heat, desensitization, transcutaneous stimulation, injections		Occasionally analgesics
Guha [69]	61-year-old woman	Reconstructive surgery of the lower orbital margin withbicortical bonegraft taken from the left ilium	At the 10 thpostoperative day, the patient presentedwith a 24-h history of a sudden onset of weakness in the left leg with pain relating to the left iliac region and the wound	Large hematoma, anterior superior iliac spine fracture. Femoral neuropathy due to pressure by the hematoma	Evacuation of the hematoma	anterior superior iliac spine and the strut supporting it appeared to be mobile	no neurological deficit and apostoperative X-ray of the iliac region showed bony union proceeding at the fracture site
van den Broecke [154]	42-year-old man	Arthrodesis of themetacarpophalangeal joint	Postoperatively, the patient immediately complained of numbness of the anterolateral aspect of the right thigh	Meralgia paresthetica caused by neurotmesis of the lateral femoral cutaneous nerve during thebonegraft harvesting was feared			Follow-up proved this condition to be permanent
	40-year-old woman	Arthrodesis of metacarpophalangeal joints of both thumbs	Postoperatively, she noted a tingling sensation of the anterolateral aspect of the right thigh	Meralgia paresthetica caused by neurotmesis of the lateral femoral cutaneous nerve was feared			The tingling sensation subsided, and complete loss of sensibility was the permanent result
Yamamoto et al. [155]	81-year-old man	Fracture of the right calcaneus 490 years before, managed with osteosynthesis of the calcaneus and bone grafting from the right anterior iliac crest	Pain, dysesthesia, and hypesthesia in the anterolateral aspect of the right thigh	Meralgia paresthetica secondary to heterotopic ossification after iliac bone graft harvesting	Neurolysis of the lateral femoral cutaneous nerve and excision of the abnormal bony excrescence	The nerve was adherent to the bony excrescence, forming a pseudoneuroma	No symptoms at 6 month follow-up

Mahli [156]	21-year-old female	L2–3 fracture. Fusion performed with bone grafts harvested from the iliac crest using a transverse incision	Pain localized in the incision area throughout the iliac wing and radiating 10–12.5 cm distally to this area	Superior cluneal nerves injury	Alcohol neurolysis 4 month postoperatively		VAS 0 4 year postoperatively
	20-year-old female	Scoliosis. Correction and fusion per-formed with bone grafts harvested from the iliac crest using a transverse incision	Pain localized in the incision area throughout the iliac wing and radiating 10–12.5 cm distally to this area	Superior cluneal nerves injury	Alcohol neurolysis 5 month postoperatively		VAS 0 4 year postoperatively
	43-year-old male	L2 fracture. Fusion performed with bone grafts harvested from the iliac crest using a transverse incision	Pain localized in the incision area throughout the iliac wing and radiating 10–12.5 cm distally to this area	Superior cluneal nerves injury	Alcohol neurolysis 7 month postoperatively		VAS 0 4 year postoperatively
	27-year-old male	Scoliosis. Correction and fusion per-formed with bone grafts harvested from the iliac crest using a transverse incision	Pain localized in the incision area throughout the iliac wing and radiating 10–12.5 cm distally to this area	Superior cluneal nerves injury	Alcohol neurolysis 6 month postoperatively		VAS 0 4 year postoperatively

Table 17.6 Case reports on vascular injury following iliac bone graft harvesting

Study	Patient	Index surgery	Symptoms	Diagnosis	Management	Intraoperative findings	Outcome
Escalas [45]	15-year-old skeletally mature girl	Idiopathic thoracolumbar scoliosis. spine fusion with Harrington-rod instrumentation and autogenous iliacbone grafts. During the operation, a Taylor retractor was used for exposure toremove the iliacbone grafts. As the grafts were being removed, the tip of the retractor was accidentally dislodged and penetrated suddenly into the sciatic notch	Nine days after surgery, the patient vomited after eating, mild abdominal distention developed, and an arterial bruit in the right lower abdominalquadrant was noted	A right renal arterial and venous angiogram, done subsequently, showed normal renal vessels and an arteriovenous fistula in the proximal portion of the right superior gluteal artery	Conservative		Seventeen months after fusion she remained asymptomatic. Intravenous pyelography 5 months after surgery had demonstrated normal right kidney function and a normal excretory system
Kahn [46]	40-year-oldwoman	Laminectomy and two-level fusion were done from L4 to sacrum. pseudoarthroses at both L4, L5 and L5, SI levels requiring revision surgery	During revision surgery, The left posterior ilium, site of previous donor bone, was approached via the midline and the superior gluteal artery lacerated		Attempts to clamp the vessel were unsuccessful and the area packed with a lap sponge. When the lap sponge was later removed, brisk bleeding was encountered. Another lap sponge was packed into the bleeding area, a new incision was made over the left posterior iliac crest, and finally the vessel was clamped and ligated		

	19-year-oldwoman	Laminectomy and fusion from L4 to sacrum	The patient felt a sharp pain in his left buttock. The pain and swelling became progressive. Active, brisk bleeding was encountered and the patient was immediately taken to surgery		Surgery: The incision was extended and the vessel finally clamped and ligated	
Catinella [44]	32-year-old woman	Harrington rod placement with iliac crest bone for scoliosis	Threemonths postoperatively she noticed a firm mass under the rim of the cast in the left gluteal region	Aneurysm supplied by the superior gluteal branch of the left hipogasrtic artery	Surgery: Thesuperior gluteal branch was identified and ligated	The patient recovered uneventfully
Lim [47]	33-year-old woman	L4–L5 posterior decompression and fusion with corticocancellous iliac crest bone graft	Inspection of the wound revealed the bleeding to be coming from the sciatic notch. The source could not be identified clearly. Angiography showed extravasation of contrast material from the superior gluteal artery with arterio-venous shunting indicating the presence of a traumatic injury to the superior gluteal vein		Selective coil embolization of the superior gluteal artery was performed	The patient's recovery was otherwise uneventful, and she obtained a solid fusion
Shin 1996 [49]	15-year-old man	Severe, progressive scoliosis. anterior discectomy and fusion from T4–T11	Laceration of the superior gluteal artery during the procurement of posterior iliac crest bone graft		Time to obtain hemostasis was only several minutes with minimal blood loss	After operation, the patient did well without any complications. Six-month follow-up evaluation showed no residual deficits or reports regarding his posterior iliac crest or gluteus maximus

(*continued*)

Table 17.6 (continued)

Study	Patient	Index surgery	Symptoms	Diagnosis	Management	Intraoperative findings	Outcome
	13-year-old woman	L1 spina bifida with progressive thoracolumbar scoliosis. anterior diskexcision plus bone grafting from T9 to the sacrum by way of a right anterior thoracoabdominal approach. Luque-type spinal instrumentation and fusion extending from the upper thorax to the sacrum	Superior gluteal vessels were injured by the placement of a retractor in the sciatic notch, and immediate marked bleeding occurred.Multiple efforts were made to tie off the bleeding vessels, including the use of suture ties as well as surgical hemoclips. Partial hemostasis was obtained, and the wound was packed with a sponge and the surgical procedure completed. The area then was reinspected, and it was thought that the bleeding had been adequately controlled	8 hafter surgery, the child began to bleed profusely	Surgery. for exploration to control the bleeding. The actively bleeding superior gluteal artery was identified and tied off with silk sutures with the bleeding quickly and readily controlled		The patient had no further bleeding, and the spine wound healed without difficulty
Neo [157]	70-year-old man	Cervical myelopathy underwent anterior cervical decompression and fusion with an anterior iliac bone graft	Fracture displacement of the anterior superior iliac spine at the donor site was noted 1 week after a second operation, which was performed to reduce the displaced grafted bone. Five months after the second operation, he reported pain and swelling at the donor site. Removal of a hematoma was attempted, which led to massive bleeding that was difficult to control	Angiography demonstrated a pseudoaneurysm of the deep circumflex iliac artery	Selective embolization of the artery was performed		The patient recovered uneventfully

Chou [158]	76-year-old man	Anterior cervical decompression and fusion with a left anterior iliac bone graft for cervical myelopathy	A painful left inguinal mass was noted 1 month later	Angiography of the left external iliac artery showed pseudoaneurysm of the deep circumflex iliac artery	Selective transarterial coil embolization of the artery was performed, and bleeding was arrested	He was symptom-free for 2 months after discharge from the hospital
Kong [159]	57-year-old man	Total laminectomy and posterolateral fusion with pedicle screw fixation and autogenous iliac bone graft for neurogenic claudication secondary to spinal stenosis at L3–L5	During bone graft harvesting from the left posterior iliac crest through a separate incision, the tip of the retractor was dislodged and penetrated into the sciatic notch	Suddenly, massive arterial bleeding occurred from the sciatic notch. Bleeding was adequately controlled by packing a large amount of gel foam and gauze into the sciatic notch and applied direct pressure for about 15 min. Six weeks postoperatively, however, the patient returned to the outpatient clinic complaining of a fist-sized painful swelling at the bone graft donor site. 3D-CT angiography, an AV fistula of the superior gluteal artery was identified, extending from the sciatic notch to the pelvic cavity	Arterial embolization was performed through the right femoral artery	At the 1-year follow-up examination, the patient was doing well without any further sequelae

Table 17.7 Case reports on fractures following iliac bone graft harvesting

Study	Patient	Index surgery	Symptoms	Diagnosis	Management	Intraoperative findings	Outcome
Reynolds [160]	52-year-old woman	A double-level anterior discectomy and fusion at C5–6 and C6–7 was performed using the Smith-Robinson 2 technique. The donor bone was removed from the right iliac crest with a Stryker saw, cutting from the superior aspect of the crest into theilium	On the twelfth postoperative day, while chasing a cat, she lunged forward and felt a slight twinge in her iliac incisional area, which cleared. The next day she stumbled backward over a hassock, requiring a maximum contraction of her leg muscles to prevent afall	X-ray films of the pelvis revealed a fracture of the right anterior superior iliac spine	Bedrest for 2 weeks		Not reported
Reale [161]	51 year-old woman	Cloward anterior approachat at C5–C6 and C6–C7. Autologous bone plugs taken with a Cloward drill from the crest of the right ilium	Fourdays after the operation, while leaning on a window-sill and rotating the pelvis to start walking, she had a"turning and pulling"sensation at the site of the iliac crest wound followed by severe pain radiating to the groin	Fracture of the crest of the right ilium at the site of the drill holes	Fifteen days of bedrest		Six months after the operation the was free from pain and neurological deficits
Blakemore [162]	57 year-old man	Cloward decompression and fusion for severe cervical spondylosis	Sudden increase of oain at the bone frat donor site while climbing stairs at home	Radiographs showed fracture of the ilium	Analgesics		The pain subsided
Guha [69]	61-year-old woman	Reconstructive surgery of the lower orbital margin with bicortical bonegraft taken from the left ilium	At the 10th postoperative day, the patient presented with a 24-h history of a sudden onset of weakness in the left leg with pain relating to the left iliac region and the wound	Radiographs showed large haematoma, anterior superior iliac spine fracture. femoral neuropathy due to pressure by the haematoma	Evacuation of the haematoma	anterior superior iliac spine and the strut supporting it appeared to be mobile	no neurological deficit and apostoperative X-ray of the iliac region showed bony union proceeding at the fracture site

Kuhn [163]	50 year-old woman	Cervical discectomy and fusion C5–C6 for cervical spondylosis with bicortical iliac crest graft	One week after discharge she was unable to walk because of pain	Radiographs showed avulsion of the anterior superior iliac spine without displacement	Restriction of activities	Asymptomatic in 4 weeks
	50 year-old woman	L3–L4 and L4–L5 fusion for spondylolisthesis with bicortical iliac crest graft	One week postoperatively acute onset of pain at the donor site	Radiographs showed avulsion of the anterior superior iliac spine with displacement	Restriction of activities	Asymptomatic in 4 weeks
Porchet [164]	56-year-old man	Anterior cervical discectomies and fusion at C5–C6 and C6–C7 for spondylotic radiculopathies. Graft was harvested from the iliac crest using osteotomes	Nine days after the operation, while walking outside, the patient suddenly developed significant pain in the right inguinal region	Plain X-rays of the pelvis showed a fracture of the anterior iliac crest on the right side	After 1 day of bed rest, the patient was remobilized and left the hospitalon the 2nd day	One month later, the patient did not complain of any pain at the bone graft donor site
	48-year-old man	Mandibular reconstruction for squamous cell carcinoma. Graft was harvested from the iliac crest using osteotomes	The postoperative course was uneventful until the 3rd day, when the patient was first mobilized On his first attempt to bear weight on the left leg, he suddenly heard a noise and felt a considerable pain in his groin. Local examination revealed severe tenderness at the iliaccrest graft donor site.	A plain X-ray of the pelvis showed a laterally dislocated fracture of the anterosuperior iliac spine	Conservative treatment was used, without bed rest	The patient was asymptomatic and walking after 10 days

(continued)

Table 17.7 (continued)

Study	Patient	Index surgery	Symptoms	Diagnosis	Management	Intraoperative findings	Outcome
Fernando[165]	52-year-old woman	L4–L5 lumbar fusion, which was performed with pedicle screw fixation, an implanted electrostimulator, and autograft bone harvested fromthe right posterior iliac crest	Three days after surgery, the patient had a sharp increase in Pain and a pelvic radiograph showed a fracture through the iliac crest bone graft site.The pain worsened over the next 2 years, and the patient was unable to walk without significant pain	Radiographs e years later showed bilateral iliac wing fractures, fragmentation, partial resorption of the pubic rami. The right iliac crest fracture communi-cated with the iliac crest bone graft defect.CT scandemonstrated nonunion of the iliac wing fractures. The left acetabulum showed a fragmented left anterior column with a fracture extending to the articular surface. There were bilateral inferior pubic rami fractures with several areas of fragmentation. The pubic symphysis demonstrated multiple small fractures with nonunited bony fragments	Surgical stabilization		At the 2-month follow-up, radio-graphs showed no indication of hardware failure, and the right posterior pain was gone
Nocini[166]	49-year-old man	Mandibular alveolar crest augmentation with iliac crest bone grafting	22 days postoperatively acute pain near the ASIS	Radiographs showed a fracture of the lateral surface of the left iliac bone involving the ASIS	Restriction of activities and non weight bearing		Sixmonths after the patient was pain free and able to return to normal daily activities

ligaments. Sacroiliac joint violation may involve the ligamentous or synovial parts of the joint, resulting in arthritic changes and subsequent persistent sacroiliac joint pain. It can be the consequence of the complicated anatomy of the area, the large amount of harvested bone graft, thin cortices, and limited visualization because of bleeding from exposed cancellous bone. Chan et al. [73] reported the imaging findings in nine patients who developed pelvic instability after bone graft harvest from the posterior aspect of the iliac crest. They concluded that pelvic instability is manifested by insufficiency fractures of the ilium or sacrum, or both, subluxation of the sacroiliac joint, and fracture or dislocation of or about the pubic symphysis.

Ebraheim et al. [74] conducted a retrospective study of 24 sacroiliac joint computed tomographic (CT) scans of patients with persistent donor site pain. The authors found a high prevalence of inner table disruption in patients with persistent sacroiliac joint pain after posterior iliac bone graft harvesting. The CT scan showed that involvement of the synovial part caused more severe degenerative changes than involvement of the ligamentous part.

Injuries to the sacroiliac joint can be either overt, or insidious, necessitating CT scan for diagnosis. The diagnosis of sacroiliac joint pain after violation requires an index of suspicion, as the symptoms may be vague. Injection of local anesthetic into the sacroiliac joint may be helpful in confirming the site of pain.

Coventry and Tapper [55] described three useful physical examination tests to examine these patients:

1. With the patient side-lying, the examiner applies lateral pelvic pressure in an attempt to reproduce posterior sacroiliac joint pain.
2. With the patient side-lying, flexion of one hip causes contralateral sacroiliac joint pain.
3. With the patient supine, a leg is crossed over and pushed into abduction. This maneuver reproduces sacroiliac joint discomfort.

Initial management of symptomatic pelvic instability after iliac crest bone graft harvest is conservative.

Fusion of the sacroiliac joint may be necessary if the pain is persistent. In some patients, resection or fusion of the symphysis pubis may be required. The most relevant case reports on violation of the sacroiliac joint following iliac bone graft harvesting are reported in Table 17.8.

17.5.1.6 Hernia

Herniation of abdominal contents through an iliac bone graft donor site is not an uncommon complication, as it may occur in up to 5% of patients [53, 75–78]. Risk factors include advanced age, female sex, obesity, and a graft larger than 4 cm [40, 52, 53].

Symptoms include vague lower abdominal pain related to the iliac crest donor site, and, typically, a sensation of fullness in the donor site. Occasionally, bowel sounds can be auscultated over the mass. Plain radiographs are suggested in the assessment of these patients. CT scan commonly is able to clearly show the hernia, confirming the diagnosis. In some patient, conservative management with manual reduction and close observation may be successful.

Surgical management follows the principles of surgery for hernias (reduction of the hernia and obliteration of the defect). Available surgical options include a soft tissue repair with the advancement of the muscles and fascia, imbrication, and fascial flaps, eventually supplemented with a mesh. Bosworth [79] described another surgical technique, which consists in changing the profile of the involved iliac crest to recontour the bone defect produced by graft harvesting. The iliac crest is straightened removing the remaining parts on both sides of the defect, and then mobilization of the fascial insertion of the transverse and the external and internal oblique muscles is performed to attach it directly to the ilium along the new crest. The ASIS must also be transported distally and posteriorly, drawing the muscular, ligamentous, and fascial structures tightly across the defect [79].

Donor site herniation can determine serious complications, such as strangulated hernia requiring resection of necrotic bowel [80]. The most relevant case reports on herniation following iliac bone graft harvesting are reported in Table 17.9.

17.5.1.7 Hematoma

Hematoma formation has been reported as a complication in patients whose donor site wounds were not drained. The reported incidence of hematoma formation is up to 10%, even though it is very low in recent series [41, 42]. The ilium is endowed with a rich vascular supply. Therefore, bleeding from the cancellous

Table 17.8 Case reports on violation of the sacroiliac join following iliac bone graft harvesting

Study	Patient	Index surgery	Symptoms	Diagnosis	Management	Intraoperative findings	Outcome
Lichtblau [167]	33-year-old woman	Revision surgery with left posterior iliac crest for ulnar radial non union	Two and one-half months later she complained of back pain with radiation to the right groin and left sacro-iliac regions	Roentgenograms revealed a marked left sacro-iliac dislocation with stress fractures of both right pubic rami. In addition there was a subluxation of the symphysis pubis	Arthrodesis of the sacro-iliac joint was attempted by Smith–Petersen technique		no complaints
Coventry and Tapper [55]	41-year-old woman	Fusion of the fourth lumbar to the fifth lumbar vertebra was carried out. The left posterior iliac crest was used as the donor site Laminectomy at the fourth lumbar vertebra was performed. and spine fusion from the fourth lumbar vertebra to the sacrum. using iliac bone grafts from the right posterior iliac crest	Ten months later, in addition to low-back pain, the patient began to notice pain in the left groin and a limp. The pain in the groin increased when she stood, and on movement of the region she felt pain and heard a slight clicking Three years later the patient again fell, with increased severity of pain in the night sacro-iliac area	Roentgenograms revealed a stress fracture through the superior and inferior pubic rami on the left Roentgenograms showed this joint to he sclerotic. and on comparison with the opposite joint. the ilium showed slight displacement cephalad	Fusion of the left sacro-iliac joint was then attempted. using bone from the right iliac crest,the sacro-iliacjoint on the right was hone-grafted	At operation. The joint was not demonstra-bly hypermo-bile. but it contained a seeming excess of fibrous	At the time of latest follow-up, however, she continued to have some midline lumbar pain and a feeling of numbness in the back of her thighs and into her feet; her activities were not limited, but she took analgesics for her discomfort Fusion developed at the fourth and fifth lumbar vertebrae and also in the right sacro-iliac joint and she was relieved of pain
	35-year-old woman	Posterior fusion was done from the fourth lumbar to the second sacral vertebra using the right posterior iliac crest as a donor area	Eight years after hen lumbosacral fusion, pain in the right buttock and thigh was constant and severe and extended to the right calf. It increased with sitting and straining and decreased with standing or lying on one side	Roentgenograms demonstrated instability at the symphysis pubis as well as increasing sclerosis of the right sacro-iliac joint	Right sacro-iliac fusion		Subsequent roentgenograms. made 16 months later. showed evidence of solid fusion of the sacro-iliac joint

36-year-old woman	Bonegrafting of the last true lumbar vertebra, the transitional vertebra, and the sacrum was carried out. The left sacro-iliac joint also was fused at the same operation. Bone for grafting was removed from the left posterior ilium, and right posterolateral gutter and transverse process fusions were done	The clicking sensation, which she had experienced before operation. continued for several months, and on repeated examination it was found to he located at the symphysis pubis and not at the sacro-iliac joint	RX: sacro-iliac joint dislocation		Symphyseal dislocation remained but was no longer clicking or painful.The patient led an active life
38-year-old woman	Pseudoarthrosis L4–L5 repaired with bone from the left posterior ilium	Within the year, however, she began to notice pain in the region of the ischial tuberosity, in the perineum, and down the posteromedial aspect of both thighs, and she was becoming increasingly disabled by her new symptoms	Roentgenograms showed evidence of subluxation of the symphysis pubis with cystic and degenerative changes	Wedge resection of the symphysis pubis	
39-year-old woman	Right hemilaminectomy at the fifth lumbar vertebra was done as well as transverse process fusion from the fourth lumbar vertebra to the sacrum, using bone from the right iliac crest	Eightmonths postoperatively pain in her leg and especially in the region of the ischial tuberosities	Instability was demonstrated on roentgenograms made with the patient standing first on one limb and then on the other	Resection of the symphysis with maintenance of the anterior ligament was carried out	Recent evaluation indicated that the clicking had ceased but pain had developed in the left sacro-iliac area and noentgenograms showed evidence of possible widening of the sacro-iliac joint and increased sclerosis

Table 17.9 Case reports on herniation following iliac bone graft harvesting

Study	Patient	Index surgery	Symptoms	Diagnosis	Management	Intraoperative findings	Outcome
Oldfield [168]	52-year-old man	Three iliacbone grafts for the repair of an extensive bone loss of the margins of the orbit and malar region	He had noticed a lump beneath his"first scar."The swelling had been there about a month and had gradually increased. It had caused no pain and it disappeared when he pressed his hand on it or lay on the opposite side	Landslide hernia of the caecum through a bone defect in the right iliac crest, following a graft	Surgery		The patient suffered no disability
Bosworth [79]	NR	Spine fusion for spondylolisthesis with autologous bone graft	Disability due to a hernia through the iliac crest	Hernia through the iliac crest	Surgery		There was no recurrence of herniation and no symptoms
	NR	Fracture of the jaw. iliac crest and a moderate portion of the body of the ilium were removed to repair the defect	Totally disabled with severe pain, but only amoderate-sized hernia	Hernia through the iliac crest	Surgery: obliteration of the hernial opening through the iliac crest		He returned to his regular work as a farmer
Pyrtek and Kelly [169]	43-year-old	Spinal fusion was performed. The bone graft was obtained from the right iliac crest	An orange-sized mass in the right lumbar region. When this mass was compressed, he complained of pain at the site of the swelling as well as a referred pain to the epigastrium	Posttraumatic hernia through the iliac bone containing cecum, appendix and terminalileum	Surgery		Free of any symptoms referable to the hernia
	59-year-old woman	Spinal fusion. with iliac autograft	Mass appearing in the left lumbar region through the scar from which the bone had been obtained	Herniation through the left iliac bone containing distal descending colon and loops of jejunum, with these viscera projecting into the left flank	Surgery		Free of any symptoms referable to the hernia
Reid [78]	59-year-old woman	Posterior lumbosacral fusion with bicortical iliac autograft	Initially the hernia caused no symptoms. Increasing local pain after standing	Hernia through an iliac bone graft donor site	Surgery. A lateral flap of the aponeurosis of the external oblique muscle was rotated over the defect and attached to the iliacus fascia		No recurrence of the hernia

Challis et al. [80]	88-year-old female	Arthrodesis of the left wrist was performed using the right iliac crest	Twenty-four days after operation the patient developed abdominal pain with vomiting but no change in bowel habit	small bowel volvulus and strangulated iliac hernia	Laparotomy	The patient made a slow but uneventful recovery
Cowley and Anderson [52]	61-year-old female	Femoral osteotomy	NR	NR	Surgery	NR
	68-year-old female	Open reduction of tibial plateau fract	NR	NR	Surgery	NR
	59-year-old female	Open reduction of femoral fract	NR	NR	Surgery	NR
	51-year-old female	Lumbar spine fusion	NR	NR	Surgery	NR
Ramirez [170]	61-year-old female	C1–C2 spinal fusion with iliac bone autograft	Soft tissue mass	Herniation of large and small bowel at bone graft donor	Surgery	NR
Ubhi and Morris [171]	37-year-old male	Open fracture of tibia and fibula. Iliac bone autograft	The 9th day the wound opened and the small bowel came out	Herniation of bowel at bone graft donor	Surgery	Uneventful recovery
Stevens and Banuls [172]	40-year-old man	Posterior lumbar fusion. Iliac bone autograft	Soft reducible swelling over the bone donor	Iliolumbar hernia	Surgery	uneventful recovery
Auleda et al. [75]	57-year-old female	Nonunion of the tibia	NR	Herniation of bowel at bone graft donor	Surgery	NR
	56-year-old female	Nonunion of the tibia	NR	Herniation of bowel at bone graft donor	NR	NR
	63-year-old female	Hip arthrodesis	NR	Herniation of bowel at bone graft donor	Surgery	NR
	81-year-old female	Knee arthrodesis	NR	Herniation of bowel at bone graft donor	Not operated on because of her poor general condition	NR
Velchuru et al. [173]	65-year-old female	Iliac bone graft harvest for anonunion of a humeral shaft fracture	Six weeks after the procedure with progressive swelling and minimal discomfort at the graft donor site	Iliac crest hernia	Surgery	The patient's postoperative recovery was uneventful

bone with harvesting can be significant. Bleeding can also arise from the vessels adjacent to the anterior ilium (the deep circumflex iliac, the iliolumbar, and the fourth lumbar vessels). Measures that can help one to decrease the risk of bleeding include restricting the exposure to a strictly subperiosteal location obtaining hemostasis before closure, and using a suction drain.

Postoperative hematomas often necessitate surgical debridement and closure, because the later complication of hematoma is infection.

Arrington et al. [81] reported on four patients with hematoma requiring revision surgery. At the time of the index procedures, topical hemostatic agents and closed suction drains were not applied in any patients. To decrease the incidence of postoperative hematoma, Banwart et al. [76] reported a four-layer hemostatic closure combined with topical hemostatic agents. The most relevant case reports on hematoma following iliac bone graft harvesting are reported in Table 17.10.

17.5.1.8 Gait Disturbance

Gait disturbance is a potential problem of harvesting bone graft from the posterior iliac region [40, 54]. It is caused by extensive stripping of the gluteus maximus muscle from the ilium, and it can result in difficulty in climbing stairs or rising from a sitting position. This complication can be avoided by securely re-approximating the gluteal fascia to the periosteum of the iliac crest. Robertson and Wray [82] reported on a patient with significant soft tissue defect caused by a detached gluteus maximus origin requiring a gluteus maximus reattachment.

17.5.1.9 Infections

Infections at the donor site occur with the same frequency as for other clean orthopedic procedure <1% of patients) [40]. Management of infections include irrigation, debridement, and the administration of antibiotics. Occasionally, deep infections can cause osteomyelitis [83].

Prophylactic antibiotic administration, use of separate instruments to avoid, meticulous hemostasis, and use of closed suction drainage are measures that can reduce the risk of infection.

17.5.1.10 Other Complications

Another potential donor site complication of iliac bone graft harvesting is urethral injury [45] Escalas and DeWald [45] reported on a patient with abdominal distension, fever, and hydronephrosis after posterior iliac bone graft harvesting. Conservative management was effective to solve patient symptoms. The mechanism of injury postulated by the authors was the attempt to cauterize a vessel bleeding through the sciatic notch.

The ureter is closer to the superior gluteal artery and the sciatic notch in women. Therefore, great care should be taken in female patient undergoing posterior iliac bone graft harvesting. Genitourinary tract injuries should be suspected in patients with postoperative hematuria, ileus, abdominal distention, and fever. Conservative management is often sufficient to resolve minor urethral injuries.

17.5.1.11 Cosmetic Deformity

Development of cosmetic deformities after iliac crest bone grafting is related to removal of the superior surface of the ilium or to the development of an unsatisfactory scar [40]. Several techniques have been proposed to avoid the defect of preserving the superior pelvic brim, or using ceramic spacers, calcium sulfate, and bone morphogenetic protein [45, 84].

17.5.1.12 Tumor Transplantation

Tumor transplantation is an uncommon, but potential complication of bone grafting. Cardacci [85] reported on a patient with transplantation of Paget's disease from an affected ilium to the tibia at the time of a bone grafting procedure to the tibia. Cole and Sindelar [86] reported on a patient in whom an osteogenic sarcoma was transplanted to the ilium at the time a tibial lesion was bone grafted. A hemipelvectomy was required to manage the lesion that developed in the ilium.

Table 17.10 Case reports on hematoma following iliac bone graft harvesting

Study	Patient	Index surgery	Symptoms	Diagnosis	Management	Intraoperative findings	Outcome
Ziccardi et al. [174]	49 year-old man	Reconstruction of zigomatico-maxillary-orbital complex fracture	Ecchymotic area along the flank and the abdomen, extended down to the groin. Testicular pain, hip discomfort, mild abdominal cramping, continual urinary urgency	Retroperitoneal haematoma	Bed rest and local ice application		Symptoms fully resolved during the next few days
Brazaitis et al. [175]	73 year-old man	Anterior cervical decompression and fusion with anterior iliac bone autograft	Over the next 12 h, congestive heart failure and pulmonary oedema. Distended abdomen and absent bowel sounds. Olyguric with increased creatinine	Retroperitoneal haematoma. Pelvic arteriogram showed active bleeding from a muscular branch of the left deep circumflex artery	The vessel was occluded with gelfoam and a single Gianturco Coil (Cook, Inc, Bloomington, IN)		The patient died on the 14th postoperative day
Stevens and Banuls [172]	27-year-old woman	Posterior L5–S1 intertransverse fusion for dysplastic facet joint arthropathy. unicortical cancellous bone graft from the posterior aspect of the right iliac crest	Immediately postoperatively, the patient presented with an area of anesthesia over the lateral aspect of the right lower leg and foot, together with a right foot drop	Large hematoma infiltrating the gluteal muscles and extending caudally to the region of the sciatic nerve at the level of the ischial tuberosity	The hematoma was evacuated		Three months postoperatively the patient had fully recovered

17.6 Bicortical Cylindrical Graft as Required by the Cloward Instrumentation

The use of Cloward instrumentation obtains full arthrodesis at the operative level following anterior decompression. The graft must therefore have good mechanical characteristics. The size of the graft and the thickness of its cortical components are important features. The graft should be taken from the medial portion of the iliac wing, which at this point has a slight posterior curvature. This is the site where the bone is at its thickest [87]. The graft should be removed carefully from under the iliac crest with the appropriate instrumentation. Bone taken more distally will be of lesser thickness, and will not be suitable for use as a dowel graft that will achieve arthrodesis in distraction. Another feature that is of practical importance is the angle at which the graft is separated from the ilium. The drill should always be applied at right angles to the external cortical surface of the iliac wing. To achieve this, it must be tilted downward by 30–40°. This orientation of the drill is necessary to avoid an oblique surface along one edge of the graft, a feature which would make the graft unsuitable as a dowel to slot into the host site. Once it has been released from its bony attachment, the graft must be cleared of all soft tissues and shaped and filed along its sides into an elliptical shape. The hole drilled between the two adjacent vertebral bodies is spherical, but, when distraction is applied, it also assumes an oblique elliptical shape. The graft must therefore be shaped to fit the elliptical shape of the drill hole, which can be achieved in distraction. In addition, the graft should be approximately 5 mm larger in diameter than the drill bit used to produce the drill hole in the vertebrae, so that distraction is maintained after the distractor has been released and the graft is in place. A technical trick that we use is to drill a hole through the full thickness of the center of the graft. This is done to ensure that any bleeding that occurs posteriorly (behind the graft) may be drained through this hole, avoiding the development of a fully contained hematoma [88].

Once the graft has been obtained, it should be mounted on the carrier, which is used to insert the graft at the host site. This graft carrier has two lateral wings that come to rest on the lateral arms of the distractor, thus limiting the advancement of the graft and avoiding its being inserted too deeply [88].

17.6.1 Errors

The graft removed may be too small if it is taken from the more distal portion of the iliac wing where the bone is thinner. Because of the mechanical and biological inappropriateness of such a graft, an additional graft must be obtained from a more suitable and better selected area [4].

If the graft is of the same size as the drill holes in the vertebral bodies, it will provide very little stability and will lead to failure of the arthrodesis because it may be easily mobilized postoperatively and will lead to collapse of the two adjacent vertebral bodies [1].

The graft may be placed too deeply in the drill hole if it is too small, either because the depth was inappropriately assessed or because the instrumentation used was inadequate. This may have serious consequences, particularly if the graft protrudes posteriorly into the canal. If this happens, the graft should be removed immediately. In most instances, this can be achieved using relatively simple techniques. Without distraction, a self-tapping screw is threaded into the center of the graft. This is relatively easy because this is an area with spongy bone. With a pair of sturdy pliers, the screw is firmly gripped. Distraction is applied and the graft can then be removed [2].

17.7 Tricortical Rectangular Graft for Smith–Robinson-Type Vertebral Fusion

To obtain a tricortical bone graft, a full thickness resection of a portion of the iliac crest must be undertaken, aiming to obtain a graft of uniform thickness. Since saws generate heat that may produce necrosis and tissue denaturing, it is better to use chisels, which must be sharp. The iliac crest is stripped of all soft tissues. The technique involves driving the first chisel into the bone approximately 2 cm from the crest. This first chisel is left in place and a second chisel is inserted into the bone more distally. This is followed by a third chisel yet more distally to complete the separation at the base [3]. A modification that is sometimes practical is the use of drill holes along the resection margin on both cortices so that the chisel can more easily and less traumatically transect the bone. This may well avoid disruption of the graft and result in a straight linear margin of resection. Once the graft has been obtained, it is shaped and filed. Here again, it must be emphasized that the diameter of the graft must be larger than that of the drilled hole, and the graft must be shaped to maintain the distraction between the two opposing vertebral bodies after its insertion [39, 88].

17.7.1 Errors

The major error is harvesting a graft from the more anterior part of the iliac wing where the bone is too thin. Other errors involve inaccuracies in the size of the graft and the insertion of the graft too deeply in the drill holes with a risk of posterior protrusion into the canal [3].

17.8 Tricortical Graft for Multiple Subtotal Vertebrectomies and Reconstruction

A tricortical graft for multiple vertebral resections must be 4–8 cm long. To obtain a graft of such size, the skin incision must be proportionally longer. This can only be achieved with an incision parallel to the iliac crest and placed approximately 1 cm below the superior surface of the crest. Muscles must be detached from the abdominal surface and from the external surface of the iliac wing to expose the entire iliac crest. At this stage, care should be taken to avoid damage to the sensitive branch of the musculocutaneous nerve, which crosses the iliac crest. The central iliac crest is the preferred zone for harvest. The graft is obtained using chisels. The chisels, one at each end of the graft being harvested, must reach a depth of approximately 1–2 cm into the bone. The graft length must exceed the length of the host trench in the vertebrae by at least 2 cm to meet the requirements of the final preparation and shaping prior to insertion. Saws should be avoided to preclude unnecessary tissue damage [2, 39, 87, 88].

Once the graft has been harvested, its bed must be subjected to careful and complete hemostasis. This will require packing with ample bone wax. Closure must be undertaken scrupulously in well-approximated layers to avoid the formation of potential cavities in the abdominal wall, which all too frequently result in hematomas and fluid cysts in the wound if the deep muscular layers have been closed too loosely. The muscles must be reattached to the bone through transosseous sutures. Suction drainage is essential postoperatively. Very often patients continue to complain of pain and discomfort in the donor area in the iliac region long after the surgery. The final preparation of the graft is important. All soft tissues have been stripped from the bone. The bone will be curved and asymmetrical and will vary in thickness depending on the exact source on the iliac crest. The steps for shaping the graft must be carried out by hand [2]. The use of a vice made out of sterilizable steel, and either placed on or anchored to the instrument table will be of particular use during these steps. Once the graft is well anchored, files of different sizes and coarseness may be used to shape the walls in such a way as to straighten the graft. In addition, the shape and configuration that is achieved should assure that the length exceeds the undistracted bony groove in the vertebral bodies by 10–15 mm. Particular care must be used in the shaping the interlocking ends. The ends must obviously be shaped to interlock with the appropriate portions of the prepared vertebral bodies. During distraction, the dowel graft is slotted to interlock perfectly with the vertebral bodies. This assures that the graft is well seated and fully stable [88].

17.8.1 Errors

Should the graft be obtained from the anterior portion of the iliac wing, it will be excessively curved, too thin, and impossible to accurately shape to fit the requirements of the host site. In patients who require extensive posterior multilevel fusions, the medio-posterior iliac crest is a good donor site. Strips of tricortical grafts may be obtained through tangential resection of the iliac crest [1, 87].

17.9 Fibula

The fibula, composed of solid, primarily cortical bone, is quite advantageous when mechanical strength and support are required in a graft. However, it is straight and very difficult to model and, therefore is not fully adaptable to maintain the existing cervical lordosis [4, 87].

Nevertheless, it is the preferred type of graft when immediate mechanical support is required. As such, it is primarily used in the management of vertebral destruction by tumor. Even though the achieved fusion produces a straight cervical spine, fibular grafts have been successfully used as described in the literature [89].

The neurovascular structures surrounding the fibula include the peroneal nerves and the anterior tibial and peroneal vessels. The common peroneal nerve in the region of the knee courses obliquely from posterior to anterior over the fibular neck and divides into superficial, deep, and recurrent branches.

In harvesting the graft, great care must be taken to avoid the all too frequent injuries to the external popliteal branch of the sciatic nerve [2, 87]. This complication can be avoided as follows:

1. Obtain the graft from the metaphysis and away from the head and neck of the fibula where the nerve crosses (Fig. 17.2).
2. Avoid penetrating into the muscular structures of the anterior compartment of the leg during the stripping of the bone.
3. It is preferable at this site to use a Gigli saw and avoid the use of oscillating saws, which may produce contusions of the nerve with the final "give" as the bone is divided.

17.9.1 Fibular Donor Site Complications

Potential complications of fibular graft harvesting include neurovascular injury, compartment syndrome, weakness of the extensor hallucis longus, and ankle instability [89, 90]. In the proximal third of the fibula, the peroneal nerves and their muscular branches are at primary risk. The extensor hallucis longus is susceptible to denervation because it is generally supplied by only one branch from the deep peroneal nerve [90]. The major structures at risk in the middle third of the fibula are the peroneal vessels. Harvesting the distal 10 cm of the fibula should be avoided, as it will result in ankle instability. Vail and Urbaniak [89] studied donor site morbidity after harvesting of vascularized fibular grafts. Muscle weakness was noted in 25 (10%) of the 247 limbs at 3 months after graft harvesting and in 2 (3%) of the 74 limbs that were evaluated at 5 years or more. The incidence of pain at the ankle joint was 1.6% at 3 months but increased to 11.5% at 5 years. The prevalence of subjective sensory abnormalities increased from 4.9% at 3 months postoperatively to 11.8% at 5 years.

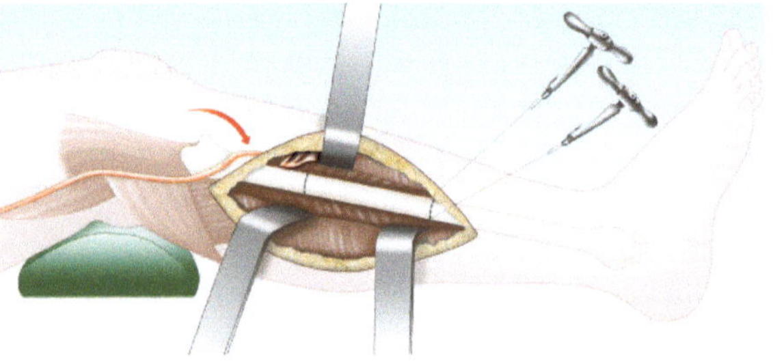

Fig. 17.2 Fibular grafts are relatively easy to obtain. After cutting through the soft tissue, the surgeon strips the periosteum, taking care of not to injure the external popliteal nerve, which crosses the neck of the fibula from back to front

17.10 Tibia

The proximal metaphysis of the tibia is a well-known source of bone graft. This site provides primarily cortical bone, although corticocancellous bone can also be obtained. The anteromedial surface is a good donor site [91]. The surgical procedure is well established. The perimeter of the graft is first outlined with drill holes after the bone has been stripped. Chisels are used to elevate the bone. This type of graft is such as to be well suited in the management of vertebral destruction by tumor and in cases requiring solid support and immediate stability [88].

17.11 Recipient Site Complications

Successful incorporation of bone graft material depends on formation of new bone, structural incorporation of host bone, and adaptive remodeling of the skeleton in response to mechanical stress [92]. These events proceed in sequential phases, similar to fracture healing. The length of time to incorporation is multifactorial, and in part reliant on overall patients' conditions, native bone environment, and properties of the specific graft material [11–13, 28, 29, 93].

Both autogenous and allograft bone are incorporated into the developing fusion mass following to a well-defined series of biologic events, consisting of hemorrhage, inflammation and vascular invasion, culminating in the replacement of graft material with new bone. However, with allograft this remodeling process occurs more slowly, and there is greater resorption of the graft compared with autograft [94].

Intervertebral graft complications are rare in single-level fusions. The incidence of graft complications appears to be associated with the length of the graft and the number of levels involved in the surgery. Long strut grafts are vulnerable to graft migration, displacement, angulation, fracture, nonunion, and instrumentation failure [95, 96]. Patients with significant fracture or displacement of the graft require a revision of the strut graft and instrumentation or additional fusion and fixation [95].

Autograft is superior to allograft in promoting multisegmental cervical fusion [13, 20]. Equivalent results were found when using allograft or autograft for single-level fusions, but the incidence of nonunion was 62% among patients receiving allograft for two-level anterior cervical fusion, compared with only 17% of those using autologous bone [26]. In another series of patients managed with multilevel cervical arthrodesis, 85% of those implanted with autograft successfully healed, whereas only 50% in the allograft group fused [97]. A nonunion frequently leads to unsatisfactory resolution of clinical symptoms [98, 99], and usually results in greater medical costs and morbidity, as well as the need for additional surgeries [100]. The most common clinical approach to favor unions has been the use of rigid internal fixation. In the past 15 years, we observed that anterior cervical plates can prevent pseudoarthrosis, graft collapse, graft migration, as well as reduce the time of use of a postoperative collar, improve anatomical and functional results, and facilitate a speedy return to work [15, 88, 101–107].

The incidence of graft displacement after cervical spine surgery is not well defined. Graft dislodgment is reported in 5–50% of multilevel corpectomy patients when stand-alone grafts have been placed without plating [108, 109].

In patients with nonunion, before the revision surgery, it is advisable to immobilize the cervical spine with orthoses, and biophysical stimulation, as in non-union of fractures of the limb [110–113].

The clinical symptoms depend on the cause of the strut graft failure. Many patients with nonunion remain asymptomatic. Pain is the most common presenting symptom in patients with symptomatic nonunion. Continued or worsening axial pain 6 months after the initial procedure and relevant radiographic appearances are consistent with nonunion [114] (Fig. 17.3a–d).

Nonunion in the presence of an anterior cervical fixation device carries the additional risk of metalwork fracture or migration with associated esophageal penetration, mediastinitis, and death [115, 116]. Posterior migration of the graft can lead to compression of the spinal cord, and result in paralysis or neural injury. Anterior dislocation of the dislodged graft may cause compression or perforation of the esophagus, and tracheal impingement with airway obstruction.

The diagnosis and management of patients with a nonunion should be pursued aggressively. Patients with early- or late-onset graft fracture usually present with neck pain. Patients with anterior graft dislodgment may complain of difficulty while swallowing or breathing. With posterior graft displacement, the patient may present with new-onset neurological deficits [95].

17.12 Cervical Nonunion

Fusion is defined, as absence of abnormal motion and lucency, and presence of bony trabeculation at the operative site [117]. As stated above, nonunion is a potential complication after attempted arthrodesis of the cervical spine, and can be distinguished in non-union without motion (fibrous) and nonunion with motion.

Nonunion can be the consequence of several factors, including the type of bone graft, the number of vertebral levels involved (see below), the type of instrumentation, errors of technique (inadequate surface area of decorticated host bone), the patient's post-operative course, compliance with activity restriction and orthosis, general conditions of the patient (see Chap. 1), assumption of drugs.

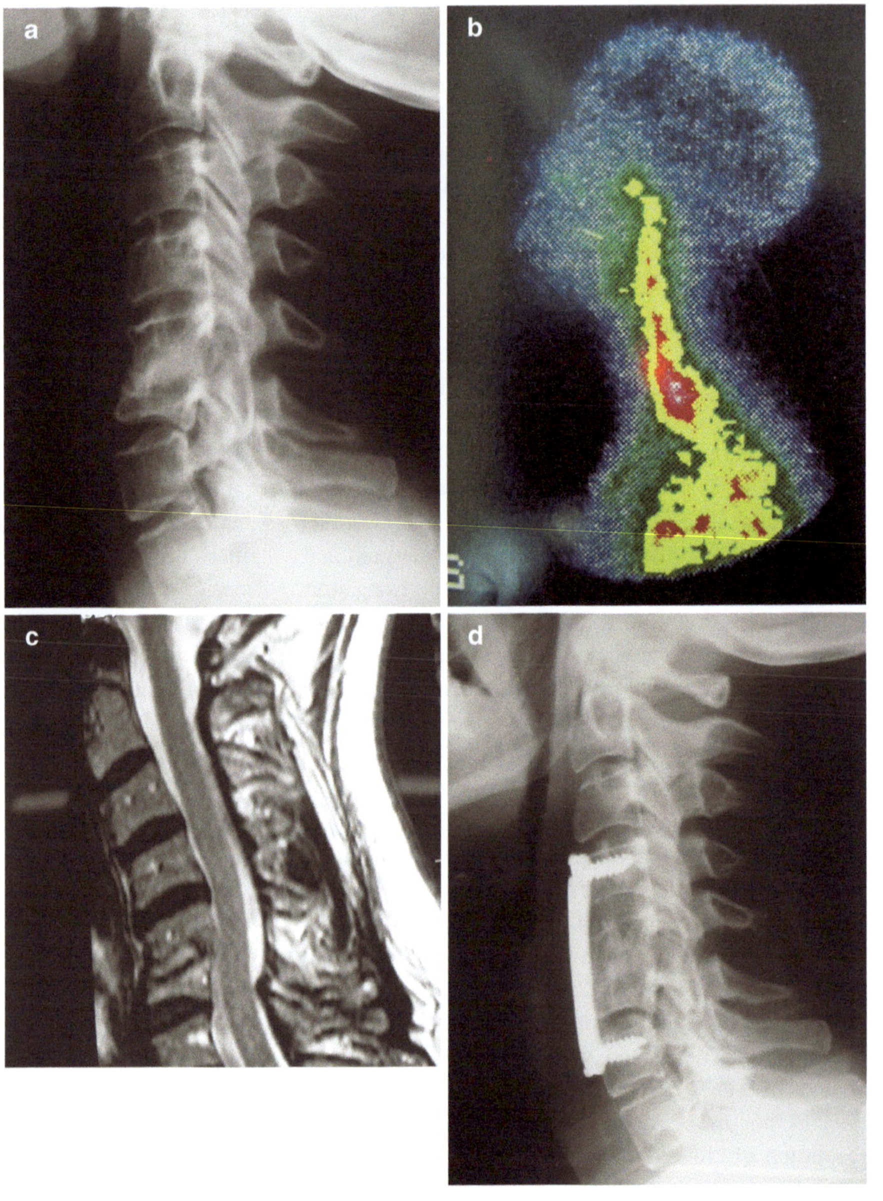

Fig. 17.3 (**a**) A 52-year-old woman with 5-year neck pain was referred to our clinic. Three years before the patient had undergone an anterior C5–C6 fusion with allograft at another hospital. (**a**) Radiographs showed a C5–C6 nonunion with segmental kyphosis. (**b**) Abnormal focal tracer uptake was detected at the bone scan. (**c**) MRI showed the C5–C6 nonunion and the osteolysis with graft resorption. (**d**) The patient underwent a multiple subtotal somatectomy with autologous iliac bone graft, plates, and screws, obtaining a restoration of the cervical lordosis

The diagnosis of nonunion has been traditionally based on the clinical triad of pain, loss of correction or fixation, and radiographic evidence of instability (spine's loss of ability to maintain normal vertebral relationships under physiological load, in such a way that the spine no longer prevents damage to the cord or nerve roots or prevents incapacitating deformity or pain) [117].

A diagnosis of delayed union is made after anterior cervical discectomy and arthrodesis, if fusion has not occurred after 6 months. Nonunion is diagnosed if fusion has not occurred after 12 months.

Not all the patients diagnosed with nonunion or union complain of pain. Asymptomatic patient with radiological signs of nonunion should be followed with serial imaging.

Revision surgery should be considered when alternative modalities of management failed to improve patient's symptoms.

17.13 Failure of Long Strut Graft for Multilevel Cervical Corpectomy

Patients with cervical stenosis from multilevel disk herniations and spondylosis causing neural compression require surgery, with the universally recognized aim to adequately decompress the myeloradicular structures. Controversy lies in the method to be used for decompression. We described the multiple subtotal somatectomy for the management of patient with canal stenosis caused by posterior protrusions of the anterior wall of the spinal canal involving three or more cervical segments [7]. Recently, in these patients, to avoid the complications related to the graft, and the morbidity related to this quite aggressive surgery, we prefer to perform a posterior approach performing wide laminectomies of the involved segments, associated to stabilization in lordosis of the cervical spine to allow the back shift of the spinal cord.

Worldwide, multilevel cervical corpectomy using long strut graft is still a commonly performed procedure for patients with multilevel involvement of the cervical spine by degenerative disease, tumors, trauma, or infection [95].

The number of levels to be decompressed determines the length of the strut graft. Generally, the iliac crest is preferred for one-and two-level corpectomies, whereas fibula graft is used for longer fusions.

One of the most troublesome pitfalls of this procedure is the migration or displacement of the graft, with a reported incidence, ranging from 2 to 60% of the patients [95]; 30–50% of the complications in these multilevel procedures arise from graft- and instrumentation-related causes with a significant rate of revision surgery [95].

When migration of the graft occurs, it may have devastating consequences for the patient, such as direct injury to trachea, esophagus, and myeloradicular structures of the anterior neck, progressive vertebral collapse and kyphosis with further neurological damage, damage to the normal intervertebral disk spaces above and below the reconstruction with cavitation of the construct. Riew et al. [118] described profound airway compromise and death from catastrophic multilevel corpectomy reconstruction failure.

Long strut graft morbidity include migration, displacement, angulation, fracture, and nonunion.

Two forms of graft displacement must be highlighted, namely complete displacement and incomplete displacement of the graft. The former, which generally is an elementary radiographic diagnosis, occurs during the immediate postoperative period, and require prompt revision surgery. On the other hand, incomplete displacement is the most frequent graft problem encountered in patients undergoing long strut graft for multilevel cervical corpectomy, and can be described in terms of millimeters of "migration" (associated with subsidence or angulation of the graft), potential painful pseudoarthrosis, and pose problems in terms of therapeutic strategies. In fact, patients without complete displacement or fracture can be initially managed with more rigid postoperative immobilization by the placement of a halo fixator until there is evidence of osseous healing. In case of failure to nonoperative management, surgery is required.

Graft fracture is another potential pitfall of long strut graft, and it has been reported more likely when the graft is harvested with an osteotome instead of a saw [119].

In our setting, we have never encountered this complication, and we prefer to use cutting osteotomes for the iliac crest, or the Gigli saw for the fibula, rather than oscillating saws, which can produce necrosis of the cells on the cutting plane.

Patients with significant fracture require revision of the strut graft and instrumentation with eventual additional posterior fusion and fixation.

As stated above, complete displacement may be easily diagnosed by standard radiographs. CT scans with sagittal and coronal reconstructions are helpful in detecting signs of nonunion at the graft–host surface and fracture of the long strut graft. Signs of failure include migration of graft in relation to the position of plate and screws, and the inferior screws migrating caudally in the vertebral body [120].

Nonunion at the graft–host surface may be asymptomatic, but if a solid biological fusion does not occur, instrumentation may fail. Long strut grafts may also fracture despite healing at the graft–host junctions. Other complications of multilevel corpectomy reconstructions include plate fracture, screw fracture or dislodgment, and uncoupling of the screw–plate interface.

The incidence of graft morbidity in patients undergoing long strut graft has been associated with the length of the graft and the number of levels involved in the surgery. The lowest incidence of graft migration has been observed in patients undergoing single-level corpectomies, with the incidence increasing with each additional level.

Wang et al. proposed that this occurred despite the use of a more rigid and stable postoperative immobilization in halo vests for the four-level procedures, when compared with the two-poster braces for one-, two-, and three-level surgeries [95, 96].

Together with graft length, another risk factor for long strut graft morbidity seems to be the actual level fused. Wang et al. [96] performed a retrospective review of 249 consecutive patients who had undergone anterior cervical corpectomy and fusion with autogenous strut grafting for cervical stenosis with multilevel disk herniations and spondylosis causing neural compression. Of the 16 patients with graft migration, 14 involved C6 as the caudal corpectomy, with the fusion extending to the C7 vertebral body. Two-level corpectomies extending to C7 have a higher rate of migration than three-, four-, and five-level corpectomies that did not extend to C7. No long fusion (two levels or more) had a problem with graft migration when it extended only down to C6. The authors suggested that the association of a fusion extending down to C7 with graft displacement is most likely related to the biomechanical features of the cervicothoracic junction, with increased stress at the graft endplate interface, and higher probability of graft morbidity.

Technical errors can also be the cause of strut graft failure following anterior cervical fusion, such as improper preparation of fusion bed or faulty choice of surgical procedure.

A technical tip to increase the chances of fusion is to preserve as much as possible the anterior cortex of the lower vertebral body to resist fracture and allow for a strong inferior anchor.

Moreover, the aggressive removal of the endplate must be avoided to prevent graft migration into the vertebral body. The graft must be positioned before the intervertebral distractor is released.

Other factors can be considered to decrease the rate of graft morbidity for those fusions that end at C7, such as more rigid postoperative immobilization (halo fixator or cervicothoracic orthosis) or the addition of posterior cervical fusion.

Patients with minimally displaced fracture and satisfactory graft position without kyphosis are likely to heal with the application of a halo fixator, with associated close observation.

In the study from Wang et al. [96], of the 16 graft migrations, 11 were not associated with complete dislodgement or fracture, and were successfully managed with careful observation and continued immobilization. One of the 16 patients was managed with halo fixator for more rigid immobilization.

Significant displacement, kyphosis, or loss of contact of the graft and vertebral body requires revision surgery.

Revision surgery, when needed, aims to restore the physiological lordosis of the cervical spine and obtain stable internal fixation to promote biological bony fusion. The appropriate approach, procedure, and timing remain crucial aspect of revision surgery [120]. Unsolved questions such as whether or not the plate and strut graft should be replaced, whether or not the posterior instrumentation be placed (if the latter is the case, which should be performed first), and the type of postoperative orthoses to be used remain. Revision surgery of long anterior cervical strut graft requires extensive expertise in circumferential approaches.

Wang et al. [96] proposed that patients presenting with increased pain, but no breathing problems or signs of neurological impairment can be managed successfully with revision of the lower vertebral endplate or extension of the corpectomy beyond the fractured segment to the next lowest level with additional grafting. Subsequent posterior cervical stabilization with interspinous process wiring or lateral mass plating and posterior cervical fusion also should be performed.

A simple posterior stabilization is usually more effective in patients in whom early radiographic evidence of failure of anterior long construct is noticed. Posterior approach is only possible in patients without significant loss of sagittal alignment and absence of displacement of the anterior construct into the retropharyngeal space [120].

Anterior revision surgery followed by a posterior stabilization can be a possible option for patients with failure of long anterior construct, replacing the anterior strut graft with or without application of an anterior cervical plate. Additional posterior fixation could be an option that prevents subsequent failure [120].

In patients with kyphotic deformity, preoperative traction can be attempted to reduce the kyphosis to determine the best surgical approach.

In patients with fixed kyphotic deformity because of healing of the long strut graft in a kyphotic position or engagement of the screws into solid bone, Sasso [120] proposed a back–front–back technique (posterior cervical release followed by anterior revision surgery of the long strut graft and successive posterior fixation). The laminectomy allows excellent visualization of the spinal cord during the reduction maneuver. When reduction of a kyphotic deformity is attempted without direct visualization of the neural elements, spinal cord monitoring is required.

The anterior approach allows greater reduction of the kyphotic deformity during the posterior manipulation. An anterior strut graft must be implanted after posterior instrumentation to allow adequate anterior load sharing, increasing the fusion rate.

Revision surgery of long strut graft is associated with high rate of intra- and postoperative complications. The rate of infection is higher, as the approach is through a previously operated surgical field. Neurological injuries can occur as a consequence of cord draping over the apex of a failed collapsed kyphotic anterior construct [120]. As the spinal cord in these patients is already damaged from long-standing myelopathy, new intraoperative damages may have catastrophic sequalae.

17.13.1 Prevention of Failure

Prevention is the better management of strut graft failure. In long strut grafts, the process of fusion may require 1–2 years to heal [95], and occurs by "creeping substitution," beginning at the endplates and extending toward the midportion of the graft. Bone resorption precedes new bone formation, and, therefore, the strut grafts are relatively weak and susceptible to delayed fracture with normal loading of the cervical spine when external bracing is discontinued. At the index procedure, the use of plates and screws providing an "internal orthosis" can significantly reduce the incidence of long graft morbidity in cervical corpectomy [95].

However, unsolved questions remain, as no superiority of any type of instrumentation has been demonstrated in comparison with the others (constrained plate–screw systems vs. semiconstrained dynamic plate, and in the field of semiconstrained plates the choice of rotational, translational, or a combination of both).

The type of anterior plate may affect the success of the anterior-only construct. Anterior plate should share the load with the graft to facilitate fusion and to protect the graft from stresses, which may cause collapse. Rigid plate designs, in which the screws are locked to the plate, resist any settling of the construct and may hold the construct in some distraction delaying or preventing fusion.

Experience with management of long-bone fractures suggests that cyclical micromotion delivered to a fracture site enhances union rates after initial stability, although excessive motion may promote nonunion. Dynamic plating systems, in which the screws may slide when the graft is settling, have the theoretical advantage to share the load with the graft, protecting it from high loads, which can cause collapse. On the one hand, dynamic cervical plates address the perceived biomechanical deficiencies of rigid cervical plates, and on the other hand settling associated with dynamic plates could lead to segmental kyphosis or foraminal narrowing [121].

To date, there are no prospective studies comparing the outcome of rigid vs. dynamic plating for multilevel corpectomy and reconstruction.

Pitzen et al. [122] conducted a prospective, controlled, randomized, multicenter study to compare implant complications, fusion, loss of lordosis, and outcome after anterior cervical plating with dynamic or rigid plates in patients undergoing a routine anterior cervical discectomy with tricortical iliac crest autograft. They concluded that dynamic cervical plate designs provide less implant complications (no patient) when compared with rigid plate designs (four patients). Speed of fusion was faster in the presence of a dynamic plate. However, loss of segmental lordosis was significantly higher if dynamic plates were used, which did not result in differences regarding clinical outcome between dynamic and constrained plates after 2 years.

Junctional plating is a technique in which a small anterior cervical plate is fixed at one end of the construct. It overlaps the end of the strut graft–vertebra junction and is able to block the end of the graft so that it does not dislodge anteriorly. It has the advantage to allow load sharing by the graft and permits the graft to settle gradually into the endplates .

Vanichkachorn et al. [123] reported on 11 patients with cervical myelopathy undergoing a multilevel (average 3.36 levels) corpectomy followed by the placement of a fibular or iliac crest strut graft. An anterior short-segment locking or buttress plate was then placed in the vertebral body, either inferior or superior to the seated graft. Posterior segmental fixation was performed in all patients during the same procedure. No patient in this series experienced graft- or construct-related complications. The authors concluded that the use of a junctional plate anteriorly along with posterior segmental fixation and fusion may prevent or decrease the incidence of graft and internal fixation dislodgement after a long-segment cervical reconstruction procedure.

Sasso [120] recommended to associate posterior instrumentation to multilevel corpectomy reconstructions until these issues are resolved.

Biomechanical data support the addition of posterior fusion for added stabilization of plated multilevel anterior cervical fusions.

DiAngelo et al. [108] and Foley et al. [124] showed that anterior multilevel cervical plating effectively increases stiffness and decreases local cervical motion after corpectomy. However, anterior cervical plating also reverses graft loads and excessively loads the graft in extension, which may promote pistoning and failure of multilevel constructs.

Therefore, anterior cervical plating may promote "pistoning" of the graft through the caudal vertebral endplate and the plate subsequently kicking out of the lower vertebral body. The addition of posterior instrumentation moves the instantaneous axis of rotation posteriorly, thus approximating its normal location in the posterior aspect of the vertebral body, protecting the graft from excessive loads during extension.

Meticulous preparation of the bone graft–host bone interface and secure placement of the graft with plating is essential for success of long-segment anterior cervical fusions. Also, attention to proper graft placement is crucial. If the plate is not properly contoured, it can act as a distraction device, and can prevent intimate bone contact between the graft and vertebra, inhibiting healing.

17.14 The Future

At present, there is little evidence to support the use of alternatives to autologous bone for cervical interbody fusion. Early enthusiasm for some implants has been overshadowed by unacceptably high complication rates. A combination of techniques and certain porous formulations may provide surgeons who fuse the cervical spine with the best option. However, the cost of such technology may be prohibitive, and the health economic implications cannot be ignored. It remains to be seen whether this approach is in the best long-term interests of patients [36, 125–127].

Core Messages

- The presence of any detrimental condition may diminish the osteogenic potential of the fusion site. Systemic risk factors include use of tobacco or other drugs, advanced age of the patient, and metabolic comorbidities (e.g., diabetes or osteoporosis). Other factors that contribute to failure of arthrodesis are structural instability, improper preparation of the host bone, and poor vascularity.
- Autogenous grafts remain the gold standard for bone grafts, because of their biological superiority. However, these grafts carry the risk of donor site morbidity, including infections, wound drainage, hematomas, fracture, prolonged pain, sensory loss, and keloids. Moreover, the patient undergoes a second skin incision, and there are the costs of long anesthetic time and hospital stay.
- Allograft bone avoids donor site morbidity, but carries the risk of disease transmission, the costs of a bone bank, host immune response, and inconsistent graft incorporation.
- Bone graft substitutes, alternatives to allografts and autografts, have osteoconductive properties. Their use in most cases is not supported by high evidence level studies.
- General complications of all bone graft materials include osseous nonunion, delayed union, graft fracture, graft extrusion, and infection.
- Length of the graft and number of levels involved in the surgery increase the incidence of complications.
- The donor site saws generate heat that may produce necrosis and tissue denaturing: use chisels! Use drill holes along the resection margin on both cortices so that the chisel can more easily and less traumatically transect the bone.
- In iliac crest, avoid harvesting the graft too anteriorly. The muscles that insert into the bone may disrupt the bone at the anterior superior iliac spine.
- When bicortical cylindrical graft is required (Cloward instrumentation), harvest the graft from the medial portion of the iliac wing, which at this point has a slight posterior curvature. This is the site where the bone is at its thickest. Apply the drill at right angles to the

external cortical surface of the iliac wing, to avoid an oblique surface along one edge of the graft.

- Avoid damage to the sensitive branch of the musculocutaneous nerve, which crosses the iliac crest.
- Once the graft has been harvested, its bed must be subjected to careful and complete hemostasis: apply bone wax.
- Close scrupulously in well-approximated layers to avoid formation of potential cavities in the abdominal wall. Reattach the muscles to the bone through transosseous sutures. Apply suction drainage.
- The fibula is the preferred type of graft when immediate mechanical support is required. Avoid damage to the external popliteal branch of the sciatic nerve obtaining the graft from the metaphysis and away from the head and neck of the fibula where the nerve crosses; avoid penetrating into the muscular structures of the anterior compartment of the leg during the stripping of the bone, use a Gigli saw; and avoid the use of oscillating saws that may produce contusions of the nerve.
- Proximal metaphysis of tibia: outlined with drill holes the perimeter of the graft before the bone is harvested. Use chisels to elevate the bone.

References

1. Boni M, Cherubino P, Denaro V (1983) The surgical treatment of fractures of the cervical spine. Ital J Orthop Traumatol 9(Suppl):107–126
2. Boni M, Denaro V (1982) The cervical stenosis syndrome with a review of 83 patients treated by operation. Int Orthop 6:185–195
3. Boni M, Denaro V (1982) Surgical treatment of cervical arthrosis. Follow-up review (2–13 years) of the 1st 100 cases operated on by anterior approach. Rev Chir Orthop Reparatrice Appar Mot 68:269–280
4. Boni M, Denaro V (1980) Surgical treatment of traumatic lesions of the middle and lower cervical spine (C3–C7). Ital J Orthop Traumatol 6:305–320
5. Whang PG, Wang JC (2003) Bone graft substitutes for spinal fusion. Spine J 3:155–165
6. Anderson DG, Albert TJ (2002) Bone grafting, implants, and plating options for anterior cervical fusions. Orthop Clin North Am 33:317–328
7. Boni M, Cherubino P, Denaro V et al (1984) Multiple subtotal somatectomy. Technique and evaluation of a series of 39 cases. Spine 9:358–362
8. Van Heest A, Swiontkowski M (1999) Bone-graft substitutes. Lancet 353(Suppl 1):SI28–SI29
9. Beaman FD, Bancroft LW, Peterson JJ et al (2006) Bone graft materials and synthetic substitutes. Radiol Clin North Am 44:451–461
10. De Long WG, Jr Einhorn TA, Koval K et al (2007) Bone grafts and bone graft substitutes in orthopaedic trauma surgery. A critical analysis. J Bone Joint Surg Am 89: 649–658
11. Bauer TW (2007) Bone graft substitutes. Skeletal Radiol 36:1105–1107
12. Bauer TW, Togawa D (2003) Bone graft substitutes: towards a more perfect union. Orthopedics 26:925–926
13. Bauer TW, Muschler GF (2000) Bone graft materials. An overview of the basic science. Clin Orthop Relat Res 371: 10–27
14. Vaccaro AR, Cirello J (2002) The use of allograft bone and cages in fractures of the cervical, thoracic, and lumbar spine. Clin Orthop Relat Res 394:19–26
15. Roy-Camille R, Judet TH, Saillant G et al (1981) Tumeurs du rachis. Techniques chirugucales, Orthopedie. Encycl Med Chir Paris 44165:4.06.04
16. Silvani V, Brambilla G, Rainoldi F et al (1987) Vertebral osteomyelitis with chronic cervical extradural abscess in a heroin addict. Neurochirurgia (Stuttg) 30:91–94
17. Brantigan JW, Cunningham BW, Warden K et al (1993) Compression strength of donor bone for posterior lumbar interbody fusion. Spine 18:1213–1221
18. Canalis E (1985) Effect of growth factors on bone cell replication and differentiation. Clin Orthop Relat Res 193: 246–263
19. Vadalà G, Di Martino A, Tirindelli MC et al (2008) Use of autologous bone marrow cells concentrate enriched with platelet-rich fibrin on corticocancellous bone allograft for posterolateral multilevel cervical fusion. J Tissue Eng Regen Med 29:515–520
20. Stevenson S, Emery SE, Goldberg VM (1996) Factors affecting bone graft incorporation. Clin Orthop Relat Res 324:66–74
21. Miyazaki M, Tsumura H, Wang JC et al (2009) An update on bone substitutes for spinal fusion. Eur Spine J 18:783–799
22. Brown MD, Malinin TI, Davis PB (1976) A roentgenographic evaluation of frozen allografts versus autografts in anterior cervical spine fusions. Clin Orthop Relat Res 119:231–236
23. Young WF, Rosenwasser RH (1993) An early comparative analysis of the use of fibular allograft versus autologous iliac crest graft for interbody fusion after anterior cervical discectomy. Spine 18:1123–1124
24. Savolainen S, Usenius JP, Hernesniemi J (1994) Iliac crest versus artificial bone grafts in 250 cervical fusions. Acta Neurochir (Wien) 129:54–57
25. Zhang ZH, Yin H, Yang K et al (1983) Anterior intervertebral disc excision and bone grafting in cervical spondylotic myelopathy. Spine 8:16–19

26. Zdeblick TA, Ducker TB (1991) The use of freeze-dried allograft bone for anterior cervical fusions. Spine 16: 726–729
27. Bishop RC, Moore KA, Hadley MN (1996) Anterior cervical interbody fusion using autogeneic and allogeneic bone graft substrate: a prospective comparative analysis. J Neurosurg 85:206–210
28. Fujishiro T, Bauer TW, Kobayashi N et al (2007) Histological evaluation of an impacted bone graft substitute composed of a combination of mineralized and demineralized allograft in a sheep vertebral bone defect. J Biomed Mater Res A 82: 538–544
29. Kanayama M, Hashimoto T, Shigenobu K et al (2006) A prospective randomized study of posterolateral lumbar fusion using osteogenic protein-1 (OP-1) versus local autograft with ceramic bone substitute: emphasis of surgical exploration and histologic assessment. Spine 31:1067–1074
30. Thalgott JS, Fritts K, Giuffre JM et al (1999) Anterior interbody fusion of the cervical spine with coralline hydroxyapatite. Spine 24:1295–1299
31. An HS, Simpson JM, Glover JM et al (1995) Comparison between allograft plus demineralized bone matrix versus autograft in anterior cervical fusion. A prospective multicenter study. Spine 20:2211–2216
32. Baskin DS, Ryan P, Sonntag V et al (2003) A prospective, randomized, controlled cervical fusion study using recombinant human bone morphogenetic protein-2 with the CORNERSTONE-SR allograft ring and the ATLANTIS anterior cervical plate. Spine 28:1219–1224; discussion 1225
33. Shields LB, Raque GH, Glassman SD et al (2006) Adverse effects associated with high-dose recombinant human bone morphogenetic protein-2 use in anterior cervical spine fusion. Spine 31:542–547
34. Vaidya R, Carp J, Sethi A et al (2007) Complications of anterior cervical discectomy and fusion using recombinant human bone morphogenetic protein-2. Eur Spine J 16: 1257–1265
35. Brown CA, Eismont FJ (1998) Complications in spinal fusion. Orthop Clin North Am 29:679–699
36. Wigfield CC, Nelson RJ (2001) Nonautologous interbody fusion materials in cervical spine surgery: how strong is the evidence to justify their use? Spine 26:687–694
37. Zeidman SM, Ducker TB, Raycroft J (1997) Trends and complications in cervical spine surgery: 1989–1993. J Spinal Disord 10:523–526
38. Ebraheim NA, Elgafy H, Xu R (2001) Bone-graft harvesting from iliac and fibular donor sites: techniques and complications. J Am Acad Orthop Surg 9:210–218
39. Denaro V, Gulino G, Papapietro N et al (1998) Treatment of metastases of the cervical spine. Chir Organi Mov 83: 127–137
40. Kurz LT, Garfin SR, Booth RE Jr (1989) Harvesting autogenous iliac bone grafts. A review of complications and techniques. Spine 14:1324–1331
41. Sawin PD, Traynelis VC, Menezes AH (1998) A comparative analysis of fusion rates and donor-site morbidity for autogeneic rib and iliac crest bone grafts in posterior cervical fusions. J Neurosurg 88:255–265
42. Schnee CL, Freese A, Weil RJ et al (1997) Analysis of harvest morbidity and radiographic outcome using autograft for anterior cervical fusion. Spine 22:2222–2227
43. Summers BN, Eisenstein SM (1989) Donor site pain from the ilium. A complication of lumbar spine fusion. J Bone Joint Surg Br 71:677–680
44. Catinella FP, De Laria GA, De Wald RL (1990) False aneurysm of the superior gluteal artery. A complication of iliac crest bone grafting. Spine 15:1360–1362
45. Escalas F, DeWald RL (1977) Combined traumatic arteriovenous fistula and urethral injury: a complication of iliac bone-grafting. J Bone Joint Surg Am 59:270–271
46. Kahn B (1979) Superior gluteal artery laceration, a complication of iliac bone graft surgery. Clin Orthop Relat Res 140:204–207
47. Lim EV, Lavadia WT, Roberts JM (1996) Superior gluteal artery injury during iliac bone grafting for spinal fusion. A case report and literature review. Spine 21:2376–2378
48. Massey EW (1980) Meralgia paresthetica secondary to trauma of bone graft. J Trauma 20:342–343
49. Shin AY, Moran ME, Wenger DR (1996) Superior gluteal artery injury secondary to posterior iliac crest bone graft harvesting. A surgical technique to control hemorrhage. Spine 21:1371–1374
50. Weikel AM, Habal MB (1977) Meralgia paresthetica: a complication of iliac bone procurement. Plast Reconstr Surg 60:572–574
51. Hu RW, Bohlman IIII (1994) Fracture at the iliac bone graft harvest site after fusion of the spine. Clin Orthop Relat Res 309:208–213
52. Cowley SP, Anderson LD (1983) Hernias through donor sites for iliac-bone grafts. J Bone Joint Surg Am 65: 1023–1025
53. Lotem M, Maor P, Haimoff H et al (1971) Lumbar hernia at an iliac bone graft donor site. A case report. Clin Orthop Relat Res 80:130–132
54. Stoll P, Schilli W (1981) Long-term follow-up donor and recipient sites after autologous bone grafts for reconstruction of the facial skeleton. J Oral Surg 39:676–677
55. Coventry MB, Tapper EM (1972) Pelvic instability: a consequence of removing iliac bone for grafting. J Bone Joint Surg Am 54:83–101
56. Goulet JA, Senunas LE, DeSilva GL et al (1997) Autogenous iliac crest bone graft. Complications and functional assessment. Clin Orthop Relat Res 339:76–81
57. Puri R, Moskovich R, Gusmorino P et al (2000) Bupivacaine for postoperative pain relief at the iliac crest bone graft harvest site. Am J Orthop 29:443–446
58. Duncan RW, McGuire RA, Meydrech EF (1994) Pneumatic gouge versus standard method for iliac crest harvesting. Orthop Rev 23:672–675
59. Steffen T, Downer P, Steiner B et al (2000) Minimally invasive bone harvesting tools. Eur Spine J 9(Suppl 1): S114–S118
60. Burstein FD, Simms C, Cohen SR et al (2000) Iliac crest bone graft harvesting techniques: a comparison. Plast Reconstr Surg 105:34–39
61. Tanishima T, Yoshimasu N, Ogai M (1995) A technique for prevention of donor site pain associated with harvesting iliac bone grafts. Surg Neurol 44:131–132
62. Tayapongsak P, Wimsatt JA, LaBanc JP et al (1994) Morbidity from anterior ilium bone harvest. A comparative study of lateral versus medial surgical approach. Oral Surg Oral Med Oral Pathol 78:296–300

63. Murata Y, Takahashi K, Yamagata M et al (2002) Injury to the lateral femoral cutaneous nerve during harvest of iliac bone graft, with reference to the size of the graft. J Bone Joint Surg Br 84:798–801
64. Shamsaldin M, Mouchaty H, Desogus N et al (2006) Evaluation of donor site pain after anterior iliac crest harvesting for cervical fusion: a prospective study on 50 patients. Acta Neurochir (Wien) 148:1071–1074; discussion 1074
65. Seiler JG III, Johnson J (2000) Iliac crest autogenous bone grafting: donor site complications. J South Orthop Assoc 9:91–97
66. Lu J, Ebraheim NA, Huntoon M et al (1998) Anatomic considerations of superior cluneal nerve at posterior iliac crest region. Clin Orthop Relat Res 347:224–228
67. Xu R, Ebraheim NA, Yeasting RA et al (1996) Anatomic considerations for posterior iliac bone harvesting. Spine 21:1017–1020
68. Fernyhough JC, Schimandle JJ, Weigel MC et al (1992) Chronic donor site pain complicating bone graft harvesting from the posterior iliac crest for spinal fusion. Spine 17:1474–1480
69. Guha SC, Poole MD (1983) Stress fracture of the iliac bone with subfascial femoral neuropathy: unusual complications at a bone graft donor site: case report. Br J Plast Surg 36:305–306
70. Smith SE, DeLee JC, Ramamurthy S (1984) Ilioinguinal neuralgia following iliac bone-grafting. Report of two cases and review of the literature. J Bone Joint Surg Am 66:1306–1308
71. Brumback RJ (1990) Traumatic rupture of the superior gluteal artery, without fracture of the pelvis, causing compartment syndrome of the buttock. A case report. J Bone Joint Surg Am 72:134–137
72. Friend KD, Koval KJ, Mirovsky Y et al (1995) Fracture of the iliac crest following bone grafting: a case report and literature review. Bull Hosp Jt Dis 54:49–51
73. Chan K, Resnick D, Pathria M et al (2001) Pelvic instability after bone graft harvesting from posterior iliac crest: report of nine patients. Skeletal Radiol 30:278–281
74. Ebraheim NA, Elgafy H, Semaan HB (2000) Computed tomographic findings in patients with persistent sacroiliac pain after posterior iliac graft harvesting. Spine 25:2047–2051
75. Auleda J, Bianchi A, Tibau R et al (1995) Hernia through iliac crest defects. A report of four cases. Int Orthop 19:367–369
76. Banwart JC, Asher MA, Hassanein RS (1995) Iliac crest bone graft harvest donor site morbidity. A statistical evaluation. Spine 20:1055–1060
77. Froimson AI, Cummings AG Jr (1971) Iliac hernia following hip arthrodesis. Clin Orthop Relat Res 80:89–91
78. Reid RL (1968) Hernia through an iliac bone-graft donor site. A case report. J Bone Joint Surg Am 50:757–760
79. Bosworth DM, Bosworth DM (1955) Repair of herniae through iliac-crest defects. J Bone Joint Surg Am 37-A: 1069–1073
80. Challis JH, Lyttle JA, Stuart AE (1975) Strangulated lumbar hernia and volvulus following removal of iliac crest bone graft. Acta Orthop Scand 46:230–233
81. Arrington ED, Smith WJ, Chambers HG et al (1996) Complications of iliac crest bone graft harvesting. Clin Orthop Relat Res 329:300–309
82. Robertson PA, Wray AC (2001) Natural history of posterior iliac crest bone graft donation for spinal surgery: a prospective analysis of morbidity. Spine 26:1473–1476
83. Younger EM, Chapman MW (1989) Morbidity at bone graft donor sites. J Orthop Trauma 3:192–195
84. Dosoglu M, Orakdogen M, Tevruz M et al (1998) Enterocutaneous fistula: a complication of posterior iliac bone graft harvesting not previously described. Acta Neurochir (Wien) 140:1089–1092
85. Cardaci GT (1994) Translocation of Paget's disease to the tibia in an iliac crest bone graft. Clin Nucl Med 19:742
86. Cole GW Jr, Sindelar WF (1995) Iatrogenic transplantation of osteosarcoma. South Med J 88:485–488
87. Denaro V, Denaro L, Gulino G et al (1998) Complicanze nella chirurgia cervicale. Giornale Italiano di Ortopedia e Traumatologia 24:681–688
88. Denaro V (1991) Stenosis of the cervical spine. Springer, Berlin
89. Vail TP, Urbaniak JR (1996) Donor-site morbidity with use of vascularized autogenous fibular grafts. J Bone Joint Surg Am 78:204–211
90. Rupp RE, Podeszwa D, Ebraheim NA (1994) Danger zones associated with fibular osteotomy. J Orthop Trauma 8:54–58
91. Chen YC, Chen CH, Chen PL et al (2006) Donor site morbidity after harvesting of proximal tibia bone. Head Neck 28:496–500
92. Greenwald AS, Boden SD, Goldberg VM et al (2001) Bone-graft substitutes: facts, fictions, and applications. J Bone Joint Surg Am 83-A(Suppl 2 Pt 2):98–103
93. Bauer TW, Smith ST (2002) Bioactive materials in orthopaedic surgery: overview and regulatory considerations. Clin Orthop Relat Res 395:11–22
94. Burchardt H, Jones H, Glowczewskie F et al (1978) Freeze-dried allogeneic segmental cortical-bone grafts in dogs. J Bone Joint Surg Am 60:1082–1090
95. Thongtrangan I, Balabhadra RS, Kim DH (2003) Management of strut graft failure in anterior cervical spine surgery. Neurosurg Focus 15:E4
96. Wang JC, Hart RA, Emery SE et al (2003) Graft migration or displacement after multilevel cervical corpectomy and strut grafting. Spine 28:1016–1021; discussion 1021–1012
97. Zhang ZH, Yin HF, Yang KQ et al (1980) Anterior route intervertebral disc excision and bone grafting in cervical spondylitic myelopathy. Chin Med J (Engl) 93: 865–868
98. Ferlic DC, Clayton ML, Leidholt JD et al (1975) Surgical treatment of the symptomatic unstable cervical spine in rheumatoid arthritis. J Bone Joint Surg Am 57:349–354
99. Zoma A, Sturrock RD, Fisher WD et al (1987) Surgical stabilisation of the rheumatoid cervical spine. J Bone Joint Surg Br 69:8–12
100. Boden SD (2002) Overview of the biology of lumbar spine fusion and principles for selecting a bone graft substitute. Spine 27:S26–S31
101. Aebi M, Zuber K, Marchesi D (1991) Treatment of cervical spine injuries with anterior plating. Indications, techniques, and results. Spine 16:S38–S45
102. Bohler J, Gaudernak T (1980) Anterior plate stabilization for fracture-dislocations of the lower cervical spine. J Trauma 20:203–205

103. Bose B (2001) Anterior cervical instrumentation enhances fusion rates in multilevel reconstruction in smokers. J Spinal Disord 14:3–9
104. Connolly PJ, Esses SI, Kostuik JP (1996) Anterior cervical fusion: outcome analysis of patients fused with and without anterior cervical plates. J Spinal Disord 9:202–206
105. Gassman J, Seligson D (1983) The anterior cervical plate. Spine 8:700–707
106. Wang JC, McDonough PW, Endow K et al (1999) The effect of cervical plating on single-level anterior cervical discectomy and fusion. J Spinal Disord 12:467–471
107. Wang JC, McDonough PW, Endow KK et al (2000) Increased fusion rates with cervical plating for two-level anterior cervical discectomy and fusion. Spine 25:41–45
108. DiAngelo DJ, Foley KT, Vossel KA et al (2000) Anterior cervical plating reverses load transfer through multilevel strut-grafts. Spine 25:783–795
109. Zdeblick TA, Bohlman HH (1989) Cervical kyphosis and myelopathy. Treatment by anterior corpectomy and strut-grafting. J Bone Joint Surg Am 71:170–182
110. Emery SE, Bohlman HH, Bolesta MJ et al (1998) Anterior cervical decompression and arthrodesis for the treatment of cervical spondylotic myelopathy. Two to seventeen-year follow-up. J Bone Joint Surg Am 80:941–951
111. Fernyhough JC, White JI, LaRocca H (1991) Fusion ratcs in multilevel cervical spondylosis comparing allograft fibula with autograft fibula in 126 patients. Spine 16: S561–S564
112. Hanai K, Fujiyoshi F, Kamei K (1986) Subtotal vertebrectomy and spinal fusion for cervical spondylotic myelopathy. Spine 11:310–315
113. Herman JM, Sonntag VK (1994) Cervical corpectomy and plate fixation for postlaminectomy kyphosis. J Neurosurg 80:963–970
114. Lowery GL, Swank ML, McDonough RF (1995) Surgical revision for failed anterior cervical fusions. Articular pillar plating or anterior revision? Spine 20:2436–2441
115. Smith MD, Bolesta MJ (1992) Esophageal perforation after anterior cervical plate fixation: a report of two cases. J Spinal Disord 5:357–362
116. Yee GK, Terry AF (1993) Esophageal penetration by an anterior cervical fixation device. A case report. Spine 18:522–527
117. Welch WC, Gerszten PC, Nestler AP, et al (2005) Management of symptomatic cervical pseudarthrosis. In: Clark CR (ed) The cervical spine. Springer, Berlin, pp 1205–1211
118. Riew KD, Sethi NS, Devney J (1999) Complications of buttress plate stabilization of cervical corpectomy. Spine 24:2404–2410
119. Jones AA, Dougherty PJ, Sharkey NA et al (1993) Iliac crest bone graft. Osteotome versus saw. Spine 18:2048–2052
120. Sasso RC (2005) Salvage of long strut graft failure following multilevel cervical corpectomy and arthrodesis. In: Clark CR (ed) The cervical spine. Springer, Berlin, pp 1212–1217
121. Rhee JM, Riew KD (2007) Dynamic anterior cervical plates. J Am Acad Orthop Surg 15:640–646
122. Pitzen TR, Chrobok J, Stulik J et al (2009) Implant complications, fusion, loss of lordosis, and outcome after anterior cervical plating with dynamic or rigid plates: two-year results of a multi-centric, randomized, controlled study. Spine 34:641–646
123. Vanichkachorn JS, Vaccaro AR, Silveri CP et al (1998) Anterior junctional plate in the cervical spine. Spine 23:2462–2467
124. Foley KT, DiAngelo DJ, Rampersaud YR et al (1999) The in vitro effects of instrumentation on multilevel cervical strut-graft mechanics. Spine 24:2366–2376
125. Cloward RB (1988) The anterior surgical approach to the cervical spine: the Cloward Procedure: past, present, and future. The presidential guest lecture, Cervical Spine Research Society. Spine 13:823–827
126. Lees F, Turner JW (1963) Natural history and prognosis of cervical spondylosis. Br Med J 2:1607–1610
127. Shono Y, McAfee PC, Cunningham BW et al (1993) A biomechanical analysis of decompression and reconstruction methods in the cervical spine. Emphasis on a carbon-fiber-composite cage. J Bone Joint Surg Am 75:1674–1684
128. Laurie SW, Kaban LB, Mulliken JB et al (1984) Donor-site morbidity after harvesting rib and iliac bone. Plast Reconstr Surg 73:933–938
129. Keller EE, Triplett WW (1987) Iliac bone grafting: review of 160 consecutive cases. J Oral Maxillofac Surg 45: 11–14
130. Kreibich DN, Scott IR, Wells JM et al (1994) Donor site morbidity at the iliac crest: comparison of percutaneous and open methods. J Bone Joint Surg Br 76:847–848
131. Hutchinson MR, Dall BE (1994) Midline fascial splitting approach to the iliac crest for bone graft. A new approach. Spine 19:62–66
132. Colterjohn NR, Bednar DA (1997) Procurement of bone graft from the iliac crest. An operative approach with decreased morbidity. J Bone Joint Surg Am 79:756–759
133. Beirne JC, Barry HJ, Brady FA et al (1996) Donor site morbidity of the anterior iliac crest following cancellous bone harvest. Int J Oral Maxillofac Surg 25:268–271
134. Kalk WW, Raghoebar GM, Jansma J et al (1996) Morbidity from iliac crest bone harvesting. J Oral Maxillofac Surg 54:1424–1429; discussion 1430
135. Hill NM, Horne JG, Devane PA (1999) Donor site morbidity in the iliac crest bone graft. Aust NZ J Surg 69: 726–728
136. Skaggs DL, Samuelson MA, Hale JM et al (2000) Complications of posterior iliac crest bone grafting in spine surgery in children. Spine 25:2400–2402
137. Ahlmann E, Patzakis M, Roidis N et al (2002) Comparison of anterior and posterior iliac crest bone grafts in terms of harvest-site morbidity and functional outcomes. J Bone Joint Surg Am 84-A:716–720
138. Heary RF, Schlenk RP, Sacchieri TA et al (2002) Persistent iliac crest donor site pain: independent outcome assessment. Neurosurgery 50:510–516; discussion 516–517
139. Cricchio G, Lundgren S (2003) Donor site morbidity in two different approaches to anterior iliac crest bone harvesting. Clin Implant Dent Relat Res 5:161–169
140. Mazock JB, Schow SR, Triplett RG (2003) Posterior iliac crest bone harvest: review of technique, complications, and use of an epidural catheter for postoperative pain control. J Oral Maxillofac Surg 61:1497–1503
141. Silber JS, Anderson DG, Daffner SD et al (2003) Donor site morbidity after anterior iliac crest bone harvest for single-level anterior cervical discectomy and fusion. Spine 28:134–139

142. Joshi A, Kostakis GC (2004) An investigation of post-operative morbidity following iliac crest graft harvesting. Br Dent J 196:167–171; discussion 155
143. DeOrio JK, Farber DC (2005) Morbidity associated with anterior iliac crest bone grafting in foot and ankle surgery. Foot Ankle Int 26:147–151
144. Kessler P, Thorwarth M, Bloch-Birkholz A et al (2005) Harvesting of bone from the iliac crest–comparison of the anterior and posterior sites. Br J Oral Maxillofac Surg 43:51–56
145. Kager AN, Marks M, Bastrom T et al (2006) Morbidity of iliac crest bone graft harvesting in adolescent deformity surgery. J Pediatr Orthop 26:132–134
146. Pollock R, Alcelik I, Bhatia C et al (2008) Donor site morbidity following iliac crest bone harvesting for cervical fusion: a comparison between minimally invasive and open techniques. Eur Spine J 17:845–852
147. Eufinger H, Leppanen H (2000) Iliac crest donor site morbidity following open and closed methods of bone harvest for alveolar cleft osteoplasty. J Craniomaxillofac Surg 28:31–38
148. Mirovsky Y, Neuwirth MG (2000) Comparison between the outer table and intracortical methods of obtaining autogenous bone graft from the iliac crest. Spine 25: 1722–1725
149. David R, Folman Y, Pikarsky I et al (2003) Harvesting bone graft from the posterior iliac crest by less traumatic, midline approach. J Spinal Disord Tech 16:27–30
150. Sandor GK, Rittenberg BN, Clokie CM et al (2003) Clinical success in harvesting autogenous bone using a minimally invasive trephine. J Oral Maxillofac Surg 61:164–168
151. Sasso RC, LeHuec JC, Shaffrey C (2005) Iliac crest bone graft donor site pain after anterior lumbar interbody fusion: a prospective patient satisfaction outcome assessment. J Spinal Disord Tech 18(Suppl):S77–S81
152. Delawi D, Dhert WJ, Castelein RM et al (2007) The incidence of donor site pain after bone graft harvesting from the posterior iliac crest may be overestimated: a study on spine fracture patients. Spine 32:1865–1868
153. Singh K, Phillips FM, Kuo E et al (2007) A prospective, randomized, double-blind study of the efficacy of postoperative continuous local anesthetic infusion at the iliac crest bone graft site after posterior spinal arthrodesis: a minimum of 4-year follow-up. Spine 32:2790–2796
154. van den Broecke DG, Schuurman AH, Borg ED et al (1998) Neurotmesis of the lateral femoral cutaneous nerve when coring for iliac crest bone grafts. Plast Reconstr Surg 102:1163–1166
155. Yamamoto T, Nagira K, Kurosaka M (2001) Meralgia paresthetica occurring 40 years after iliac bone graft harvesting: case report. Neurosurgery 49:1455–1457
156. Mahli A, Coskun D, Altun NS et al (2002) Alcohol neurolysis for persistent pain caused by superior cluneal nerves injury after iliac crest bone graft harvesting in orthopedic surgery: report of four cases and review of the literature. Spine 27:E478–E481
157. Neo M, Matsushita M, Morita T et al (2000) Pseudoaneurysm of the deep circumflex iliac artery: a rare complication at an anterior iliac bone graft donor site. Spine 25:1848–1851
158. Chou AS, Hung CF, Tseng JH et al (2002) Pseudoaneurysm of the deep circumflex iliac artery: a rare complication at an anterior iliac bone graft donor site treated by coil embolization. Chang Gung Med J 25:480–484
159. Kong CG, Park JB, Won YD et al (2009) Arteriovenous fistula of the superior gluteal artery as a complication of posterior iliac crest bone graft harvesting: 3D-CT angiography and arterial embolization. Eur Spine J 18(Suppl 2): 250–253
160. Reynolds AF Jr, Turner PT, Loeser JD (1978) Fracture of the anterior superior iliac spine following anterior cervical fusion using iliac crest. Case report. J Neurosurg 48: 809–810
161. Reale F, Gambacorta D, Mencattini G (1979) Iliac crest fracture after removal of two bone plugs for anterior cervical fusion. Case report. J Neurosurg 51:560–561
162. Blakemore ME (1983) Fractures at cancellous bone graft donor sites. Injury 14:519–522
163. Kuhn DA, Moreland MS (1986) Complications following iliac crest bone grafting. Clin Orthop Relat Res 209: 224–226
164. Porchet F, Jaques B (1996) Unusual complications at iliac crest bone graft donor site: experience with two cases. Neurosurgery 39:856–859
165. Fernando TL, Kim SS, Mohler DG (1999) Complete pelvic ring failure after posterior iliac bone graft harvesting. Spine 24:2101–2104
166. Nocini PF, Bedogni A, Valsecchi S et al (2003) Fractures of the iliac crest following anterior and posterior bone graft harvesting. Review of the literature and case presentation. Minerva Stomatol 52(441–448):448–452
167. Lichtblau S (1962) Dislocation of the sacroiliac joint: a complication of bone grafting. J Bone Joint Surg Am 44: 193–198
168. Oldfield MC (1945) Iliac hernia after bone grafting. Lancet 1:810–812
169. Pyrtek LJ, Kelly CC (1960) Management of herniation through large iliac bone defects. Ann Surg 152:998–1003
170. Ramirez H Jr, Bennett WF, Peters V (1985) CT diagnosis of hernia through iliac bone-graft donor site. J Comput Assist Tomogr 9:411–412
171. Ubhi CS, Morris DL (1984) Fracture and herniation of bowel at bone graft donor site in the iliac crest. Injury 16:202–203
172. Stevens KJ, Banuls M (1994) Iliolumbar hernia following bone grafting. Eur Spine J 3:118–119
173. Velchuru VR, Satish SG, Petri GJ et al (2006) Hernia through an iliac crest bone graft site: report of a case and review of the literature. Bull Hosp Jt Dis 63:166–168
174. Ziccardi VB, Lalikos JF, Sotereanos GC et al (1992) Retroperitoneal hematoma as a complication of anterior iliac crest harvest: report of a case. J Oral Maxillofac Surg 50:1113–1116
175. Brazaitis MP, Mirvis SE, Greenberg J et al (1994) Severe retroperitoneal hemorrhage complicating anterior iliac bone graft acquisition. J Oral Maxillofac Surg 52:314–316

Pitfalls Related to Inadequate or Incomplete Surgical Technique and Errors of Level

18

Luca Denaro, Rocco Papalia, Nicola Maffulli, and Vincenzo Denaro

Contents

18.1 Incomplete or Inadequate Surgical Technique

Insidious pitfalls of cervical spine surgery include the incomplete or inadequate surgical technique. Inadequate decompression is one of the most common reasons for failed spinal surgery [11]. Both traditional and the more recent minimally invasive techniques may be not sufficient to obtain adequate decompression of the myeloradicular structures [9]. In particular, increased rates of incomplete decompression have been demonstrated with minimally invasive procedures [12,14].

Understanding the common sites where neural impingement occurs in the cervical spine, correlating patient's symptoms to these changes recognized on imaging studies help provide a preoperative template for thorough decompression [11]. A thorough preoperative assessment of the patient, evaluation of the sagittal alignment of the cervical spine, of any static and dynamic causes of compression, instability (if present), identification of the location of the compression, and diagnosis of the compressive lesion help the surgeon to minimize technical errors [11]. The most important concept regarding inadequate decompression is to avoid it with careful preoperative planning of the index procedure [11]. Before considering surgical intervention, the surgeon should have a complete understanding of the indications for surgery and should have conducted a thorough physical examination and evaluation of radiologic and electrophysiological studies.

Patients who have had surgery and present with persistent neurologic symptoms, or who do not recover as expected, pose a unique challenge [11]. Some examples can be reported to explain the relevance of the problem. In the field of traditional techniques, in patients with cervical degenerative disease, anterior

L. Denaro (✉)
Department of Neuroscience, University of Padua, Via Giustiniani 5, 35128 Padua, Italy
e-mail: lucadenaro@hotmail.com

L. Denaro et al. (eds.), *Pitfalls in Cervical Spine Surgery*,
DOI: 10.1007/978-3-540-85019-9_18, © Springer-Verlag Berlin Heidelberg 2010

trans-discal decompression cannot be considered to have been performed if the posterior and postero-lateral osteophytes have not been completely removed if a complete decompression of the myeloradicular structures is not obtained [7,16].

Frequently, in patients with severe posterior osteophytosis and associated ossification of the posterior longitudinal ligament, it is difficult to remove the bar of osteophytes and/or the ossified posterior longitudinal ligament itself, and therefore, as a true decompression is not performed, the cause of compression persists. When an arthrodesis follows the decompression, the suppression of the movement can determine the resorption of the posterior osteophyte, but this can occur only after a long time. Therefore, in the postoperative period, neurologic damages may persist when an incomplete decompression is performed. The correct behavior must be the direct intra-operative removal of the cause of compression with immediate clinical benefit.

The incomplete removal of the posterior and postero-lateral osteophytes can become a severe pitfall with impairment of the neurological status of the patient when an arthrodesis is not performed, and eventually a cervical disc arthoplasty is implanted [10].

Failure to provide full stabilization of the involved segments at the end of the surgical procedure is one of the major factors in determining failure of technically well-performed and complete decompression. The need for internal stabilization should always be anticipated and planned preoperatively [9].

Another important pitfall may be to perform an arthrodesis, which is not able to restore the physiological lordosis of the operated segment, frequently from the use of underdimensioned cage or graft, or from the use of hardware to stabilize the cervical spines, which are not modeled in lordosis. The consequences of such error (stabilization in kyphosis of the operated segment) will result in a major alteration of biomechanical forces acting on the neck, with functional overloads to the adjacent intervertebral discs, with consequent intervertebral disc degeneration. Cervical kyphosis results in a pathological shift in the normal sagittal vertical axis of the head. The clinical consequence is often severe axial neck pain and progressive neurological compromise.

Furthermore, when performing a discal decompression, it is important to evaluate the status of the intervertebral discs adjacent to the fusion to avoid that functional overloads resulting from arthrodesis may accelerate the progression of intervertebral disc degeneration. In selected patients, it may be indicated to perform a preventive arthrodesis of the adjacent spinal level.

In posterior procedures, examples of failure may be decompression of the canal by laminectomy without a wide decompression of the laminae and yellow ligaments (in particular in patients with constitutional stenosis), or inadequate decompression of the root canal (foraminotomy) in patients with myeloradiculopathy [9]. These are some examples of pitfalls from incomplete surgery. On the other hand, pitfalls may arise also from too extensive decompression, especially when multi-level surgery is performed. The excessive removal of the apophyseal joints (often not necessary), and of two important posterior stabilizing structures (ligamentum nuchae and spinous apophyses) may result in the long-term development of severe neck deformity (such as Swan neck deformity) and severe instability, which can result in increased spinal mobility leading to further disc deterioration and/or facet spondylosis, and further cord compromise [28].

For this reason, in the past, for many years the systematic laminectomy has been abandoned for the management of patients with cervical spondylotic myelopathy. Today, these problems have been solved in patients undergoing wide multi-level laminectomies by stabilization and fusion in lordosis of the operated cervical spine, which allow the back-shift of the cord.

The surgeon must stabilize above all patients with instability (trauma, rheumatoid arthritis, degenerative spondylolisthesis), young patients, particularly those with hypermobile vertebrae, when a wide decompression is performed, when the lateral masses are weakened by the dissection or disease, because they produce deformity after laminectomy (swan neck with progressive kyphosis). These circumstances may lead to cord injury, and the consequences may be even more serious than the symptoms that led to the original procedure. The indication for internal stabilization very seldom occurs intraoperatively, and usually this occurs with destructive processes, such as tumors. If in doubt, stabilize! [9].

One of the most common pitfall is constituted by the use of instrumentation to stabilize the cervical spine without the addition of bone graft to realize a biological fusion. The rates of failure increase when long plates are used without bone graft, especially in older patients with osteoporotic bone, in whom the poor quality of the bone will not allow fusion. The use of bone auto- or allograft will allow one to obtain a definitive biological fusion in 5–6 weeks, also allowing one to reduce the time of bracing. Recently, we used autologous bone marrow cells concentrate enriched with platelet-rich fibrin on corticocancellous bone allograft to enhance postero-lateral multilevel cervical fusion [22].

Disadvantages in the field of minimally invasive spine surgery can include the inability to obtain a full exposure to pathological processes, impossibility to adequately decompress even single level, when performed at multiple levels, without clinical benefits for the persistence of the pathology.

These are typical examples of correct indication to surgery with poor outcome because of incomplete and inadequate surgical correction of the disease process. Often, the clinical symptoms do not improve after such incomplete procedures [3–6].

A successful operation may be expected if a correct surgical indication has been made. A wrong surgical indication, in fact, is probably the most important factor responsible for poor surgical outcomes. This is particularly true in degenerative spinal pathologies, since the condition may be asymptomatic, and thus not requiring any management, or causes a wide spectrum of symptoms. As a result, in any patient in whom surgery may be indicated, a careful clinical and radiologic evaluation should be performed to confirm patient's symptoms (see Chap. 4).

Inadequate surgical technique may be the cause of pitfall in every patient in whom technically correct surgery has been performed, but an incorrect surgical indication was posed. Judicious choice of anterior or posterior approach should be made after individualizing each case. An example can be represented by a patient with circumferential stenosis with anterior osteophytes and hypertrophic yellow ligaments and laminae, with clinical features of pathology of the spino thalamic tract, in whom an anterior segmental decompression may not allow benefits to the patients for the persistence of the posterior compression.

Pitfalls related to incomplete or inadequate surgical technique from traumatic and tumoral pathology are described in Chaps. 11 and 12, respectively.

18.2 Errors of Level

One the most common pitfalls in cervical spine surgery is related to errors in identification of the correct level where surgery must be performed. These pitfalls may arise from technically perfect executed surgery, failed because surgery did not address specifically the cause of the disease. These pitfalls may arise from the inadequate radiographic visualization of the intervertebral level where surgery should be performed. Difficulties in recognizing the correct level may also arise from the presence of congenital malformations, which the surgeon must study preoperatively correlating the patient's symptoms with imaging and electrophysiological studies (i.e., Klippel–Feil syndrome, basilar invagination, congenital synostosis, etc.). The metal marker should be checked after the surgical approach when the dissection is on the vertebral plan, and it should be repeated in dubious cases (Fig. 18.1).

This topic is complex and carries shocking consequences for the surgeon, for the patient, and for the public, with terrible medico-legal consequences. The errors of level have been extensively studied by many of the most important medical societies. Therefore, we dedicated a focus on this topic by a revision of the literature, which is reported below.

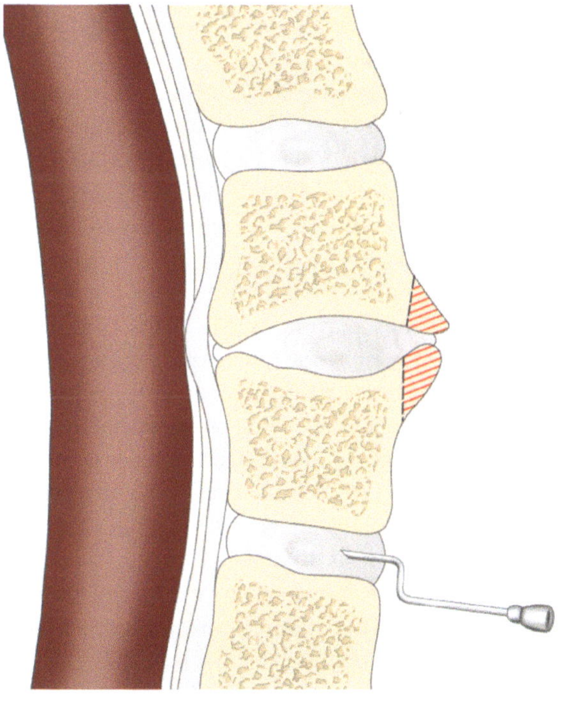

Fig. 18.1 The metal marker should be checked after the surgical approach when the dissection is on the vertebral plan

18.2.1 To Prevent the More Common Errors of Level: Revision of the Literature and General Considerations

In cervical spine surgery identifying the specific patient, and proper surgical sites are crucial patient safety concerns [18]. The term wrong-site surgery typically encompasses surgery on the wrong person, the wrong organ or limb, or the wrong vertebral level [26]. Wrong-site surgery is an overwhelming problem affecting the patient and surgeon, which may result from inadequate preoperative planning, inadequate care of the surgeon, absence of institutional controls, or errors in communication between patient and surgeon and between members of the surgical team [1]. Wrong-site surgery is an unacceptable rare pitfall of cervical spine surgery, but shocking to the public and receiving a great deal of media attention.

Consequences can be catastrophic to patients, healthcare professionals, and institutions. Therefore, an approach that balances simplicity, safety, and efficiency is mandatory. Safety is of crucial importance for quality spine care. Endeavors of physician and researchers aim to advance the science of patient safety, understand its epidemiology, implement scientifically sound yet feasible interventions, and develop measures to evaluate progress [26].

Wrong-site surgery is not just an orthopedic surgery problem that occurs because the surgeon operates on the wrong limb. This is a system problem that affects other surgical specialties as well. While the number of reported orthopedic surgery cases is not high relative to the total number of orthopedic professional liability insurance claims, a retrospective study of a sample of insurers across the country provides evidence that 84% of the cases involving wrong-site orthopedic surgery claims resulted in indemnity payments over a 10-year period, compared with all other types of orthopedic surgery claims where indemnity payments were made in 30% of orthopedic surgery claims during this same time period.

Although the problem appears to be rare, the incidence of these errors is difficult to measure. About 1 in 4 orthopedic surgeons is involved in a wrong site surgery in their practice lifetimes, as estimated by the Wrong Site Surgery Task Force [1]. In 2008, wrong site surgery was reported to be the first most common sentinel event (13%) by the Joint Commission on Accreditation of Healthcare Organizations (JCAHO) [20]. The prevalence of wrong level surgery on the spine is almost nine times more than the prevalence of wrong site operation in hand surgery [17], probably because of the unique features of spine.

In a survey of site-verification protocols, among 2,826,367 operations at insured institutions during the study period (1985–2004), 15 spine wrong-site operations were identified [15]. The authors concluded that current site-verification protocols could have prevented only two-thirds of the examined cases. Mody et al. [19] conducted a questionnaire study to evaluate the prevalence of wrong level surgery among spine surgeons and the preventive measures they undertook to avoid its occurrence. An anonymous, 30-question survey with a self-addressed stamped envelope was sent to all members ($n = 3{,}505$) of the American Academy of Neurologic Surgeons. Four hundred and fifteen (12%) surgeons responded, with 64 (15%) of them reporting that, at least once, they had prepared the incorrect spine level, but noticed the mistake before making the incision. 207 (50%) stated that they had performed 1 or more wrong level surgeries lifetime. From an estimated 1,300,000 spine procedures, 418 wrong level spine operations had been performed (prevalence 1 in 3,110 procedures). The majority of the incorrect level procedures were performed on the lumbar region (71%), followed by the cervical (21%), and the thoracic (8%) regions. One wrong level surgery led to permanent disability, and 73 cases resulted in legal action or monetary settlement to the patient (17%).

In another study [2], the authors asked neurosurgeons to complete an anonymous survey to report the number of cervical discectomies performed during the previous year, as well as whether wrong site surgery had occurred. There was a 75% response rate and a 68% survey completion rate. Participating neurosurgeons performed 2,649 cervical discectomies. Based on this self-reporting, the incidence of wrong-level cervical discectomies was estimated to be 7.6 occurrences per 10,000 operations. Neurosurgeons recognized fatigue, unusual time pressure, unusual patient anatomy, and a failure to verify the operative site by radiography and emergent operations as factors contributing to wrong site surgery.

The JCAHO performed a root cause analysis of 126 patients, and identified potential risk factors, that included emergency operations, unusual patient characteristics (including morbid obesity, physical deformity, or congenital variations), unusual time pressures to start or complete the procedure, and involvement of multiple surgeons or multiple procedures in a single surgical visit [15]. Wrong-site surgery can be the result of failure in communication between the surgeon and the patient (with the patient not involved in identifying the site), and/or incomplete or inaccurate communication between surgical team members.

In 1999, the Institute of Medicine (an arm of the National Academy of Sciences, an agency of the United States Federal Government) published a landmark document on medical errors titled "To Err is Human. Building a Safer Health System" [13], focusing the public and media attention on adverse events occurring during the patient management and their prevention [27]. The report was based on two review papers of hospital data without specific data on spine and contained the assertion that at least 44,000 people, and perhaps as many as 98,000 Americans die in hospitals every year as the result of preventable medical errors [8,21]. Wong et al. [23] evidenced the lack of effective analysis before the provocative numbers were accepted by the media and published, as data on medical errors were based on only two studies (one from New York [8] and the other from Colorado and Utah [21]), and only a small random sample of patient discharge records was examined (respectively 1.7% of discharges in New York in 1984 and 2.7% of discharges in Colorado and Utah in 1992). These incidents were considered negligent, and therefore, likely preventable, in 17.7% of the New York cases [8] and in 35.1% of the cases in Colorado and Utah [21].

More spine-specific information was provided by other quality improvement databases. Wrong site surgery seemed to be the most directly preventable medical error in spine surgery [23].

The American Academy of Orthopedic Surgeons (AAOS) specifically analyzed the issue of wrong site surgery of the spine. The AAOS closed claims contained 11 cases of wrong level spinal surgery. In all instances, the claims were found to be indefensible, and the incidents related to a 1-level decompressive procedure. 10 of the 11 cases were errors in operating at the level above the true pathologic segment.

In an attempt to improve patient safety, the Canadian Orthopedic Association (COA), the American Orthopedic Association (AOA), and the AAOS have embraced a commitment to patient safety for a number of years.

The COA developed the "Sign Through Your Initials" program and the AAOS the "Sign Your Site." The AAOS Sign Your Site Program has been recently modified to include provisions for verification of the appropriate side and level in spinal surgery [1]. A checklist was provided as a systems memory aid and documentation instrument [27].

The Sign Your Site Program has always been a voluntary initiative among members of the AAOS.

The AAOS [1] proposed an effective method of eliminating wrong-site surgery. Briefly, before the patient is moved to the operating room, the surgeon signs his/her initials on the operative site with a permanent marking pen, then the surgeon operates through or adjacent to his/her initials. Intra-operative radiographs marking the exact vertebral level (site) of surgery can avoid spinal surgery to be performed at the wrong level.

The surgeon must sign his/her initials on the operative site with a permanent marking pen, in a way the mark will be visible after the patient has been prepped and draped immediately before surgery.

Confirmation of the correct patient, surgery, and surgical site must be executed before the patient arrives in the operating room. Operating room nurses, technicians, hospital room committees, anesthesiologists, residents should be involved in this process. Records of the patient should be available in the operating facility. Preoperatively, it is necessary to ensure that consent forms have been accurately completed and signed, the diagnosis is correct, and any reasonably anticipated blood products, devices, and special instrumentation for surgery is available and correctly matched to the patient. When the patient arrives in the operating room, the surgical team should take a time out to communicate about the correct patient name and medical record number (or social security number, date of birth, or other identifier), patient allergies, correct procedure, site, equipment and devices, and administering of antibiotics. Before surgery, all the omitted information and discrepancies must be addressed [26,27].

In patients in whom wrong-site surgery is discovered, the surgeon should always act in accordance with the best interests and well-being of the patient, and record the events in appropriate medical records. In patients receiving general anesthesia, if the surgeon discover that surgery is being performed at the wrong site, he/she should take appropriate steps, if possible, to return the patient to the preoperative condition and carry out surgery at the correct site, unless medical reasons suggest to not proceed. He/she should also advise the patient, and the family of the patient as soon as reasonably possible. If wrong site surgery is discovered postoperatively, the surgeon should discuss the error with the patient and, if appropriate, with the family of the patient and stabilize a plan to rectify the mistake [1].

The North American Spine Society (NASS) on the basis of the original Sign Your Site advisory promulgated the "Sign, Mark, and X-ray" (SMaX) campaign, a more comprehensive program for the identification of the appropriate level and side for surgery of the spine [24].

In addition to marking the incision area, SMaX requires a radiograph of the spinal level for site verification before starting surgery. Radiograph is a protective "independent check" [18]. This program outlines a series of steps and double-checks to avoid wrong-site spine surgery.

The three essential components of the Sign, Mark, and X-ray program are:

(1) Reviewing the medical records, including imaging studies, to confirm patient identification, the site of surgery, and the procedure to be performed.
(2) Specifying the side of surgery as part of the site-marking process.
(3) Radiograph the spine during surgery with the marker in place to confirm the level to which the surgery must be performed confirming the spinal level of pathology intra-operatively.

The confirmation of the level at which the surgery must be performed with a metal marker and adequate vertebral count is mandatory. The first or second cervical vertebra must always be shown on this intra-operatively check film [9].

The patient must be involved in confirming the operative site through informed consent and during the actual marking. Operative informed consent form should state the site and side of surgery and should personally be obtained by the surgeon. Copies of the informed consent should be shared with the patient, surgeon, anesthesiologist, assistant or scrub nurse, and circulating nurse.

In 2003, the JCAHO developed the Universal Protocol for Preventing Wrong Site, Wrong Procedure, Wrong Person Surgery. The Universal Protocol emphasizes three minimum requirements: preoperative verification, site marking, and a "time out" in the operating room. The latter means that no procedure is started until all questions and concerns from all individuals involved are addressed.

A decrease of threats of lawsuits and actual suits filed related to wrong site surgery has been recorded since the introduction of these methods. Before surgery, the correct patient verbal name should be checked with patient and confirmed with the ID bracelet. All medical records should be correlated (written notes, laboratory, reports, imaging studies, consent forms) [25,27].

Surgeon or credentialed provider (e.g., fellow, resident, physician assistant), who is a member of the patient's surgical team, should mark skin for first site marking with indelible ink, on the neck or torso, in the general area of surgery, and on the proper side of surgery (when a unilateral approach is planned). Final localization of surgical level intra-operatively via radiograph, bony landmark, metal marker should be performed [25,27].

Obtaining intra-operative radiographs does not guarantee correct level surgery [19]. Congenital variations, inadequate radiologic exposure, or incorrect counting of the spine level, inadequate radiologic visualization because of large body size or surgical table limitation, failure to recognize the absence of an expected lesion in the operative level can lead to misinterpretation of the radiographic image [19]. Several other methods have been proposed to identify the operation site, including intra-operative computed tomography scan, spinal neuronavigation, transligamentous ultrasound, and longitudinal grid tubes surface markers filled with halibut liver oil [19].

Several site-verification protocols are available and they vary across hospitals [25]. Many of them require multiple redundant checks. To date, there are no published evidences to offer guidance on the effectiveness of site-verification protocols [18]. In the design of patient safety-oriented protocols, there is a natural tendency to maximize redundancy in checks. No protocol will prevent all cases of wrong level surgery. Therefore, it will ultimately remain the surgeon's responsibility to ensure the correct site of operation in every case [15].

In conclusion, to err is indeed human. Intra-operative radiographs, personal marking of the intended site, and communication between the surgeon and the patient before anesthesia must be implemented. Strict adherence to the above preventive guidelines is recommended to decrease the risk of wrong level surgery.

Core Messages

- Increased rates of incomplete decompression have been demonstrated with minimally invasive procedures.
- Understanding the common sites where neural impingement occurs in the cervical spine, correlating patient's symptoms to these changes recognized on imaging studies help provide a preoperative template for thorough decompression.
- Failure to provide full stabilization of the involved segments at the end of the surgical procedure is one of the major factors in determining failure of technically well-performed and complete decompression. The need for internal stabilization should always be anticipated and planned preoperatively.
- The consequences of stabilization in kyphosis of the operated segment will result in a major alteration of biomechanical forces acting on the neck, with functional overloads to the adjacent intervertebral discs, with consequent intervertebral disc degeneration.
- When performing a discal decompression, it is important to evaluate the status of the intervertebral discs adjacent to the fusion to avoid that functional overloads resulting from arthrodesis may accelerate the progression of intervertebral disc degeneration. In selected patients, it may be indicated to perform a preventive arthrodesis of the adjacent spinal level.
- Pitfalls may arise also from too extensive decompression, especially when multi-level surgery is performed. The excessive removal of the posterior stabilizing structures may result in the long-term development of severe neck deformity (such as Swan neck deformity) and severe instability.
- Difficulties in recognizing the correct level may also arise from the presence of congenital malformations, which the surgeon must study preoperatively correlating the patient's symptoms with imaging and electrophysiological studies (i.e., Klippel–Feil syndrome, basilar invagination, congenital synostosis, etc.).
- Errors of level represent a complex topic and carry shocking consequences for the surgeon, the patient, and the public, with terrible medico-legal consequences.
- Potential risk factors, which included emergency operations, unusual patient characteristics (including morbid obesity, physical deformity, or congenital variations), unusual time pressures to start or complete the procedure, and involvement of multiple surgeons or multiple procedures in a single surgical visit.
- Wrong-site surgery can be the result of failure in communication between the surgeon and the patient (with the patient not involved in identifying the site), and/or incomplete or inaccurate communication between surgical team members.
- The COA developed the "Sign Through Your Initials" program and the AAOS the "Sign Your Site." The surgeon must sign his/her initials on the operative site with a permanent marking pen, in a way the mark will be visible after the patient has been prepped and draped immediately before surgery. Confirmation of the correct patient, surgery, and surgical site must be executed before the patient arrives into the operating room. Operating room nurses, technicians, hospital room committees, anesthesiologists, residents should be involved in this process. Records of the patient should be available in the operating facility. Preoperatively, it is necessary to ensure that consent forms have been accurately completed and signed, the diagnosis is correct, and any reasonably anticipated blood products, devices, and special instrumentation for surgery is available and correctly matched to the patient. When the patient arrives into the operating room, the surgical team should take a time out to communicate about the correct patient name and medical record number (or social security number, date of birth, or other identifier), patient allergies, correct procedure, site, equipment and devices, and administering of antibiotics. Before surgery, all the omitted information and discrepancies must be addressed.
- The North American Spine Society (NASS) promulgated the "Sign, Mark, and X-ray" (SMaX) campaign. In addition to marking the incision area, SMaX requires a radiograph of the spinal level for site verification before starting surgery. Radiograph is a protective "independent check."

- The JCAHO developed the Universal Protocol for Preventing Wrong Site, Wrong Procedure, Wrong Person Surgery. The Universal Protocol emphasizes three minimum requirements: preoperative verification, site marking, and a "time out" in the operating room. The latter means that no procedure is started until all questions and concerns from all individuals involved are addressed.
- Strict adherence to the above preventive guidelines is recommended to decrease the risk of wrong level surgery.

References

1. American Academy of Orthopedic Surgeons (AAOS) (2006) Advisory statement: wrong site surgery. American Academy of Orthopedic Surgeons, Rosemont, IL. Available at: www.aaos.org/wordhtml/papers/advistmt/1015.htm. Accessed January 10, 2009
2. Ammerman JM, Ammerman MD (2008) Wrong-sided surgery. J Neurosurg Spine 9:105–106; author reply 106
3. Boni M, Cherubino P, Denaro V (1983) The surgical treatment of fractures of the cervical spine. Ital J Orthop Traumatol 9(Suppl):107–126
4. Boni M, Denaro V (1982) The cervical stenosis syndrome with a review of 83 patients treated by operation. Int Orthop 6:185–195
5. Boni M, Denaro V (1982) Surgical treatment of cervical arthrosis. Follow-up review (2–13 years) of the 1st 100 cases operated on by anterior approach. Rev Chir Orthop Reparatrice Appar Mot 68:269–280
6. Boni M, Denaro V (1980) Surgical treatment of traumatic lesions of the middle and lower cervical spine (C3–C7). Ital J Orthop Traumatol 6:305–320
7. Bono CM, Min W (2005) Avoiding complications in patients with ankylosing spondylitis undergoing spine surgery. Curr Opin Orthop 16:178–183
8. Brennan TA, Leape LL, Laird NM et al (1991) Incidence of adverse events and negligence in hospitalized patients. Results of the Harvard Medical Practice Study I. N Engl J Med 324:370–376
9. Denaro V (1991) Stenosis of the cervical spine. Springer, Berlin
10. Denaro V, Papalia R, Denaro L et al (2009) Cervical spinal disc replacement. J Bone Joint Surg Br 91-B:713–719
11. Devin CJ, Espiritu MT, Kang JD (2009) Prevention, identification, and treatment of inadequate decompression of the cervical spine. Instr Course Lect 58:699–715
12. Hacker RJ, Miller CG (2003) Failed anterior cervical foraminotomy. J Neurosurg 98:126–130
13. Institute of Medicine (1999) To Err is Human. Building a Safer Health System. National Academies Press, Washington, DC. Available at: http://newton.nap.edu/catalog/9728.html. Accessed January 9, 2009
14. Koc RK, Menku A, Tucer B et al (2004) Anterior cervical foraminotomy for unilateral spondylotic radiculopathy. Minim Invasive Neurosurg 47:186–189
15. Kwaan MR, Studdert DM, Zinner MJ et al (2006) Incidence, patterns, and prevention of wrong-site surgery. Arch Surg 141:353–357; discussion 357–358
16. Lee JY, Lim MR, Albert TJ (2005) Inadequate decompression following anterior cervical surgery: surgical treatment options. Curr Opin Orthop 16:189–193
17. Meinberg EG, Stern PJ (2003) Incidence of wrong-site surgery among hand surgeons. J Bone Joint Surg Am 85-A: 193–197
18. Michaels RK, Makary MA, Dahab Y et al (2007) Achieving the National Quality Forum's "Never Events": prevention of wrong site, wrong procedure, and wrong patient operations. Ann Surg 245:526–532
19. Mody MG, Nourbakhsh A, Stahl DL et al (2008) The prevalence of wrong level surgery among spine surgeons. Spine 33:194–198
20. Sentinel Event Statistics as of December 31 (2008) Available at: http://www.jointcommission.org/SentinelEvents/Statistics/
21. Thomas EJ, Studdert DM, Burstin HR et al (2000) Incidence and types of adverse events and negligent care in Utah and Colorado. Med Care 38:261–271
22. Vadala G, Di Martino A, Tirindelli MC et al (2008) Use of autologous bone marrow cells concentrate enriched with platelet-rich fibrin on corticocancellous bone allograft for posterolateral multilevel cervical fusion. J Tissue Eng Regen Med 2:515–520
23. Wong D, Herndon J, Canale T (2002) An AOA critical issue. Medical errors in orthopaedics: practical pointers for prevention. J Bone Joint Surg Am 84-A:2097–2100
24. Wong D, Mayer T, Watters W (2001) Prevention of wrong site surgery: sign. mark and X-ray (SMaX). North American Spine Society, La Grange, IL. Available at: http://www.spine.org/smax.cfm. Accessed 21 Jan 2009
25. Wong DA (2006) Spinal surgery and patient safety: a systems approach. J Am Acad Orthop Surg 14:226–232
26. Wong DA, Herndon JH, Canale ST et al (2009) Medical errors in orthopaedics. Results of an AAOS member survey. J Bone Joint Surg Am 91:547–557
27. Wong DA, Watters WC III (2007) To err is human: quality and safety issues in spine care. Spine 32:S2–S8
28. Young PH, Young JP, Young JC (2007) Microsurgical posterior approaches to the cervical spine, chapter 13. In: Mayer HM (ed) minimally invasive spine surgery. Springer, Berlin, pp 107–117

Complications Due to Inadequate Cervical Spinal Immobilization

19

Luca Denaro, Domenico D'Avella, Nicola Maffulli, and Vincenzo Denaro

Contents

L. Denaro (✉)
Department of Neuroscience, University of Padua, Via Giustiniani 5, 35128 Padua, Italy
e-mail: lucadenaro@hotmail.com

19.1 Introduction

Adequate immobilization of the cervical spine is an essential part of the postoperative care of the patient [1]. Orthoses are external applied devices that offer a safe way to immobilize the cervical spine, to increase fusion success, to decrease the rate of graft migration and instrumentation failure, to relieve postoperative pain, to give the patient a sense of security and comfort after surgery, and to improve the postoperative scar [2]. Historically, patients undergoing cervical spine surgery were immobilized in plaster, which was regarded as the only external immobilization device able to provide true postoperative immobilization of the cervical spine. The introduction of the internal fixation has provided a useful tool to increase fusion rates, maintain alignment, and decrease subsidence and dislodgement of the graft. Internal fixation acts as an internal brace, limiting motion between the graft and vertebral bodies, decreasing axial forces, reducing the tendency for graft failure.

Recent decades have been characterized by great advances in material engineering, which deeply changed the bracing industry. Today, a large variety of different orthoses for the cervical spine are available, and new thermoplastic, so-called breathable, lightweight, durable, magnetic resonance imaging compatible materials are used for the production of cervical spinal orthoses. They are commonly named based on the locality of design (Philadelphia, Miami, etc.) or based on the name of their inventor (Schanz, Thomas, Guilford, etc.).

This chapter does not aim to provide a detailed description of all the commercially available cervical orthoses, for which the reader should refer to other publications. We wish to highlight the need for a correct choice of the cervical orthosis in an attempt to

L. Denaro et al. (eds.), *Pitfalls in Cervical Spine Surgery*,
DOI: 10.1007/978-3-540-85019-9_19, © Springer-Verlag Berlin Heidelberg 2010

minimize errors from inadequate postoperative cervical immobilization.

The choice of specific orthoses is crucial to allow fusion and avoid undue stress on the operated region [3, 4]. Excessive residual movement may facilitate mobilization of the graft, failure of the instrumentation, with possible myeloradicular damage. A potential pitfall may be the use of the appropriate orthotic, but not left in place for a sufficient length of time to ensure fusion [5]. Premature removal of the orthotic brace can have serious consequences, including nonunion, instability, and mobilization of the graft and instrumentation, and may lead to total disruption at the operative site [6, 7].

The ability to restrict the movement is widely variable among different types of cervical spine orthoses, and the choice of the device is highly dependent on the required degree of restriction of cervical motion. The indications to their use depend primarily on three factors: type and stability of lesion (stable, potentially stable, or instable lesions), the level of the lesion, the function that the orthoses must exert (prevalent immobilization or traction action).

For example, when using the cervical orthoses for potentially unstable types of fractures or dislocations, a high degree of restriction of cervical motion and a stable fixation of the head on the neck are required. Also, when surgery involves multilevel corporectomies with massive grafts, high degree of restriction of motion with adequate postoperative immobilization is mandatory to avoid the risk of mobilization of the graft, particularly when torsional forces are applied. On the other hand, postoperative bracing for a one-level fusion with instrumentation is probably not necessary, and increasingly the surgeons are limiting the use of a postoperative brace or even eliminating its use [2].

Campbell et al. [2] performed a randomized clinical trial to evaluate whether the use of a cervical collar after single-level anterior cervical fusion with plating increases the fusion rate and improved clinical outcomes. Two hundred and fifty-seven patients were included in the analysis, of which 149 were braced and 108 were not. The authors concluded that the use of a cervical brace does not improve the fusion rate or the clinical outcomes of patients undergoing single-level anterior cervical fusion with plating, suggesting that the use of a cervical plate, acting as an internal brace, replaces the function of the external brace in these patients.

The cervical orthoses can be generally classified as cervical or cervicothoracic orthoses; noninvasive or invasive traction devices. They can be also classified as soft braces, semi-rigid braces, and rigid braces. They can be also distinguished into devices with prevalent immobilization or traction action.

1. Soft Cervical Collars: They are flexible collars, used mostly as a transition between the more rigid collars and no collar at all. Soft Cervical Collars are inexpensive and comfortable, but are not able to provide wide restriction of motion. The primary application of these orthoses is the management of whiplash injuries. Generally, they are not used in the postoperative management of patients undergoing cervical spine surgery.
2. Semi-rigid cervical braces: They are more rigid collars and provide better motion control than the soft cervical collar. They generally consist of two semi-rigid pieces, reinforced at the front and back with plastic struts. Some semi-rigid braces have a thoracic extension, and may be used when a higher restriction of motion is required to the lower cervical spine and the cervicothoracic junction.
3. Rigid collars include Halo, SOMI, and Minerva Braces.

Halo is the most rigid cervical brace (see below). It allows the most rigid fixation of the cervical spine and is used in patients with unstable cervical spine. It consists of a titanium ring (or halo) around the head of the patient, which is held in place by four screws (or pins) in the skull. The ring is attached by four bars to a vest worn on the trunk to anchor the device and hold the neck in place. This device is worn at all times until the spine heals. Patients actually find chewing and talking less awkward with this device, because it does not restrict chin movement. SOMI (sterno-occipital-mandibular-immobilization) Brace is a rigid cervical spine orthosis, consisting of an anterior chest yoke attached anteriorly to the curved rigid shoulder supports. The original Minerva Brace was a heavy, cumbersome plaster jacket, which posed significant obstacles in obtaining adequate radiographs and in providing hygiene to the patient. Successively, the thermoplastic Minerva body jacket was developed to address the problems of the plaster Minerva body jacket [8]. It consists of a bivalved polyform shell encompassing the cervical spine and thorax and is molded to provide support for the occiput and mandible. A circumferential chest strap, combined with nylon screws at the level of the neck and a rigid Polyform headband, holds the anterior and posterior sections together.

Despite the large number of new cervical spinal orthoses, few of them have been tested in well-conducted scientific studies. Therefore, the clinical application of one of them is related more to the preference of the spinal surgeon, rather than to the well-defined clinical recommendations.

In choosing the appropriate postoperative cervical orthoses, comfortable support and restriction of movement are two conflicting requirements that must be obtained. Generally, the compliance of the patient with the brace is highly related to the level of comfort experienced while wearing the brace.

The orthosis that perfectly immobilizes the cervical spine does not exist. Several studies have shown that all of the currently available orthoses, including the most restrictive, allow some residual motion of all cervical vertebral levels in all planes [9–12].

In particular, a brace may be effective to limit the motion of a segment of the cervical spine, but ineffective to limit it in other regions of the cervical spine.

As each patient has a particular neck anatomy, thus altering the fit and efficacy of the orthosis [13], the choice of the brace should be always carefully matched to the neck anatomy of the patient. Theoretically, the contact area should be maximized to lower the contact pressures [13].

19.2 Complications of Cervical Spinal Orthoses

Complications related to inadequate immobilization depends on the specific type of utilized devices. Orthoses with an effect of traction (i.e., SOMI brace, Halo fixator) will present a higher incidence of complications when compared with those with an immobilization action.

Patients immobilized in cervical orthoses require meticulous nursing care to prevent complications from the immobilization device. The most common complications related to cervical orthoses include pressure ulcers on the chin, mandible, ears, shoulders, laryngeal prominence and occiput, progressive neurological deterioration related to ineffective immobilization, marginal mandibular nerve palsy (a branch of the seventh cranial nerve) causing sensory disturbance and drooping of the lower lip, psychological dependence, muscle atrophy, soft tissue contracture, and pain.

The most common complication of cervical immobilization using collars is skin breakdown. Hospital-acquired pressure ulcers have been identified as a serious and preventable medical error that should never occur. Prolonged and excessive pressure of tissue against a bony prominence may determine tissue ischemia, finally resulting in pressure ulcers [14]. Pressure exerted by a cervical collar is a possible cause of pressure ulcers. Capillary closing pressure sustained above 32 mmHg at these sites may be responsible for skin breakdown [15].

Despite only 1% of all pressure ulcers occurring in correspondence to the occipital area [14], in patients wearing a cervical collar the incidence of pressure ulcers ranges from 23.9 to 44% [16–18]. Obviously, the incidence of pressure ulcers is higher in patients wearing cervical collar for longer periods of time [16]. Skin complications are often difficult to avoid in patients in intensive care units, particularly when they have concomitant head injuries and are unable to communicate cervical pain.

Severity of skin complications in patients wearing a cervical collar are variable. Davis et al. [17] classified 55% of the pressure ulcers that developed under a cervical collar as full thickness wounds. Skin breakdown and macerated skin in patients wearing cervical collars occur especially at the level of the occipitut, chin, mandibula, ears, and shoulders [15], with the most serious wounds occurring in the occipital area [18], because of the little subcutaneous tissue overlying the bone at the level of the occiput. When skin breakdown is quite severe, plastic surgery for repair and reconstruction of the damaged skin may be required [19], causing patient morbidity with consequent increased length and cost of hospitalization [20, 21].

Powers et al. [22] evaluated the incidence of tissue breakdown associated with cervical immobilization in 484 patients. Skin breakdown was noted in 33 (6.8%) patients.

Rodgers et al. [23] reported on a patient who developed a pressure area associated with nerve palsy on the mandible after wearing a cervical collar for 5 days. Two days after the removal of the collar, the nerve damage was resolved.

Skin complications related to the use of cervical collars can be minimized when standard protocols for cervical collar management are used and staff education on techniques for changing cervical collars, measuring for proper fit, skin assessment, skin care, and collar maintenance is performed [22]. This is a particularly important aspect, as routine skin assessment and care are not always performed by nurses because of the fear in removing the cervical collar due to the risk of spinal injury. If adherence to strict care with skin cleansing, inspecting, and changing of pads is not performed meticulously, the associated problems and incidence of skin breakdown may become a challenge.

When these complications occur, a practical measure of management is to remove the orthosis and to apply another one with different skin regions of contact.

Risk factors for developing occipital pressure ulcers include shock, use of vasopressors, long-term cervical spine immobilization, long prehospital transport, massive fluid overload, agitation, excessive moisture, and poorly fitting collar [24].

There are no studies in literature comparing pressure exerted by cervical collars and the risks of skin complications among different cervical braces.

Cervical immobilization may also impair the respiratory function. Kreisler et al. [25] described airway obstruction due to a semi-rigid cervical collar. The authors postulated that the tight-fitting cervical collar interfered with normal lymphatic and venous drainage.

19.3 Halo Vest Immobilization

The halo immobilization, first used by Perry and Nickel [26] for the immobilization of unstable cervical spines in 19 patients with poliomyelitis based on the work of Bloom during the Second World War [27], provides the most rigid fixation of the cervical spine. It is therefore indicated in patients in whom the pathology determines a high level of instability. Although halo fixator provides the most rigid immobilization of any currently available orthoses, it does not absolutely immobilize the cervical spine. In the past, it has been used for many years as a firstline tool to stabilize the cervical spine, before the development of internal fixation [28]. Today, the halo immobilization continues to reserve a well-defined place in the management of pathologies in whom a high degree of instability is determined, including acute trauma, preoperative gradual correction of spinal deformity, and postoperative immobilization after complex cervical surgeries. Example of procedures requiring postoperative halo immobilization include sagittal plane correction surgeries (i.e., corrective osteotomy for ankylosing spondylitis), multilevel corpectomy (three or more levels), fixation of unstable upper cervical injury, stabilization of injuries with circumferential instability, and patients with unstable cervical spine from infections or tumors [28].

In patients with massive destruction of the cervical bodies from tumors (primitive or secondary), infections, and unstable cervical fracture, the halo fixator is a useful tool preceding, allowing, and following the surgery. Application of halo fixator in these patients is mandatory to safely perform the surgery.

Absolute contraindications to halo immobilization are cranial fracture, local bone deficiency (as in patients with severe osteomalacias, bony fragility from cranial localization of plasmocytoma, localized cranial osteolysis), and sepsis or severe soft-tissue injury. Patient requiring a craniotomy for the management of intracranial condition (i.e., subdural hematoma) may not be the ideal candidates for halo immobilization [28]. Relative contraindications are severe chest trauma for the impossibility to adequately dress the jacket, obesity, and advanced age for the high rates of respiratory complications.

The halo fixator consists of ring, skull pins, vest, vest lining/padding, upright longitudinal struts, and anteroposterior fixation rods [28].

To position the halo fixator, the patient is placed flat in the supine position. Head and neck are manually stabilized and maintained in neutral position. Several sizes are generally available to allow the appropriate choice of the halo ring, which should not be >1 cm away from the skin and not contact the skin or the ears at any point [28].

When the ring is too large, the pins may not reach the cranium, or may loose. Both partial and full circumferential halo ring are available. Advantages of a partial ring include that it opens posteriorly, facilitating ring positioning in the supine decubitus.

The anterior pin trajectories must be directed toward the safe zone, which is the 1 cm width of bone above

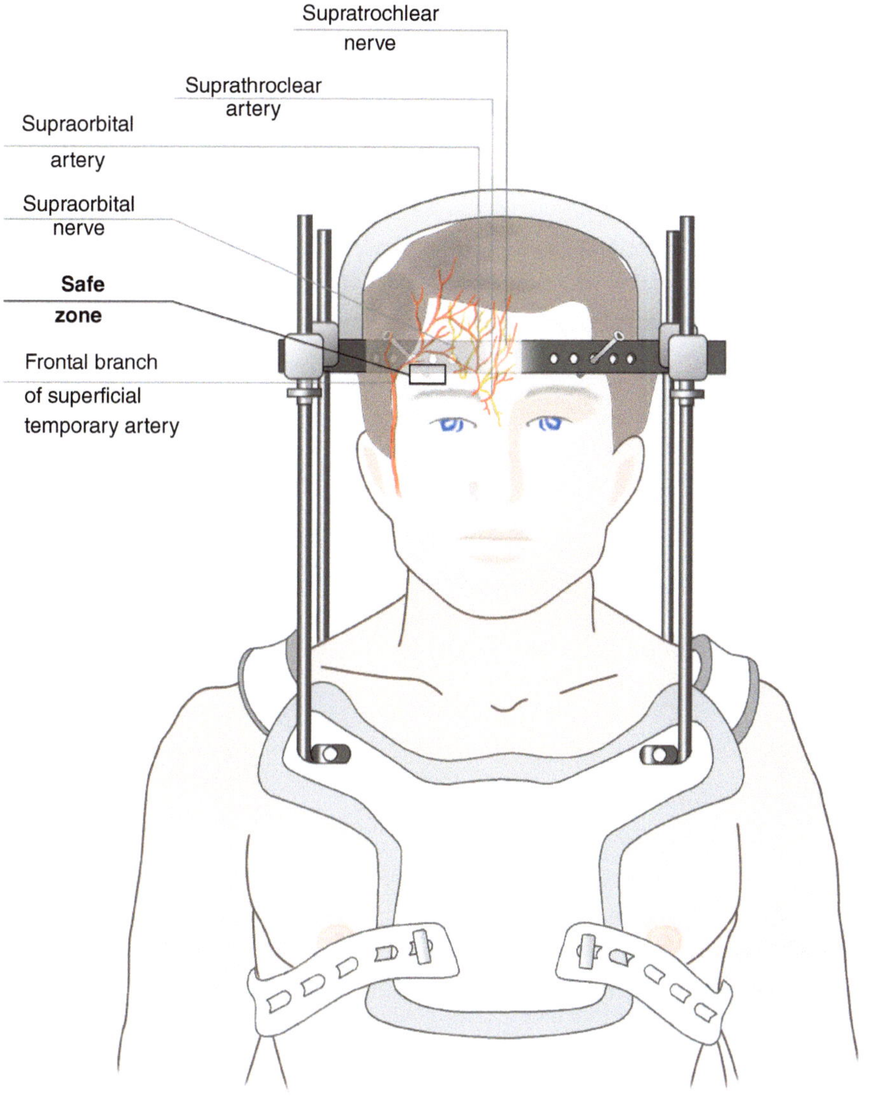

Fig. 19.1 Frontal view of the components of a Halo device in place. The safe zone for anterior pin insertion is located approximately 1 cm just above the lateral one-third of the orbit (eyebrow). Awareness of the safe zone avoids pin placement too far lateral within the thin temporal bone (deep to the temporalis muscle) and avoids injury to medial structures, including the supraorbital and supratrochlear nerve and artery, and frontal sinus

the lateral border of the eyebrow (Fig. 19.1). The thin temporal bone may be damaged when more lateral pin insertion is performed, whereas supraorbital and supratrochlear arteries and nerves may be injured in the case of medial pin positioning. The pins must engage the bone close to or at a 90° angle. One of the most common complications when placing the pins at angle different from 90° is that the pins may dislodge more easily.

The safe zone for the posterior pins is wider. The ring should be parallel to the transverse plane of the head. As even slight pressure can determine soft-tissue necrosis, ring should not contact the ears. The skin is prepared with a chlorhexidine or iodine-impregnated solution. Local anesthesia is injected to the site of pin insertion. The ring is placed into its ideal position and stabilized with temporary position blockers. The pins are screwed into their respective holes on the halo ring. During the positioning of the anterior pins, the patient is asked to close the eyes to avoid the orbicularis oculi muscles to be entrapped in the open position. Also, it is necessary to avoid the penetration of temporalis muscle because halo pin at this level may determine pain and impede mandibular motion during mastication or talking.

The vest is constituted by two halves. The posterior half is placed first by rolling the patient to one side, at the same time as maintaining the neck in neutral position, with the inferior border approximately at the level of T11 or T12 vertebra. The patient is then log rolled back to the supine position, and the anterior half is applied with the inferior border reaching the level of the xiphoid process. The two halves are then strapped to each other. At the end, the ring is fixed to two connectors on the right and left side that are supported by two longitudinal posts arising from the anterior and posterior parts of the vest. Once the Halo is positioned, a fluoroscopic control is mandatory to ensure the appropriate positioning of the device.

Vieweg et al. [29] conducted a review of 35 relevant studies involving a total of 682 patients with 709 different types of injuries to determine the outcomes after immobilization in a halo vest for various injuries to the upper cervical spine between 1962 and 1998. They concluded that bony upper cervical spine injuries managed with Halo fixator had healing rates between 85 and 96%. Reports of injuries involving multiple levels with or without primarily ligamentous injury showed less favorable results.

19.3.1 Complications of the Halo Immobilization

Advantages of the halo immobilization include precise cervical spine positioning, effective immobilization, ease of application, success in maintaining reduction, less interference with mandibular function when compared with other types of orthosis, and the ability to allow early mobilization of the patient [30].

Although the halo is an effective form of cervical immobilization, complications with its use are encountered periodically. Familiarity with the design rationale and proper method of application can help one to minimize the morbidity of this commonly used device. The use of a halo fixator has been associated with several device-related complications, including pin loosening, pain, pin-site neurovascular damages, bleeding, infection and cosmetically disfiguring scars at the pin site, intraparenchymal, epidural, or subdural abscesses related to pin penetration, difficulty in swallowing, pressure sores to the ears (from inadequate positioning of the Halo) and to the trunk (from inadequate positioning and nursing of the jacket), loss of reduction or progression of the spinal deformity, and, rarely, cranial nerve palsies from excessive traction.

Garfin et al. [31] conducted a study on the osteology of the skull in 27 cadaver and 20 CT scans of skulls to determine the optimal placement of halo pin sites. They confirmed previously recommended halo pin insertion sites, anterolaterally and posterolaterally, where the bone is very thick and the thinner frontal sinus and temporal fossae are avoided. The halo device should not be used in patients with associated skull fractures, existing scalp infections, pathologically soft bone such as in plasmocytoma [32], rheumatoid arthritis [33], and previous cranioplasty [30].

The most common complication in adults is pin loosening [31, 34, 35], occurring in up to 36% of patients, with slightly higher rate in anterior pins when compared with posterior pins [31] (Figs. 19.2 and 19.3). In children, anterior pin loosening occurs in up to 87% of pins [36]. Pain of new onset at the pin site should lead the physician to suspect pin loosening or infection.

The second most common complication is infection at the pin site. Infections in adults occurs in up to 20% [37], and in children 39 and 57% [34, 36]. Infections may be classified as superficial and deep. Superficial infections can be managed with oral antibiotics with or without pin removal. Deep infection may be associated with osteomyelitis or, rarely, intracranial abscess [36, 37]. Deep infection can be a challenge, as it requires pin removal, insertion of a new pin at a new site, debridement, and systemic antibiotics. In patients in whom pin drainage develops, bacterial cultures must be taken to determine the pathogen responsible for infection and to establish the appropriate antibiotic management regime. If cellulitis develops, or the infection fails to respond to the

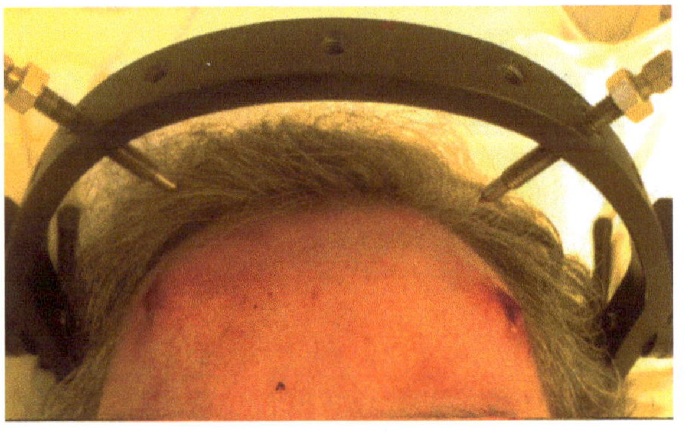

Fig. 19.2 Clinical picture of a patient with pin loosening

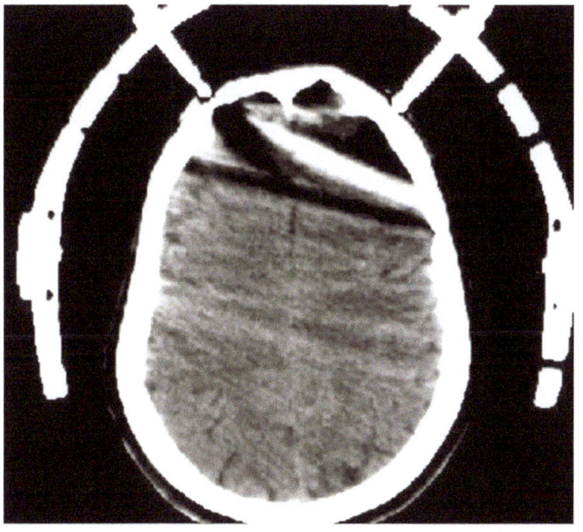

Fig. 19.3 A CT scan performed the day before pin loosening in the same patient showed osteolysis around the tip of the left-anterior pin. The right-anterior pin did not engage the cranial bone

antibiotics, pin replacement is indicated, using an adjacent hole in the ring, avoiding to place pins through areas of cellulitis, and placing it prior to remove the infected pin to avoid shift of the head within the halo ring [13].

Long-term complications of the pins include cosmetically disfiguring scars at the anterior pin sites (9–13%) and pain at the pin sites (13–18%) [36, 37]. Tightening the halo pins to 6-in./lbs of torque at 24-h and 1-week after application is associated with the least pin site complications [38]. Pressure necrosis of the skin is more common in children, and it has an incidence from 2 to 11% [35, 37].

Intracranial penetration is an insidious complication of pins, with dural puncture ranging from 1 to 4% and may result from a fall while wearing a halo orthosis [35–37]. The most serious complications associated with the use of halo device occur when pins penetrate the inner table of the skull, resulting in cerebrospinal fluid leak and rarely in an extradural hematoma and intracranial abscess.

Papagelopoulos et al. [30] reported on a patient with an epidural abscess after halo pin intracranial penetration at the site of a previous cranioplasty. The pins and the halo vest were removed, the pin site was cleaned, and a Philadelphia cervical collar was applied. The patient was subjected to immediate intravenous antibiotic management for 2 weeks, followed by oral antibiotics for 2 additional weeks. The patient had a gradual improvement of his symptoms within the first 48 h. At the latest follow-up visit, he had fully recovered and his fracture had healed.

Intracranial abscess as complication of the use of the halo immobilization is not usual [37, 39–45]. Orthopedist should suspect brain abscess in any patient presenting with a cerebrospinal fluid leakage and systemic signs of infection or central nervous system dysfunction. Symptoms that should alert the physician are loose pins, scalp or pin-site cellulitis, headache, eye pain, fever, seizures, and neurologic changes. Intracranial propagation of skin bacteria from pins may be the cause of epidural abscess. The dura mater is normally resistant to infection, but it may be damaged or inflamed by the pressure or penetration of the inner table. Staphylococci are the most common pathogens. The management of intracranial abscess consists in craniotomy and surgical debridement [39]. Supraorbital nerve injury may occur in up to 3% of patients [36, 37].

Dysphagia may occur in up to 2% of patients [36, 37]; in some patients, it occurs as a result of overextension of the neck, and can be alleviated by adjusting the halo, generally flexing the neck or translating the head anteriorly.

The use of the halo device in the elderly has been associated with a higher rate of complications [46, 47]. On the other hand, in a retrospective review conducted among children aged 3 years and younger managed with halo ring fixation, Halo ring fixation was demonstrated to be safe and with a complication rate similar to that in older children [48]. Unique to this age group, toddlers may be more prone to falls than older children, and limited ambulation should be recommended.

Core Messages

- The specific choice of orthotic immobilization is crucial to the immobilization of the spine to allow fusion and avoid undue stress on the bone grafts.
- The indications to their use depend primarily on three factors: type and stability of lesion (stable, potentially stable, or instable lesions), the level of the lesion, and the function that the orthoses must exert.

- Premature removal of the orthotic brace can have serious complications, including non-union, instability, and mobilization of the graft.
- Patients immobilized in cervical orthoses require meticulous nursing care to prevent complications from the immobilization device.
- The most common complications related to cervical orthoses include pressure ulcers on the chin, mandible, ears, shoulders, laryngeal prominence and occiput, progressive neurological deterioration related to ineffective immobilization, marginal mandibular nerve palsy (a branch of the seventh cranial nerve) causing sensory disturbance and drooping of the lower lip, psychological dependence, muscle atrophy, soft tissue contracture, and pain.
- The halo immobilization provides the most rigid fixation of the cervical spine, and is therefore indicated in patents in whom the pathology determines a high level of instability.
- Absolute contraindications to halo immobilization are cranial fracture, bone deficiency, sepsis, or severe soft-tissue injury.
- When positioning the halo fixator, the patient is asked to close the eyes to avoid the orbicularis oculi muscles to be entrapped in the open position. Also, it is necessary to avoid the penetration of temporalis muscle because halo pin at this level may determine pain and impede mandibular motion during mastication or talking.
- The most common complications reported with the use of a halo fixator are pin loosening, pain, pin-site bleeding, infection and cosmetically disfiguring scars at the pin site, difficulty in swallowing, pressure sores, loss of reduction or progression of the spinal deformity, and cranial nerve palsies.

References

1. Bible JE, Biswas D, Whang PG et al (2008) Postoperative bracing after spine surgery for degenerative conditions – a questionnaire study. Spine J 9:309–316
2. Campbell MJ, Carreon LY, Traynelis V et al (2009) Use of cervical collar after single-level anterior cervical fusion with plate: is it necessary? Spine 34:43–48
3. Boni M, Denaro V (1982) The cervical stenosis syndrome with a review of 83 patients treated by operation. Int Orthop 6:185–195
4. Boni M, Denaro V (1980) Surgical treatment of traumatic lesions of the middle and lower cervical spine (C3–C7). Ital J Orthop Traumatol 6:305–320
5. Maeda T, Arizono T, Saito T et al (2002) Cervical alignment, range of motion, and instability after cervical laminoplasty. Clin Orthop Relat Res (401):132–138
6. Denaro V (1991) Stenosis of the cervical spine. Springer, Berlin
7. Denaro V, Denaro L, Gulino G et al (1998) Complicanze nella chirurgia cervicale. Giornale Italiano di Ortopedia e Traumatologia 24:681–688
8. Millington PJ, Ellingsen JM, Hauswirth BE et al (1987) Thermoplastic Minerva body jacket–a practical alternative to current methods of cervical spine stabilization. A clinical report. Phys Ther 67:223–225
9. Cline JR, Scheidel E, Bigsby EF (1985) A comparison of methods of cervical immobilization used in patient extrication and transport. J Trauma 25:649–653
10. Denaro V (1982) Tutele ortopediche per il rachide cervicale. Convegno internazionale di aggiornamento sulla patologia e chirurgia del rachide cervicale. Pavia 33-28 Maggio
11. Fisher SV (1978) Proper fitting of the cervical orthosis. Arch Phys Med Rehabil 59:505–507
12. Graziano AF, Scheidel EA, Cline JR et al (1987) A radiographic comparison of prehospital cervical immobilization methods. Ann Emerg Med 16:1127–1131
13. Clarck CR (2005) The cervical spine, 4th edn. Lippincott Williams &Wilkins, Philadelphia
14. Barczak CA, Barnett RI, Childs EJ et al (1997) Fourth national pressure ulcer prevalence survey. Adv Wound Care 10:18–26
15. Webber-Jones JE, Thomas CA, Bordeaux RE Jr (2002) The management and prevention of rigid cervical collar complications. Orthop Nurs 21:19–25; quiz 25–17
16. Chendrasekhar A, Moorman DW, Timberlake GA (1998) An evaluation of the effects of semirigid cervical collars in patients with severe closed head injury. Am Surg 64:604–606
17. Davis JW, Parks SN, Detlefs CL et al (1995) Clearing the cervical spine in obtunded patients: the use of dynamic fluoroscopy. J Trauma 39:435–438
18. Molano Alvarez E, Murillo Perez Mdel A, Salobral Villegas MT et al (2004) Pressure sores secondary to immobilization with cervical collar: a complication of acute cervical injury. Enferm Intensiva 15:112–122
19. Hewitt S (1994) Skin necrosis caused by a semi-rigid cervical collar in a ventilated patient with multiple injuries. Injury 25:323–324
20. Plaisier B, Gabram SG, Schwartz RJ et al (1994) Prospective evaluation of craniofacial pressure in four different cervical orthoses. J Trauma 37:714–720
21. Powers J (1997) A multidisciplinary approach to occipital pressure ulcers related to cervical collars. J Nurs Care Qual 12:46–52
22. Powers J, Daniels D, McGuire C et al (2006) The incidence of skin breakdown associated with use of cervical collars. J Trauma Nurs 13:198–200
23. Rodgers JA, Rodgers WB (1995) Marginal mandibular nerve palsy due to compression by a cervical hard collar. J Orthop Trauma 9:177–179

24. Jacobson TM, Tescher AN, Miers AG et al (2008) Improving practice: efforts to reduce occipital pressure ulcers. J Nurs Care Qual 23:283–288
25. Kreisler NS, Durieux ME, Spiekermann BF (2000) Airway obstruction due to a rigid cervical collar. J Neurosurg Anesthesiol 12:118–119
26. Perry J, Nickel VL (1959) Total cervical spine fusion for neck paralysis. J Bone Joint Surg Am 41:37–43
27. Sawers A, Dipaola CP, Rechtine GR II (2008) Suitability of the noninvasive halo for cervical spine injuries: a retrospective analysis of outcomes. Spine J 9(3):216–220
28. Bono CM (2007) The halo fixator. J Am Acad Orthop Surg 15:728–737
29. Vieweg U, Schultheiss R (2001) A review of halo vest treatment of upper cervical spine injuries. Arch Orthop Trauma Surg 121:50–55
30. Papagelopoulos PJ, Sapkas GS, Kateros KT et al (2001) Halo pin intracranial penetration and epidural abscess in a patient with a previous cranioplasty: case report and review of the literature. Spine 26:E463–E467
31. Garfin SR, Botte MJ, Centeno RS et al (1985) Osteology of the skull as it affects halo pin placement. Spine 10:696–698
32. Abitbol JJ, Botte MJ, Garfin SR et al (1989) The treatment of multiple myeloma of the cervical spine with a halo vest. J Spinal Disord 2:263–267
33. Lipson SJ (1989) Rheumatoid arthritis in the cervical spine. Clin Orthop Relat Res (239):121–127
34. Baum JA, Hanley EN Jr, Pullekines J (1989) Comparison of halo complications in adults and children. Spine 14:251–252
35. Glaser JA, Whitehill R, Stamp WG et al (1986) Complications associated with the halo-vest. A review of 245 cases. J Neurosurg 65:762–769
36. Dormans JP, Criscitiello AA, Drummond DS et al (1995) Complications in children managed with immobilization in a halo vest. J Bone Joint Surg Am 77:1370–1373
37. Garfin SR, Botte MJ, Waters RL et al (1986) Complications in the use of the halo fixation device. J Bone Joint Surg Am 68:320–325
38. Vertullo CJ, Duke PF, Askin GN (1997) Pin-site complications of the halo thoracic brace with routine pin re-tightening. Spine 22:2514–2516
39. Dennis GC, Clifton GL (1982) Brain abscess as a complication of halo fixation. Neurosurgery 10:760–761
40. Garfin SR, Botte MJ, Triggs KJ et al (1988) Subdural abscess associated with halo-pin traction. J Bone Joint Surg Am 70:1338–1340
41. Goodman ML, Nelson PB (1987) Brain abscess complicating the use of a halo orthosis. Neurosurgery 20:27–30
42. Graziano GP, Herzenberg JE, Hensinger RN (1993) The halo-Ilizarov distraction cast for correction of cervical deformity. Report of six cases. J Bone Joint Surg Am 75:996–1003
43. Humbyrd DE, Latimer FR, Lonstein JE et al (1981) Brain abscess as a complication of halo traction. Spine 6: 365–368
44. Kameyama O, Ogawa K, Suga T et al (1999) Asymptomatic brain abscess as a complication of halo orthosis: report of a case and review of the literature. J Orthop Sci 4:39–41
45. Muller EJ, Wick M, Muhr G (1998) Subdural abscess as a complication of halo fixator. Unfallchirurg 101:655–657
46. Horn EM, Theodore N, Feiz-Erfan I et al (2006) Complications of halo fixation in the elderly. J Neurosurg Spine 5:46–49
47. Tashjian RZ, Majercik S, Biffl WL et al (2006) Halo-vest immobilization increases early morbidity and mortality in elderly odontoid fractures. J Trauma 60:199–203
48. Caird MS, Hensinger RN, Weiss N et al (2006) Complications and problems in halo treatment of toddlers: limited ambulation is recommended. J Pediatr Orthop 26: 750–752

Index

MIX
Papier aus verantwortungsvollen Quellen
Paper from responsible sources
FSC® C105338

If you have any concerns about our products,
you can contact us on
ProductSafety@springernature.com

In case Publisher is established outside the EU,
the EU authorized representative is:
Springer Nature Customer Service Center GmbH
Europaplatz 3, 69115 Heidelberg, Germany

Printed by Libri Plureos GmbH
in Hamburg, Germany